# Habitus in Habitat II

## Other Sides of Cognition

natur, wissenschaft und die künste
nature, science et les arts
nature, science and the arts

Band 4



PETER LANG
Bern · Berlin · Bruxelles · Frankfurt am Main · New York · Oxford · Wien

Sabine Flach & Jan Söffner (eds)

# Habitus in Habitat II

## Other Sides of Cognition

PETER LANG
Bern · Berlin · Bruxelles · Frankfurt am Main · New York · Oxford · Wien

**Bibliographic information published by Die Deutsche Nationalbibliothek**
Die Deutsche Nationalbibliothek lists this publication in the Deutsche Nationalbibliografie; detailed bibliographic data is available on the Internet at ‹http://dnb.d-nb.de›.

British Library and Library of Congress Cataloguing-in-Publication Data:
A catalogue record for this book is available from *The British Library*, Great Britain

Library of Congress Cataloging-in-Publication Data

Habitus in habitat II : Other Sides of Cognition / Sabine Flach & Jan Söffner (eds). – 1st ed.
p. cm. – (Natur, Wissenschaft und die Künste ; Bd. 4)
ISBN 978-3-0343-0531-0
1. Cognition. 2. Brain–Research. 3. Thought and thinking. I. Flach, Sabine. II. Söffner, Jan.
III. Title: Habitus in habitat 2. IV. Title: Habitus in habitat two.
BF311.H24 2011
153–dc22

2010048844

The proceedings are result of a conference which was supported by the German Federal Ministry of Education and Research (promotional reference: 01UG07129).
The authors of this publication are responsible for its content.

Cover illustration: Suzanne Anker: *White Light*, 2009, digital print mounted on sintra, 96"x120" / 243.8cm x 304.8cm.

Cover design: Thomas Jaberg, Peter Lang AG

ISBN 978-3-0343-0531-0


Hochfeldstrasse 32, CH-3012 Bern
info@peterlang.com, www.peterlang.com, www.peterlang.net



Printed in Switzerland

# Contents

## *Different Minds*



## *Control and its Limits*

# Introduction

SABINE FLACH / JAN SÖFFNER

This book addresses the other sides of cognition, that is, those aspects not yet focused on as such by brain research – such as 'twilight' or scansion phenomena of consciousness, states of boredom or meaninglessness, and subliminal forms of experiencing. Drawing attention to the nuances of cognition implied in these states and processes, *Other Sides of Cognition* will specifically attempt to shed light on how the knowledge surrounding cognition can address forms and figurations of subjective, cultural and social understanding. Especially focusing on questions of environment-related forms of habitualization (the question of a *habitus in habitat*), the book searches for a different epistemology of states of minds and states of bodies, focusing on those aspects present in cognitive behaviour, which get lost all too easily, when following to strictly the endeavour of science to attain isolation and measurability.

With this second book in the series *habitus in habitat*[1] we are especially interested in a discussion that allows for crossing boundaries between historical and systematic disciplines, and between both the sciences and the knowledge of the arts. This especially affords opportunities to *conceptualise the interplay of cognition and emotion*, such as the transition zones existing to conscious processes (the not-yet conscious) or transformations of perception and the body-in-context. In analysing the interaction between artistic knowledge and the sciences, the book will focus chiefly on elaborating the specific methodological approaches in order to elucidate novel avenues and concepts within science and research. The aim is thereby to bring into view unexplained interrelations, concealed or invisible complexities, gradual shifts and intensifications occurring in cognitive processes – such as *modulations* of stimulus response schemes, which imply zones of non-knowledge or a different kind of knowledge than the one addressable while examining such schemes only. These zones seem to form a kind of background or an excluded other side of the processes measurable as discrete patterns or entities, nevertheless retaining their intrinsic identity.

The book places into new perspective the interplay of cognitive processes and emotions, as currently discussed heatedly in brain research,[2] on the basis of –

1 The others are: *Emotion and Motion* (Vol. I), *Synaesthesia and Kinaesthetics* (Vol. III), and Sabine Flach and Jan Söffner: *Emotionaler Habitus*.

2 See, among others, Roth: *Fühlen, Denken, Handeln*; Damasio: *The Feeling of What Happens*; Singer: *Ein neues Menschenbild?*; Poeppel: *Brain and Speech*; Pöppel and Edingshaus: *Ge-*

especially – a detailed investigation of European and US-American visual art and literature. When the 1990s were hailed as the "Decade of the Brain,"[3] this elevated neuro- and cognitive sciences to the status of the 'leading sciences' in explaining cognitive processes. This hegemonic claim, which entails conceptual exclusions,[4] will not simply be questioned here; rather, by explicitly assuming that the arts have their own specific knowledge, and that this knowledge is both irreducible and characteristic, the Other Sides volume focuses on how the genuine and productive achievements of the arts contribute to developing another epistemological history of cognition. Its fundamental claim is that the singular knowledge of the arts has a specific epistemic status, insofar as it articulates aspects of knowledge which are unrenderable in positive terms as an instance of knowledge production; within the scope of the book, this will not be considered to constitute sheer non-availability or revocation, but will instead be analysed with regard to those procedures to which it gives rise by virtue of its specific mediality.

In analysing the interaction between artistic knowledge and the sciences, the *Other Sides of Cognition* focuses chiefly on a non-convertible difference, albeit not with a view to demarcating the arts and the sciences, but rather to elaborating the specific approaches and epistemological procedures of visual and narrative art in order to use these for the purposes of science and research. Adopting this specific approach, this book fathoms the other sides of cognition inasmuch as the exclusions and grey areas produced by brain research occur as themes in art and literature – notably, these exclusions and grey areas form the site of complex cultural and social processes.[5] Based on the assumption that visual and narrative artistic production contributes to the enhancement of knowledge and cognition, the *Other Sides* examines nuances, exceptions, changes, and interstices in the interplay between cognition and emotions, which have been lost as a result of the endeavour of science to attain isolation, measurability, that is, definability and objectivability, and thus standardisation and regularisation. The term *Other Sides* thus designates both specific epistemological objects and a particular methodological procedure.

Unlike the privileging of the metaphor of cartography[6] or of the face in some branches of the cognitive sciences as a surface upon which the interrelation of cognitions and emotions[7] can be visualised, the *Other Sides* furthermore ex-

*heimnisvoller Kosmos Gehirn*; Klaus Herding: *Pathos, Affekt, Gefühl*; Geyer: *Hirnforschung und Willensfreiheit*; Breidbach: *Die Materialisierung des Ichs*; Hagner: *homo cerebralis*.

3 http://www.loc.gov/loc/brain/

4 See: Otniel Dror: "Fear and Loathing in the Laboratory and Clinic".

5 See for further the approaches adopted by the social studies of Science: Gibbons, Limoges and Nowotny: *The New Production of Knowledge*; Nowotny/Scott/Gibbons: *Re-Thinking Science*.

6 Toga and Mazziotta: "Introduction to Cartography of the Brain".

7 Sigrid Weigel: "Phantombilder zwischen Messen und Deuten".

plores the 'other knowledge' that the arts have with the interrelation of cognition and emotion on the basis of the manifold articulations of the *body*, that is, artistic and literary *body scenarios*.[8] These afford opportunities to *conceptualise the interplay of cognition and emotion*, such as the transition zones existing in consciousness (the not-yet conscious) or transformations of perception, which imaging procedures sometimes systematically exclude inasmuch as they are harnessed to localising cognition with isolated and well-defined entities – a premise that sometimes goes unquestioned in the use of Positron Emission Tomography (PET) and functional Magnet Resonance Tomography (fMRT).[9] Similar problems of localization and most of all stimulus-response based research arise, when we deal with narrative figurations. Especially the – often subliminally felt – temporality of the connections and transfigurations of narrative elements often escape the logic of simple events that could be isolated. Inasmuch as the Other Sides considers the phenomena in question also from the vantage point of non-scientific fields and their epistemological particularities, it aspires not merely to contribute to current debates on brain research from a stringent cultural studies perspective, but considers its endeavour as also relevant for the history of knowledge and, most prominently aesthetics as essential domains for developing a different history of cognition.

The focus of this approach lies on the complex interplay of vegetative, neuromuscular, cognitive, and emotional processes present throughout the body – and their phenomenological and cultural counterparts. The book thereby pursues the question of how embodied cognition and it examines nuances, exceptions, changes, and interstices in the interplay between cognition and emotions, between emotions and absence of emotions, between habituated/automatized actions and meaningful relations with an environment, and searches for an epistemology of states of minds and states of bodies. While these issues are difficult to address when following the scientific endeavour to isolate, define and objectify – nevertheless they cannot be neglected, even when making epistemological and philosophical claims from the results of empirical sciences. The term *Other Sides* thus designates both specific epistemological objects, and a particular openness for finding and discussing new methodological approaches, bringing together the specific strengths of various disciplines.

In methodological terms, contemporary artistic and literary works are conceived to constitute *experimental arrangements [Experimentalanordnungen]*[10] by

8 See Flach: *Körper-Szenarien*; Fischer-Lichte and Fleig: *Körper-Inszenierungen*.

9 For a critical perspective on such imaging procedures, see: Hagner: *Der Geist bei der Arbeit*, pp. 195–222.

10 For a discussion on the notion of experimental arrangements, albeit with particular regard to historical avant-garde movements, see: Schramm: *Bühnen des Wissens*. This concept also refers the envisaged *Other Sides* project to another ZfL-based project – "WissensKünste. Die Kunst zu wissen und das Wissen der Kunst" – which is conceived as an experimental laboratory for investigating the interrelation of art and science. Further, close relations exist here

which media, materials, methods, practices, staff, and locations form completely new alliances, remain flexible among each other, and hence subject to ongoing and ever-new negotiation. In contrast to focusing analysis on works and outcomes, the *Other Sides* centres on instances of the *constitution* of knowledge. This brings into view unexplained interrelations, concealed or invisible complexities.

So far, the methods of textual, iconic, and media criticism have entered the history of knowledge under various notions, such as a "poetology/poetics of knowledge,"[11] "aesthetic knowledge,"[12] and "iconic knowledge (Bildwissen)."[13] Nonetheless, these approaches obviously start out from the sciences to undertake their historical analysis of knowledge formations. *The idea for the 'Other Sides' proceeds along different lines*: It starts out from the analysis of specific procedures of knowledge production in visual and narrative arts and sets them in dialogue with the knowledge of the sciences. Although it goes without saying that the knowledge of the arts is deeply rooted in historical configurations. The *Other Sides* therefore investigates this knowledge along the lines of historical change, hoping to bring about *new perspectives* of – and a *shift* in – the histories of knowledge and cognition.

But historical transformations cannot be the only issue to be addressed. The knowledge of the relationship between outer experience and inner processing is often described through combining different iconic metaphors and metaphors of motion in an undetermined space. Metaphors of movement – as in the case of mind wandering, of air (as in the case of the atmosphere), the change from light to the absence of light (twilight) – mark and conceal the unknown and provisional in the interrelations existing between perception, emotion, and the human body, and hence become part of a phenomenological study of consciousness. This is especially intriguing, if we consider that these are metaphors drawn from embodied experiences, which means that they therefore themselves concern the interrelation of cognition and embodied experiencing. Vagueness and indecision, the precision of the imprecise in what is called 'atmospheric' and the unspecific motion of the body, thereby figure as markers for the absence of an epistemology of the subliminally embodied environmental relation. Here too, the nuanced zones of transition seem to form a kind of background to the more reflexive side of cognition. Nevertheless these background phenomena, these other sides of what becomes manifest, can provide for intrinsic orientations of consciousness.

with Hans-Jörg Rheinberger's notion of the "experimental system" (Rheinberger: *Experimentalsysteme und epistemische Dinge*).

11 See: Vogl: *Poetologien des Wissens um 1800.*

12 Stafford: *Artful Science*; Bredekamp and Werner: *Bildwelten des Wissens*; Horst Bredekamp's considerations are an exception to the rule in this respect, inasmuch as he starts out from the explicit antecedence of art towards the sciences, that is, in contrast to Foucault's discursive analysis of the art chamber as a thought model for the relationship between art and science.

13 Kemp: *Visualizations.*

They form an other side of perceptive,[14] sensorimotor,[15] existential,[16] or even ontological cognition.[17]

To give a further example: The notion of a "scansion of consciousness"[18] can be considered an alternative to the well-established narratological notion of the "stream of consciousness." Narrative theory takes up this notion, first employed by William James in *The Principles of Psychology* (1890), to describe processes of consciousness metaphorically as a continuous stream. Turning the metaphor of the 'stream' into a metaphor of 'scansion' implies addressing an important kind of conscious relation with the current urban environment. First developed by Charles Baudelaire's and Walter Benjamin's notion of the 'flaneur', a concept that is currently shifting into another direction, *scansion* focuses more on stress-induced states of consciousness related to an even more fragmented environment or reality. The notion of a scansion of consciousness, hence, may allow for better focusing on breaks and break-downs of consciousness, forming an other side of cognition as well. Moreover, by studying obsessive-compulsive disorders and paranoia, psychoanalysis has furnished essential analyses of how thought processes and compulsive behaviour are intertwined. The notion of coerced thought and action is indeed a challenge for addressing habitat-related habituations: What is the difference between coercion and habituated action patterns? What makes habitat-habituation act against its own functioning – as is the case in 'neurotic' coerced behaviour? And what does this tell us about the way embodied existence serves as a point of departure for, and a bearer of, the development of cognitive procedures/systems operating as the production site of pleasure and disquiet, and the interconnections of cognitive and emotional processes?

Talking about emotions, feelings and moods as an essential part of cognition also implies the need of talking about how – if at all – they can be absent, and how this state of non-state can be addressed. One emotional issue especially focused on in this tome is the manifold phenomenon of boredom. This issue can also be called a twilight phenomenon, since it concerns the emotion of the absence of other emotions, the inertia as the action of not acting, and a kind of resistance to environmental affordances. As such a state it has been characterized as the fundament of a phenomenology of world-openness,[19] but it also concerns the paradox emotion of apathy and phenomenologies of inattentiveness, exhaustion and especially of a kind of non-state beyond the dichotomy of sleeping and waking. By focusing on boredom, the book also addresses a cognitive notion of

14 See for example Merleau-Ponty: *Phénoménologie de la perception.*
15 See for example Siewert: "Attention and Sensorimotor Intentionality".
16 See for example Ratcliffe: *Feelings of Being.*
17 For example in Heidegger's concept of "Stimmung" as a kind of disclosedness – see his *Die Grundbegriffe der Metaphysik.*
18 See Flach in this volume.
19 See Heidegger: *Die Grundbegriffe der Metaphysik.*

emotionality to explore the other sides of cognition in two productive ways: It denotes not only an emotional state associated with a specific experience of time; described by Walter Benjamin as the "highpoint of mental relaxation" (*Höhepunkt der geistigen Entspannung*), it also affords a description in cognitive terms. Moreover, repetitive structures, discontinuous and decelerated thought processes, lack of willingness, and concomitant disorders of communicative procedures, forgetfulness, and other specific perceptual modes can be focused on – and, of course, boredom as the nearly inevitable background-mood of subjects in cognitive experiments – a subject recently broached in the novel field of 'resting-state' fMRI research.[20]

Thinking about the other sides of cognition also means to focus on the knowledge one does not have, but one can be had by. So what is the kind of cognition ecstatic practises, emotional states like rage or fury, or drug use can produce? What is their epistemology? And what is the emotionality of shared interactions, which do not seem to have a subject of knowledge? How can culturally shared practises shape our bodies and minds – and which kinds of cognition do they entail? And how can narratives be shared in a way that engages situated bodies as sites of cognition?

For discussing all these issues, habituations taking place in a culturally shaped environment are fundamental. Focusing on the other sides of cognition therefore also means to address phenomena of both emotional and sensory relations with the cultural habitat and to consider, which kinds of habitus can evolve from a sensorimotor and, most of all, an emotional relation with it. The book will accordingly address environmental relations with what is not part of 'sense data' in a strict meaning of the term. Here, once again, not only conscious products of thought and perception, but especially the zones and forms of interaction between hypertrophic and switched off consciousness will play a key role for thinking about the interplay between the construction and deconstruction of personal identity.

The chapters focus on visual and narrative art and explore temporal, processual and spatial aspects of cognition with regard to narrative structures and mediality. The various arrangements of specific materials represent *constellations*; that is, literary and artistic productions are not examined separately, but associated by means of common *structural* factors, from which the *Other Sides* strives to derive building blocks of a different epistemological history of cognition.

The book opens with a section on *Twilight* phenomena as an other side of perception, meaning and consciousness. Harold Schweizer dedicates himself to the shade in both a concrete and a metaphorical way, describing it as a "stubbornly elusive" phenomenon lacking the sharp distinctive outlines of a shadow, the reference to a concrete object (of which it would be the shadow), and rather being a tone, an affective quality of light than a graspable object of thought. This,

20 See Margulies and Callard in this volume.

in his eyes, is what makes it a "trope for poetic knowing" and allows this twilight phenomenon to be an existential intuition. Sabine Flach focuses on twilight and the knowledge of the Arts, dedicating herself to phenomena of consciousness. Investigating on phenomena of boredom and inertia, she develops a concept of vision beyond the dichotomy of a mental and a material image. How important the focus on these and similar phenomena can be for psychology and the neurosciences can be seen from the third contribution of this tome. Felicity Callard and Daniel Margulies focus on the brain activity in the so-called "resting state", that is in the absence of a specific sensory input to be computed. The emergence of these dynamics leads them to describe a different notion of the self "specified through and anchored by these dynamics."

The second section does not leave these grey areas – but turns to a specific aspect of their phenomenology. Dealing with phenomena of *Attention and Boredom* they fathom out the other side of a reflexive awareness, of conscious presence, and of a reflexive consciousness. Nicolas de Oliveira and Nicola Oxley focus on states between inattention and concentration as reflected, staged and transformed by contemporary artworks. Unifying these issues with the (non)emotional state of boredom, Oliveira and Oxley are concerned with an "aesthetics of disengagement" as a kind of other side of the aesthetic of surplus or overstatement present in the mass media. A similar point is made by Holger Schulze, who is concerned with the generative and productive qualities of boredom in art experience. In focusing on musical examples by Morton Feldman, Aphex Twin, and Einstürzende Neubauten he describes boredom's force to "draw us back from routines of perception, interpretation and even feeling", thereby allowing for shifts and breaks in the perceptive and emotional habitus. Jan Slaby, instead elaborates on a heideggarian notion of Stimmung. Departing from a notion of emotions and moods as an other side of cognition, Slaby applies his concept of "affective intentionality" to Heidegger's theory of boredom to put forth its existential analysis. Julian Klein's paper, instead, focuses on the relationship of framing and differently layered forms of attention as a ground for defining artistic knowledge and aesthetic experience. The neuroscientific correlate of phenomena discussed in this section, is approached by Alexander Thiele, who discusses the neural bases of a "biased competition model of attention."

The third section *Different Minds* addresses a variety of exemplary phenomena of how mental states and mental activity can be conceived of. This topic especially allows for opening up the dialogue about the other sides of cognition for historic dimensions. Pierre Cassou-Noguès discusses Emil Posts theory of non-linear computation leading to a model of plural minds as a challenge for Turing machines. Post argues with a co-presence of different states of mind being processed according to different rules – leading to a multitude of other sides and, potentially, to alternative kinds of breakdown situations. Gerhard Scharbert turns to a more physiological side of mental "not-normality. In focusing on the cycle of poets assembled by the French neurologist Jacques-Joseph Moreau de Tours, he compellingly argues entanglement of drug experiments and poetic knowledge plays a key role for the origin of modernity. In an insightful overview on the history of reflex theory, Yvonne Wübben focuses on the origins of both stimulus-response based theories and modern neurology. Including not just illustrations, but also images in her study, she makes the claim that experimental practices with their specific forms of know how have established and influenced theories about the brain as a center of afferent and efferent nerve activity. This offers decisive insights in practices of conceiving the habitat in terms of stimuli and theories of procedural brain and nerve activity. Isabelle Moffat, on the other hand, exposes the unitary thought of Lancelot Law Whyte, which outlines an early perspective beyond the opposition of mind and matter, thought and physiology. In describing an early work by Jean Painlevé, Jan Söffner outlines the basics of a phenomenology considering cross-species relations.

The fourth section, *Control and its Limits*, focuses on the entanglement of cognition and power. In a precise analysis of Jim Jarmush's "The Limits of Control" (2009), Fabienne Liptay argues that the "elimination or displacement of the plot [in] art cinema allows for an intensified embodied experience" due to an increased awareness of the viewer's senses. Thereby the aesthetic experience finds other sides, escaping the cinematic control over meaning production. Warren Neidich instead focuses on what he calls "Neuropower", i.e. the power exercised by the dispositives designed to work on human neuro-plasticity by developing a respective human habitat.

The conference *Habitus in Habitat II – Other Sides of Cognition* was the second major event organized by the research project *Habitus in Habitat*, primarily based in the research department "WissensKünste – Kunst und Wissenschaft" at the Zentrum für Literatur- und Kulturforschung (ZfL) in Berlin. We wish to thank all of our colleagues at the ZfL for the fruitful discussions about the topic and for participating at the conference as speakers or chairs. And we are also very grateful for the great help of Maureen Jeram, Franck Loric, Jana Wolf and Andrea Schulz for this publication.

Our special thanks go to the director of the ZfL, Prof. Dr. Dr. h.c. Sigrid Weigel, for her confidence in our research work and for engagement in the project. We are equally grateful about the collaboration of our colleagues from the Berlin School of Mind and Brain – and we are especially thanking the directors Prof. Dr. Arno Villringer and Prof. Dr. Michael Pauen, for being long-term cooperation partners on the project and for discussing the insights of the cognitive sciences, philosophy and the neuro-sciences with us, which are all of equal importance for our project.

We also thank the "Medizinhistorisches Museum der Charité", and here especially Prof. Dr. Thomas Schnalke, who provided an unforgettable conference site, namely the *Hörsaalruine*, which is located in the Museum – and who, moreover made it possible to realize the art exhibition, "Enception" within the rooms of the museum. We are very grateful that Ryan Cordell, in collaborating with Prof. Dr. Ulrich Dirnagl, has realized this project.

Very special thanks are due to our colleagues from the research group "Habitus in Habitat", which – independently from the research project at the ZfL – has been working together in regular meetings for several years now, consisting of members of the ZfL, the Berlin School of Mind and Brain and the research group "Picture Act and Embodiment" at the Humboldt Universität zu Berlin. We are grateful for the vivid, critical and enthusiastic discussions of this research group; without the existence of the forum, the topics realized in this volume would not have been possible.

## References

Bredekamp, Horst and Gabriele Werner (eds.): *Bildwelten des Wissens. Kunsthistorisches Jahrbuch für Bildkritik.* Vol. 1 ff., Berlin (Akademie Verlag) 2003 ff.

Breidbach, Olaf: *Die Materialisierung des Ichs. Zur Geschichte der Hirnforschung im 19. und 20. Jahrhundert*, Frankfurt a. M. (Suhrkamp) 1997.

Damasio, Antonio R.: *The Feeling of what Happens. Body and Emotion in the Making of Consciousness* San Diego et al. (Harcourt) 1999.

Dror, Otniel: "Fear and Loathing in the Laboratory and Clinic" in: Fay Bound Alberti (ed.): *Medicine, Emotions and Disease, 1700–1950*, New York (Palgrave) 2006.

Fischer-Lichte, Erika and Anne Fleig: *Körper-Inszenierungen. Präsenz und kultureller Wandel*, Tübingen (Attempo) 2000.

Flach, Sabine and Jan Söffner: *Emotionaler Habitus. Verkörperte Sinnlichkeit zwischen Subjektivität und Umweltrelation* (forthcoming in 2011).

Flach, Sabine: *Körper-Szenarien. Zum Verhältnis von Körper und Bild in Video-Installationen*, Munich (Fink), 2003.

Geyer, Christian (ed.): *Hirnforschung und Willensfreiheit. Zur Deutung der neuesten Experimente*, Frankfurt a. M. (Suhrkamp) 2004.

Gibbons, Michael / Camille Limoges / Helga Nowotny et al.: *The New Production of Knowledge. The Dynamics of Science and Research in Contemporary Societies*, London (Sage) 1994.

Hagner, Michael: *Der Geist bei der Arbeit*, Göttingen (Wallstein) 2006.

Hagner, Michael: *homo cerebralis. Der Wandel vom Seelenorgan zum Gehirn*, Berlin (Berlin Verlag) 1997.

Heidegger, Martin: *Die Grundbegriffe der Metaphysik. Welt – Endlichkeit – Einsamkeit* (1929/30), Frankfurt am Main (Klostermann) 2004.

Herding, Klaus (ed.): *Pathos, Affekt, Gefühl. Die Emotionen in den Künsten*, Berlin (de Gruyter) 2004.

Kemp, Martin: *Visualizations. The Nature Book of Art and Sciences*, Berkeley / Los Angeles (University of California Press) 2000.

Merleau-Ponty, Maurice: *Phénoménologie de la perception*, Paris (Gallimard) 1945.

Nowotny, Helga, Peter Scott and Michael Gibbons: *Re-Thinking Science: Knowledge and the Public in an Age of Uncertainty*, Oxford (Polity Press) 2001.

Poeppel, David (ed.): *Special Issue: Brain and Speech* (= *Cognitive Science*, 21 [2001] 5).

Pöppel, Ernst and Anna-Lydia Edingshaus: *Geheimnisvoller Kosmos Gehirn*. Munich (Bertelsmann) 1994.

Ratcliffe, Matthew: *Feelings of Being – Phenomenology, Psychiatry and the Sense of Reality*. Oxford (Oxford University Press) 2008.

Rheinberger, Hans-Jörg: *Experimentalsysteme und epistemische Dinge. Eine Geschichte der Proteinsynthese im Reagenzglas*, Göttingen (Wallstein) 2001.

Roth, Gerhard: *Fühlen, Denken, Handeln. Die neurobiologischen Grundlagen des menschlichen Verhaltens*, Frankfurt a.M. (Suhrkamp) 2001.

Schramm, Hilmar et al. (eds.): *Bühnen des Wissens. Interferenzen zwischen Wissenschaft und Kunst*, Berlin (Dahlem University Press) 2003.

Siewert, Charles: "Attention and Sensorimotor Intentionality", in: David Woodruff Smith and Amie Lynn Thomasson (eds.): *Phenomenology and Philosophy of Mind*, Oxford (Oxford University Press) 2005.

Singer, Wolf: *Ein neues Menschenbild? Gespräche über Hirnforschung*, Frankfurt a. M. (Suhrkamp) 2003.

Stafford, Barbara: *Artful Science. Enlightenment, Entertainment and the Eclipse of Visual Education*, Cambridge, MA (MIT Press) 1994.

Toga, Arthur and John Mazziotta: "Introduction to Cartography of the Brain", in: Arthur Toga and John Mazziotta (eds.): *Brain Mapping. The Methods*, Amsterdam / Boston (Academic Press) 1996.

Vogl, Joseph (ed.): *Poetologien des Wissens um 1800*, Munich (Fink) 1999.

Weigel, Sigrid: "Phantombilder zwischen Messen und Deuten. Bilder von Hirn und Gesicht in den Instrumentarien empirischer Forschung von Psychologie und Neurowissenschaft", in: Florian Steger and Bettina v. Jagow (eds.): *Repräsentationen. Medizin und Ethik in Literatur und Kunst der Moderne*, Heidelberg (Winter) 2004, 137–176.

# *Socially Shared Emotions*

# Writing in the Shade
## A Meditation

Harold Schweizer

Whereas shadow is cast by an object's shape, shade is the content of a shadow; shade lacks the outlines and measurable contours of shadow. Shade bears none of the liabilities of Plato's allegations of shadow's unreality. Shade is not a reference to a thing, it is a quality of light and darkness, and as such a trope for particular emotional and cognitive states, "a green thought" as Andrew Marvell in his poem "The Garden" so memorably puts it. Since the language needed to articulate "a green thought in a green shade" seems as elusive as shade itself, I offer not an analysis but a series of meditations on cognitive states for which shade seems an apt figure, albeit one that defines this cognitive state as nothing more determinate than an aura, an atmosphere, an ambience, a mood, a tone, an undertone. The tropical proliferation in this series of references alerts us that shade cannot be reduced to the mimetic, two-dimensional shape of a shadow. Shade is not shadow, nor is it cast by an object. Shadow is cast, shade is provided. Shade is a tone of light, a tone of darkness, just as tone is a shade of sound or color. We use the tropes of shade and tone when we apply them to those qualities of human expression by which language does not simply designate meanings, does not only refer to things, does not only function as shadow. For words perform their signifying not only as shadows of things. In their most intensive signification they convey resonance, timbre, silence, intimation, tone. What a tone is a tone of we don't know, but we know we have heard it and thereby know something – or another – more deeply. More deeply conveys more shade.

## I

The history of the term *shade* does not facilitate our speaking of it, since there shade seems synonymous with shadow, twilight, dusk, night, death, foreboding, "an ill defined patch of darker color on the wing of a moth," a variation, a ghost, a shelter, a retired spot, a shutter.[1] The word *shade* does not exist either in French or in German where *ombre* or *Schatten* represents both shadow and shade. Although the uses of the word *shade* thus attest to more than some overlap with *shadow*, shade is to be strictly distinguished from shadow. I will repeatedly in-

1 *Oxford English Dictionary.*

voke that difference only because shade is so distinctly different but its distinctness is stubbornly elusive.

II

The elusiveness of this difference between shadow and shade can be tested by assigning either of these two words certain adjectival modifiers, like *cool, dark, quiet, serene*. My contention is that the less such a quality partakes of the world of material, physical reality, the more it seems to become descriptive of the properties of shade. Shade enters into figurative combinations almost without effort – a quiet shade, a serene shade, a tranquil shade – whereas the combination of such adjectives with shadow would imply a more deliberate, almost forced metaphorical effort, as in quiet shadow, serene shadow, tranquil shadow. In the adjectival modifiers of shade, we seem to speak of our own affect rather than of objects, as if the qualities of shade reached into us. Conversely, when I speak of qualities of shadow, they seem to denote the external world. Shadow, in short, represents external reality, whereas shade denotes a fluid exchange between external and internal, physical and mental worlds.

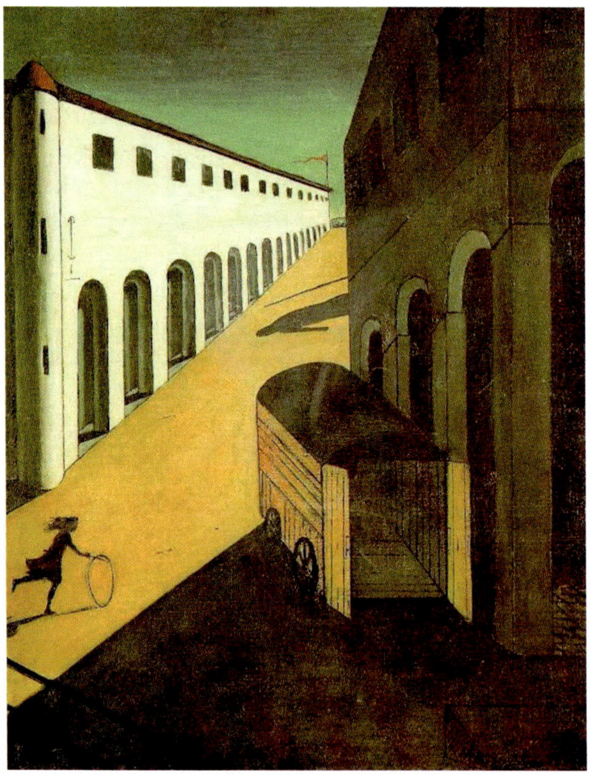

Fig. 1: Giorgio de Chirico, Mystère et mélancholie d'une rue, 1914.

III

What is so disturbing in the sharp outlines of the shadows painted by Giorgio de Chirico is that they seem violently cast onto the ground, so that de Chiroco's shadows exaggerate the definable, dimensional quality of shadows; they remain starkly external to the forlorn figures who sparsely populate de Chirico's paintings and who function like pointers of sun-dials, who seem to have their being in too bright a light, and who cannot enter the shadows cast almost always by tall, square, institutional buildings. The fluid interchange between material and mental worlds facilitated by shade seems here forcibly thwarted, so that the world of these paintings remains alien; light and darkness are too clearly separated.

IV

Although shade is always technically caused by the shadow of an object, it is the affective quality of light that we mean when we speak of shade. Shade is "a speechless cloud of light."[2] Although caused by the shadow of a tree's foliage, for example, shade does not seem thereby wholly determined or defined; shade is quality, affect, experience, whereas shadow is space, outline, silhouette. The only shadow a tree can cast is with its trunk; its foliage does not cast a shadow but rather provides shade. Hence the phrase "shade tree." Shade is not defined by the outlines or patterns of shadows on the ground but by the darkened, cool stillness of light. Thus shade is often used in figurative senses to denote a range of sentiments from the dread of death to joyful intimations of peace and shelter. The forebodings or pleasures or tranquility that shade evokes are themselves not determinable states, or shapes, or qualities: They are not shadows but shades of feeling – of calm, of cool, of rest, of peace.

2 Merwin: *Migration*, p. 389.

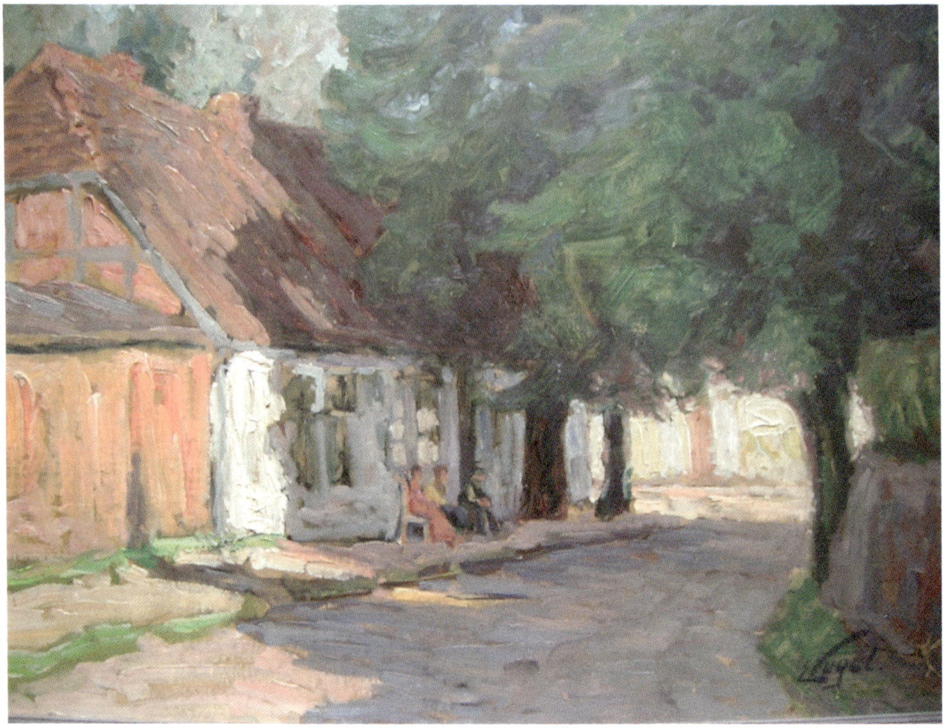

Fig. 2: Unknown German painter, title unknown, around 1930.

## V

In his book *Seeing Dark Things: A Philosophy of Shadows* (there are some books on shadow, none on shade), Roy Sorensen writes about "the *intangibility* of shadows" and admits that though he can "feel *that* there was shadow," he could not feel the shadow itself, only the objects therein.[3] Shade, I suggest, is the word that designates this feeling *that* there is shadow, a feeling of air, of light, of all the intangible, evanescent realities that air and light signify and perhaps convey as they extend themselves into our interior and thence to existential intuitions of time and of ourselves. Shade has an effect, physical and mental, on those who find themselves in it, beautifully exemplified in Andrew Marvell's "green thought in a green shade," where shade denotes the coalescence of inner and outer worlds. Shade is here a figure for a mind in repose, in rest, in delay, in waiting.

3 Sorensen: *Seeing Dark Things*, p. 118.

VI

Perhaps a slower time passes in the diminished light of shade. Objects in shade (of which I am one) seem to endure differently, without impatience, as if they were pausing, resting; as if something delayed them.

VII

I can suddenly see them (and myself among them) because I see them a little longer. I shade my eyes to see more clearly. One has to move oneself into the right measure of light; one needs to retreat from the glare of light in order to see, and yet I do not see well in shade where outlines dissolve and merge into each other. Shade calls into question my seeing and the distances that seeing implies. Shade is an intimate space.

VIII

An early poem of Wallace Stevens ends with the lines

> I never knew
> That fluttering things have so distinct a shade[4]

Distinct in this shade are the transience and fragility of fluttering things. Perhaps things flutter because they have little solidity in time, no more solidity than shade. A much later poem, one of Stevens' most important, "An Ordinary Evening in New Haven," seems to confirm this notion of fluttering things as it ends with this brief meditation:

> It is not in the premise that reality
> Is a solid. It may be a shade that traverses
> A dust, a force that traverses a shade.[5]

– as if shade were a metaphor for a reality found fluttering, insubstantial, like an ill defined patch of darker color on the wing of a moth. All of Stevens' claims in this proposition partake of the quality of shade; nothing, in fact, is claimed, reality may be nothing more solid than a shade, a shade might traverse nothing more solid than a dust; or it might be a force, also not solid, that traverses a shade, all of which assigns reality neither substance nor determinable cause, but only movement. Reality, in Stevens' lines, is a shade, a dust, a force traversing; reality is a mere duration, and all that is traversed by it is rendered itself a traversing, such as we are – transient, insubstantial, fluttering dust or shade.

4 Stevens: "Le Monocle de Mon Oncle", p. 14.
5 Ibid., p. 417.

IX

Words cast shadows, the shadows of the solid things to which they refer. But language speaks not only in shadows, imitations, references. The shadow of a word contains a shade of something of which it is not the premise that it is a solid.

X

Shade as a trope for a poetic knowing implies that literary words, such as they are, not only cast shadows with all their attendant platonic liabilities, but that when we are in the shade of words – their tones and resonances – we may experience their shade as a respite from the binaries that structure the signifying of words, and that structure our knowing: as in light and darkness, objects and shadows. Shade then is a trope for a cognitive intermission, a lull – and in the pause of light that shade provides we may acquire a different knowing, not of solid things but of a fluttering. Shade, then, is a figure for existential intuitions, intuitions of an insubstantial reality, a wing of a moth, a reality neither as definable as a shadow nor as solid as a thing.

XI

Since shade has no material essence, it is a word often used to denote comparisons, variations, nuance, indirection, foreboding, liminality: in short instability, movement. Shade is passage, traversing, for there can be no shade that is not also a location and time, as in the time and location depicted in the anonymous painting (fig. 2). Since shade cannot be sustained across time and space – because shade moves, fades, lightens, darkens – implies that we pass through it, that we leave behind intangible, unverifiable intimations – of a fluttering. Writing in the shade is to write what lies slightly outside of the signifying of words, or indeed what lies deeply inside of the shadow cast by words, just as shade lies in shadow. Writing in the shade, given the trope that it is, is writing not beyond, but very closely, very intimately, next to, words.

XII

As if words were objects that cast a transient shadow of the thing they darkly reference; as if one who writes in shade would have to move deeply inside this shadow that words cast so as to feel the intimations and pleasure that words afford as they stand between us and the blinding real.

XIII

Writing in the shade is not to write what words mean but how they resonate in their meaning-making, how they intimate, gesture, allude as they signify. In a poem by Yves Bonnefoy, the speaker urges the reader not to read (what words mean) but to listen (how they resonate):

> Passant, ce sont des mots. Mais plutôt que lire
> Je veux que tu écoutes.

And a few lines later:

> Puis sache un bruit plus faible encore, et ce que ce soit
> Le murmur sans fin de nos ombres,

which in Hoyt Roger's translation reads: "Then know an ever fainter sound, and let it be / The endless murmuring of all our shades."[6]

XIV

Maurice Blanchot describes the movements of the writer's hand as passing through "*l'ombre du temps*" which in English is "the shadow of time." The shadow of time, Blanchot goes on, is "the shadow of a hand slipping in an unreal way towards an object that has become its shadow." The writer's hand, he claims, "belongs to shadow, the hand itself is a shadow."[7] But *ombre,* like the German *Schatten,* means both shadow and shade. For Blanchot precisely seeks to overcome the implicit Platonisms of shadow – shadow that is always the unreal opposed to the elusive real. Blanchot's troping of the writer who writes through shadow alludes not to an unreal but to an unknown and provisional toward which such writing is inclined.

XV

Writing in the shade, to borrow another phrase from Blanchot, is to write of, or on, "the dark side of the day."[8] Such writing invokes a "being which protests against revelation" – "the flutter of closing wings is their speech," Blanchot adds,[9] reminding us of Stevens' fluttering things, and which in turn reminds us of "an ill defined patch of darker color on the wing of a moth." As Blanchot's writer's hand moves within the definable *shadows* of semantic conventions, these are the conventions that threaten revelation – revelation that would be deception, for it is not in the premise that reality is a solid.

6 Bonnefoy: *The Curved Planks*, p. 58–59.
7 Maurice Blanchot: *The Gaze of Orpheus*, p. 67.
8 Ibid., 48.
9 Ibid., 49.

XVI

If writing is to come into the shade of words, then writing will not assume the defined – and always implicitly deficient, indeed ominous – outlines that shadow denotes, it will not serve as reflection of an object, it will not be performed as the unreal shadow that is the representation of an object. So when I ask how can writing be a writing in the shade, I mean something other than an opposition between light and darkness, object and shadow, truth and representation. Writing in the shade is what, I think, Blanchot might have meant by his figure of *l'ombre*. All of Blanchot's metaphors of *l'ombre* lend themselves only to allude to that intangible, undefiniable quality for which we feel drawn to a writer – that which (Blanchot writes) "is still speaking when everything has been said"[10] and which is nothing other than "tone."

XVII

Shade is tone. "The tone of a work," Blanchot claims, is "what is most authentic about it"; tone is "the intimacy of the silence [the writer] imposes on speech"; tone is "what speaks in him."[11] Elsewhere Blanchot writes with reference to tone that "the language of literature is a search for [the] moment which precedes literature" or that literature "offers its language to what is murmured in the absence of speech,"[12] and which echoes Bonnefoy's "endless murmuring of all our shades." But it is not the negation of literature that evokes the moment before literature, it is not the negation of language that evokes the absence of speech. Rather it is the very movement of language that awakens that which is not language. It is not opposed to language but implied in it, just as shade is not opposed to light but within it.

XVIII

Tone is to sound what shade is to light. Tone is a shade of difference. Shade is a tone of light. Shade is where sight is closest to sound. Tone is not the defined other, the shadow, of sound; tone is the shade that sounds have. Tone is the shade words have when we hear them.

XIX

To speak of shade as a metaphor of tone, or of tone as a metaphor of shade, is to speak of those ungraspable qualities of writing (or indeed of language itself), qualities borrowed no doubt from painting and music by which writing aspires to become sound and color – something other than reference, something other than the mere shadow of things. Such writing is not writing as representation but as

10 Ibid., 68.
11 Ibid., 70, 71.
12 Ibid., 46, 58.

*experience,* not writing to produce a knowledge but a haunting, perhaps an intimation of that which speaks in us when we speak.

XX

For Blanchot, *ombre* is a metaphor for tone, tone is a metaphor for something still speaking when everything has been said, which is the intimacy of silence, the murmur in the absence of speech, that which speaks *in us*. Intimacy and murmur are denominations of shade – private, subjective – neither aspiring to publicity, understanding, or clarity, as if the resonance of tone, its intimacy and murmur, called out to the innermost of another's hearing and understanding of that which speaks in us when we speak. For another's innermost hearing is to hear in words, in the sounds they make, something that resounds beyond their function or failure, something for which words are only the occasion so that a sound could be made that would resound in another person.

XXI

Shade is the habitat of those who need rest, among them those who are waiting and those who are dying. I am assigned the shade that falls within me. I do not come into shade by appointment; I find myself in shade; perhaps in shade I find myself.

XII

And yet, our lives demand that our speech be revelation, not the flutter of closing wings. We perform our functions in the realm of shadow; but we perform our fluttering (being) in shade. Writing in the shade is writing about insubstantial, fluttering being, not a solid. Such being, as Blanchot would have understood it, is most authentically a being that fully embraces its mortality. As Bonnefoy writes in "*Une Voix*":

> Tout cela, mon ami,
> Vivre, qui noue
> Hier, notre illusion,
> À demain, nos ombres.[13]

XIII

We enter shade, it enters us, and we become the fluttering thing that casts a shadow inwardly. The inward shadow cast by the body in the body's half-light is duration – a shade insubstantial, moving, fluttering, an ill defined patch of darker color on the wing of a moth.

13 "All that, my friend, / Is how we live, tying / Yesterday, our illusion, / To tomorrow, our shades." Bonnefoy: *The Curved Planks*, p. 45.

## XXIV

And though we attempt to measure the length of it, what we call existence time and age are but movements of darkness and light. Shade has neither length nor breadth though I stand in it; it has neither length nor breadth though it lies in me.

## XXV

I am already a shade, a quality of light, a passage within which I am detained. I linger and stand like the pointer of a sundial. My body casts the shadow within which I have my being.

## XXVI

The shades of the underworld in Homer's, Virgil's, Ovid's or Dante's poems, who have their being "without flesh and bones," who remain where one cannot "hold one another,"[14] – have entered into an ontology that I already intuit in the shade that lies within me and that constitutes that immaterial thing – not a thing but a shade – that we call being, self, mortal destiny. When I try to grasp it, I am like that visitor to the underworld who attempts to embrace the shades of the dead. Hence the centrality of the Orpheus myth in Blanchot's writing, "Orpheus [who] must submit to the law of the underworld in order to produce the artwork"[15] – Orpheus who in Blanchot's work sees in the shade of Eurydice presence and absence, life and death, simultaneously.

## XXVII

Writing in the shade is to see darkly; it is to write towards that which initiated the writing in the first place, even as the writing itself is the only thing that traces that elusive initiation that Blanchot has called silence before speech. The syntax of the sentence, the form of the poem, the writing on the page, trace the outlines of shadow, in the shadow of which something happens and darkens as one keeps writing – darkens and deepens, as does a style that becomes more and more a writer's own.

14 Homer: *The Odyssey*, xi; p. 228–239.

15 Simon Critchley: *Very Little ... Almost Nothing: Death, Philosophy, Literature*, London (Routledge) 2004, p. 49.

## References

Blanchot, Maurice: *The Gaze of Orpheus and Other Literary Essays*, trans. Lydia Davis, Barrytown, NY (Station Hill Press) 1981.

Bonnefoy, Yves: *The Curved Planks*, trans. Hoyt Rogers, New York (Farrar Straus and Giroux) 2006.

Critchley, Simon: *Very Little ... Almost Nothing: Death, Philosophy, Literature*, London (Routledge) 2004.

Homer: *The Odyssey*, trans. Robert Fitzgerald, New York (Vintage Classics) 1990.

Merwin, W. S.: *Migration. New and Selected Poems*, Port Townsend (Copper Canon Press) 2005.

Sorensen, Roy: *Seeing Dark Things. The Philosopy of Shadows*, Oxford (Oxford University Press) 2008.

Stevens, Wallace: "Le Monocle de Mon Oncle", in: *Collected Poetry and Prose*, New York (The Library of America) 1997.

## List of Illustrations

Fig. 1 Giorgio de Chirico, Mystère et mélancolie d'une rue (Mystery and Melancholy of a Street), 1914, Oil on canvass, 87 x 71,5 cm (Private collection).

Fig. 2 Unknown painter, title unknown, around 1930, oil on canvas 60 x 49cm (private collection).

# On Twilight

SABINE FLACH

> People believe that scientists are there to lecture them, poets, musicians and the like to please them. *That they have to something to teach them* does not cross their minds.[1]

## I Prologue

> I have never read a comment about when, in closing one eye and 'only looking with one eye', that you cannot see the darkness (blackness) with the closed one at the same time.[2]

In a notebook from the estate of Ludwig Wittgenstein, the philosopher poses a question whose epistemic value must have so occupied him as to turn into a revenant with – as is suitable for such a ghost – such an irritating and penetrating impact on his thinking, as well as on his reflexivity about his own perception, that the question appears in two further manuscripts.[3]

This insisting question appears in the first notebook written between March 24 and April 12, 1950, between comments on color and color terms, and becomes a decisive parameter for a thinking which leads to thought passages on the relation between '*internal*' and '*external*':

The question, short but effectual, is: "Am I aware that I see?"[4]

It stands oddly alone within Wittgenstein's writings and is only seconded from afar by two more thoughts, which moreover seem to be closely related to each other. They are: "Can the sentence, 'There are people who can see' stand in a psychology? and "One would want to say, If such people were to not exist, then the term to see would also not exist."

1 Wittgenstein: *Vermischte Bemerkungen*, p.79
2 Wittgenstein: *Zettel*, p. 419.
3 The first notebook has been categorized by Georg Henrik von Wright as MS 173. In the notebooks MS 174 and 176, Wittgenstein has elaborated on the same question as exposed here (cf. the precise study by Thomas Macho: "Ist mir bekannt, daß ich sehe?").
4 Cf. for the following considerations about Wittgenstein's question the detailed arguments exposed in Macho: "Ist mir bekannt, daß ich sehe?"

In its relation to each other, the little conversation on humans and their vision circumnavigates our question, highlights and emphasizes it. Because while it seems obvious that the question of whether there are humans who can see, takes on an external perspective whose view on people and their abilities has always been a descriptive external perception, Wittgenstein's effort is directed at himself, respectively at us – insofar as we read this question and make it our own.

Thus, the question: "Am I aware that I see" implicates an eminent *self-perception*, a self-perception that includes and indicates the capability for a reflexive self-distance, and it is this self-distance, that is essential for the acquirement to not just to see but to reflect about the process of seeing while seeing.[5] This then creates a nexus between the words "Bekannt" – 'known' and "Sehen" – 'see': Because extending far beyond the meaning of 'known' in the sense of "Vertraut sein" – 'familiar with', the "Bekannt" – 'known' used by Wittgenstein here explicitly implicates its etymological root, which always combines the "Kennen" – 'known' – as a type of "Wissen" – *knowledge* – with "Erkennen" – 'recognizing' – as a form of "Wahrnehmen" – *perception.* It thus not only "bezeugen" – *attests* to the interweaving of knowledge and awareness but above all broadens the question *mind-theoretically* on the relation between 'internal' and 'external', on 'own' and 'other', on 'seeing' and 'thinking'."[6]

The question which then, however, appears, is: Of what kind *is* a seeing that constantly oscillates between 'external' and 'internal'? Which *correspondence phenomenon* of external given and internal appearance is thereby described?

The question of the *mental image* – what it is, how it appears and how one could talk about it – is encircled by it – and that is the basis of the following remarks.

As soon as it is established that humans are able to think in images, the question concerning its constitutional set-up arises in all its clarity: Does an internal and an external vision exist? And would the visual seeing – the seeing of objects and people – then be a seeing of first order, while consciousness – self-relation or reflection – would define a seeing of second order?

And if one speaks of mental images less of vision than one does of imagination[7] and with it of sensation, all these descriptions concerning the ability to produce visualized images often equal, the production of a distinction, a distinction between an "Ich-Bewußtsein" – "self-awareness" and an "Aufmerksamkeits-Bewußtsein"[8] – "attention awareness." The "self-awareness" is defined as "feeling that it is me who does something and experiences something and that I am awake and 'conscious'" and differentiates from an awareness that "concentrates on certain internal and external events, such as percipience, thinking, feeling, remembering or imagining." In contrast to the 'self-awareness', this second

5 Flach: *Lament.*

6 Macho: "Ist mir bekannt, daß ich sehe?", p. 212.

7 Cf. Roth: *Das Gehirn und seine Wirklichkeit.*

8 Cf. Macho: "Ist mir bekannt, daß ich sehe?" and Roth: *Das Gehirn und seine Wirklichkeit.*

awareness is – according to him – closely related to attention or even identical with it. The more strongly attention is concentrated upon a certain event, the more conscious it is."[9]

If one would like to resolve the question of what this is, and what our ability to create mental images is about, and to think *with* them and *through* them, then it is *neither* sufficient – and this is the *thesis* of the following remarks – to establish and maintain this distinction between an internal and external scheme of seeing; – the simple antagonism introduced here indeed does not lead to precision but to an imprecise concept of vision, since this division misses out on too much, *nor* does it suffice to relate mental images to pure visual consciousness theories and thus restrict seeing to a physiological process. This would be – so the following argumentation – a rather impermissible reduction.

Rather, it is necessary to link this seeing to a *visual* term, which – in the sense of Georges Didi-Huberman – can trace its origin back to the meaning: *visio*.

In this *imagination* of seeing, the actual "Bildsinn" – 'sense of images' is not only the eye, – as you know, but this en passant, one can also see with closed eyes – but the sense for the visual – and with it the pictorial itself, which naturally includes forms of imagination, Einbildung in the sense of Einbildungskraft, and empathy.

The mentioned distinctions, however, are *foreign* to this sense. "One would have to return to the world of the visibly reproduced (représenté), namely to the *conditions of looking*, of *presentation (présentation)* and "Gestaltbarkeit" – 'the options of forming and shaping' [...] the visual (would be) the new terminus to be introduced which raises up from the visible[10] (as an element of reproduction [représentation] in the classical sense of the word) as well from the invisible (as an element of abstraction). [...] the visual's character tends to withdraw the 'normal' (better said: usually adopted) conditions of visible cognition from us."[11]

Furthermore, it is necessary to understand the mental in an expedition, to perform a double movement: Assuming that an essential iconic structure is imminent to the mental, it is also important to revise the term of a – mental or imaginative – image. This revision detaches it from a simplifying reference to objects of the external world and leads to an image term which encompasses the images' own singularities and extends beyond the optical phenomenon of 'image'. Images of this kind are definitely neither purely retinal phenomenon nor a representation of a view of the own self that allows a glimpse of the soul in order to constitute itself as

9 Roth: *Das Gehirn und seine Wirklichkeit.* The quotation continues: "Wir wollen diesen Zustand das Aufmerksamkeits-Bewußtsein nennen. Das Bewußtsein des eigenen Ich und der personalen Identität bildet hierzu einen ständig vorhandenen Hintergrund." ("We wish to call this state the attention-awareness. The awareness of one's own Ego and one's own identity forms a background constantly present to it.")

10 Didi-Huberman: *Vor einem Bild*, p. 24 [first italicization S.F.].

11 Ibid. p. 25–26.

an organ of knowledge.[12] The point is to understand those pictures in their own dignity, in their own organization of movement, which can be described by a reflection from Paul Valéry on the *specific* abilities of images: Because sometimes, he writes, an image shows more than the objects it represents: “Une image est plus qu’une image et parfois plus que la chose même dont elle est image.”[13]

The point is to open a dimension in which *seeing* itself gains an *optical additional value* and in which the *knowledge* of the *certainty* that art does not necessarily have to reproduce what is visible but instead what one has *not yet seen.*

In this sense, an artistic undertaking not only refers to something but primarily it shows itself. The character of the image takes place within a discrepancy. It can neither be simply regarded as a piece of reality, nor can the glance simply be allowed to become lost among that which is displayed; as such, an image *always* contains an interior reflection and the approach to thematizing the issue of manners of perception. If the images’ character results from relieving the tension between the medium of representation and that which is represented, *only then* can the context be discussed concerning the specific conditions which initially create visibility, meaning the preconditions of certain constructions for visibility.[14]

If one follows these exemplifications, such an *image meaning* is always attached to a *double visibility* which sees itself as essentially governed by the iconic: the relation between ‘visible’ and ‘meant’, of the ‘show itself’ and the ‘shown’.[15] But then it is not primarily the eye that governs this pictorial sense; rather, a perception is essentially generated atmospherically, its sense would be a body that, in this case, always comprises a movens, thus an iconic kinetics.[16]

## II “Perception indeed stylizes”

How can inner imagines be thought of if one excludes that they lead to illegitimate substantializations of fundamentally immaterial objects? The assumption that the mental can be framed as an image and thus as an icon does not at all de-

12 Cf. Macho: “Ist mir bekannt, daß ich sehe?”, p. 221–222.

13 Paul Valéry quoted in: Dagognet: *Philosophie de l’image* (without pagination). What Paul Valéry describes is the additional value of each picture, the art’s additional value, which goes beyond the mere reproduction of the world. For Valéry, those genuine and productive achievements of art take center stage themselves, meaning the reality of the arts which goes beyond simply reproducing the world. A *special* demand is made of art: it should not simply confirm what we already know but rather, we expect exactly this additional value, *increase being or awareness*.

14 Cf. Flach: *‘Körper-Szenarien’*. For the relation of the specific media of the image and the construction of visibility, cf. Spielmann: “Schichtung und Verdichtung”.

15 Gottfried Boehm: “Augenmaß”, p. 33.

16 Flach and Söffner: *Emotionaler Habitus*.

termine that the consciousness is a small box into which the act of seeing inserts small material images that have to be looked at as perceptions as in a gallery, must be hung and viewed as paintings on a wall. Even if there is no doubt that ideas of perceptions are immaterial, this still does not imply that perceptions as ideas do not possess structural features known from images.

Whoever wishes to give an image to the mind (or soul) needs to first tie the mind to the structural moments of this image; the same goes for a moving image that is tied to pulse, processes, rhythm and tact. The property common to ideas and representations does not exist with reference to a *material* picture – still, the common point of reference needs to be looked for in the *visual context*:

Because *by* and *through* looking at something, one does not see images in one's mind, but rather a visual perception is primarily the awareness of something seen – and this can be pictorial. If one does not use inner images to explain that we see something, then one can easily explain with them *how* one sees something in the perception of it.[17]

Perceptions are, this is common knowledge, results of the action of a subject.[18] If one understands inner pictures as the products of a subject, then this individual subject is a very particular one in a specific condition; *which is shown in those pictures the subject itself produces*. This is an *active creation* in which a perception can only be directed towards an object that has been presented in a pictorial form: thus, it is *not* about *content* but about the comparison between a "Darstellung" – 'image-presentation' and "Wahrnehmung" – 'a perception' or a "Vorstellung" – 'imagination', that refers to the structural mode of "Anschauung" – 'perceiving'.

This means that ideas of perceptions in their immanent composition exhibit stylistic structures known from images. If you will, it is all about specific stylistic properties of an extended seeing, without which perception would be impossible. Or, as put by Maurice Merleau-Ponty: "Perception indeed stylizes!"

This allusion to the structural resemblance between images and perceptions hints at a condition that is constitutive of the *mental ability to shape images*: There is a mutuality between the type of perception – i.e. that which Merleau-Ponty calls 'stylize' – and the perceiving subject, i.e. the beholder. *This* form of perception transcends the notion of perception in the classic phenomenology in so far as it offers more than just the explanation of a uniquely *intentional reference*. Such forms of perception are not only perceptions *of* something, but are autonomous vis-à-vis the intentionality, which means – on the one hand – that *the way in which* one perceives something is independent of the phenomenon *of what* one perceives.

On the other hand this type of perception has always been *dynamic*, i.e. one not only sees changing objects, but these in their ever-changing stylized appear-

17 Cf. Wiesing: "Vom Cogito zum Video", p. 140.
18 Cf. ibid., p. 141.

ance.[19] Such seeing cannot be thought of without a personal subject – and vice versa. This relationship shows that something "can only be seen if one sees in stylized fashion and when a personal self is expressed by it, because the stylistic way results from the constitution and approach, from contingent conditionality and the attitude of the one who sees. Seeing always implies structures (…) and giving weight to objects."[20]

The conclusion is that in this stylized manner of perception, the subject shows itself, i.e. "the current and individual self of a person"[21] – so that we may well negate the distinction between an 'external' and 'internal' sphere that I made in the beginning, *without* confusing them totally. That means that the seeing subject determines and chooses the way in which an inner picture is built. As such, the way of perceiving simultaneously represents a statement concerning the properties of a person. Consequently, a mental image – and this would be my definition – may be described as a process. A mental image would be a distinct oscillation, a vibration creating a space for the echo, produced by pendulum-like movements between a perceiving subject and the explorations of its inner sensations.

This definition of the mental image shall now be discussed against the background of a prominent example: the state of the twilight that is not only of great epistemological importance – as well as important in terms of its spatial and temporal nature –, but which also found its way into the arts. In particular, video art offers a preferred point of reference insofar as the processuality, the temporally bound nature and the spatiality of video works is interpreted in analogy to brain processes as put forward by Curtis L. Carter: "Consequently, the establishment of a fuller understanding of video styles requires a clarification of the relationships between the functioning of the *human mind and the image-producing capabilities of video*." However, they also lay claim to a form of autonomy that the traditional representational relationship forfeits in order to make this structure more dynamic. Images are thus processes that do not reproduce reality, but render it visible.[22]

This visibility, which is always generated by a process, characterises specifically to generate an *intermediate space* between the viewer and the image of the Video. Temporary, transitory, and unfolding in the interplay between perception, imagination, remembrance and feeling,[23] this space defies any attempt to determine its location. On the contrary – it *marks out the space* in which perceptions – with and through the concisely Space-Time-Constellation that is typical for all video-works – could occur first of all – and with that a perceptual impression is formed in a very special way: the network of relations in a stimulus pattern – not its individual parts – are recognised as a structural whole, or Gestalt. This is pre-

19 Ibid. p. 141–142.
20 Ibid., p. 143.
21 Ibid. p. 142.
22 Boehm: "Die Wiederkehr der Bilder", p. 33.
23 Contrary to the concept of Platonic Ideas, modern science ascribes the ideas to the plasticity of the brain.

cisely how Rudolf Arnheim describes it in his study *Kunst und Sehen*: "The forces that identify the meaning of events also come to life within the viewer and result in that kind of excited participation that distinguishes artistic experience from the mere passive intake of information."[24]

It needs to be understood that – according to the given hypothesis – these works are of interest not due to their motive-like negotiation of neurological processes or the representation of history of modern brain research, but rather to their examination of scope. They model cognitive processes in a specific way. Thus, representations of space and movements as well as of light and shadow are used for the analysis and subtle differentiation of processes of thinking and states of consciousness. The structural frame of the artistic work, in which the topic of the action expresses itself, arouses – following Arnheim – corresponding powers in the recipient. One of the most prominent examples of a blend between a neurological and a narrative-theoretical concept is the "stream of consciousness". The narrative theory adopts the notion first introduced by William James in *The Principles of Psychology*,[25] which describes conscious processes metaphorically as a continuous stream.

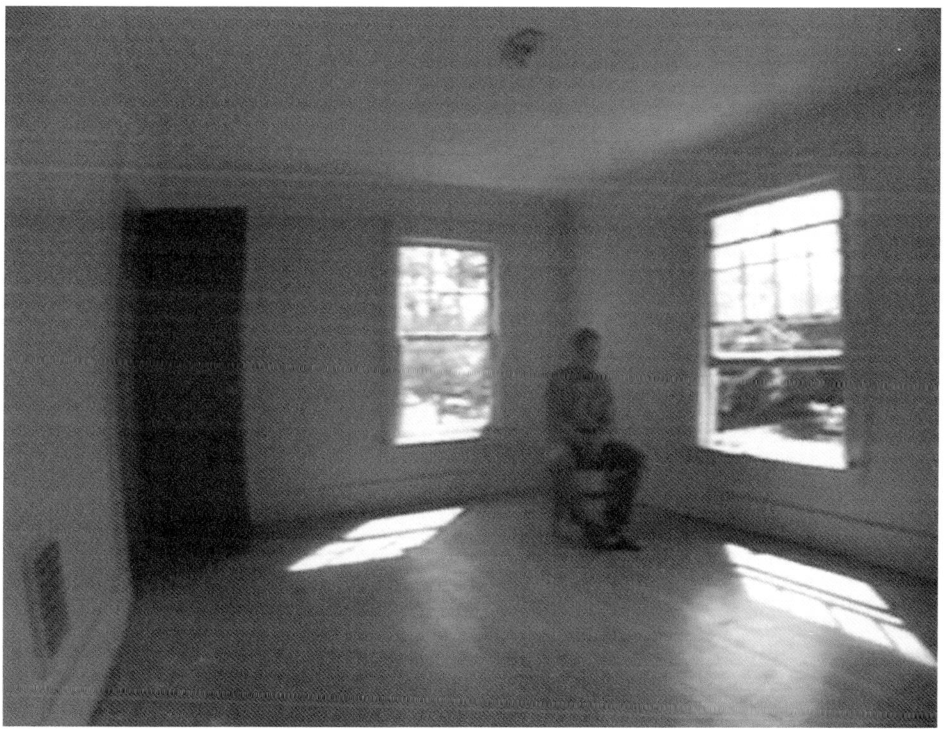

Fig. 1. Bill Viola, Reasons for Knocking at an Empty House, video still, 1983.

24 Arnheim: *Kunst und Sehen*, p. 15.
25 James: *The Principles of Psychology*, Vol. 1, p. 239.

The first chosen example hangs on exactly this potential of the narrative concept. With respect to conceptions of perception and consciousness, I *shift* the emphasis away from the "stream" towards "scansions of consciousness" in order to analyze specific types of rhythm and interruption as the interface between cognitive and visceral processes. Only then – I argue – can moments of *boredom and inertia be found* that may accompany the state of Bill Viola in the physical condition of paralysis. The analysis concentrates on repetitive structures, discontinuity and deceleration of thought and bodily processes, as well as deficiencies in the mode of perception induced thereby.

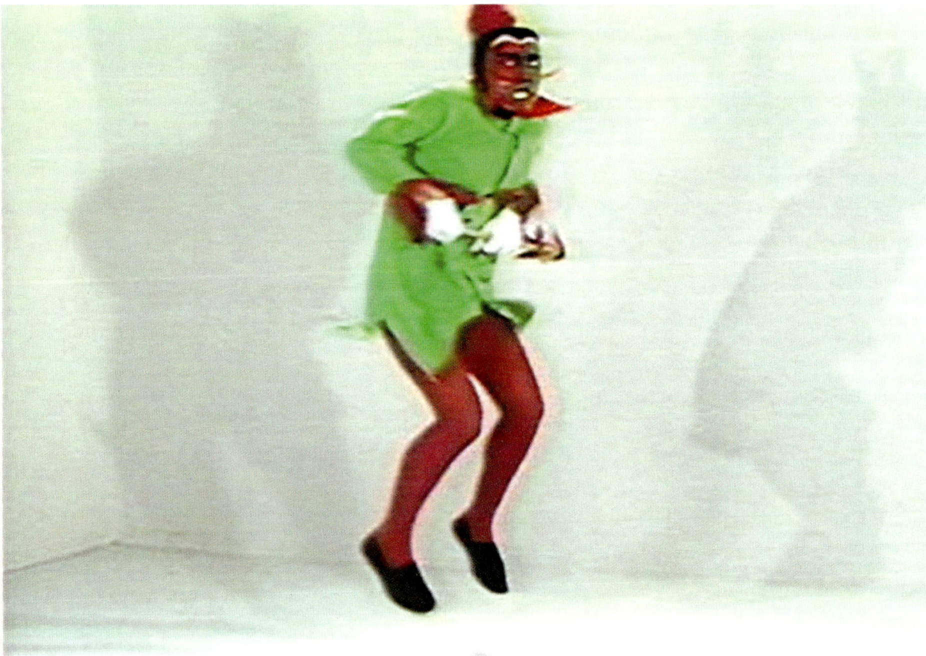

Fig. 2: Bruce Nauman, Clown Torture, video still, 1987.

My second example highlights the twilight not resulting from structures of slow-down but, in direct opposition, from those of density, the *thought coercion.* Again, this is about bodily investigations of thought systems and their irregularities. In the work of Bruce Naumann presented here, the body takes on the function of performing systematic orders on the one hand and represents the starting point and holder of the development of cognitive processes and systems on the other.

## III Perception over time equals thought[26]

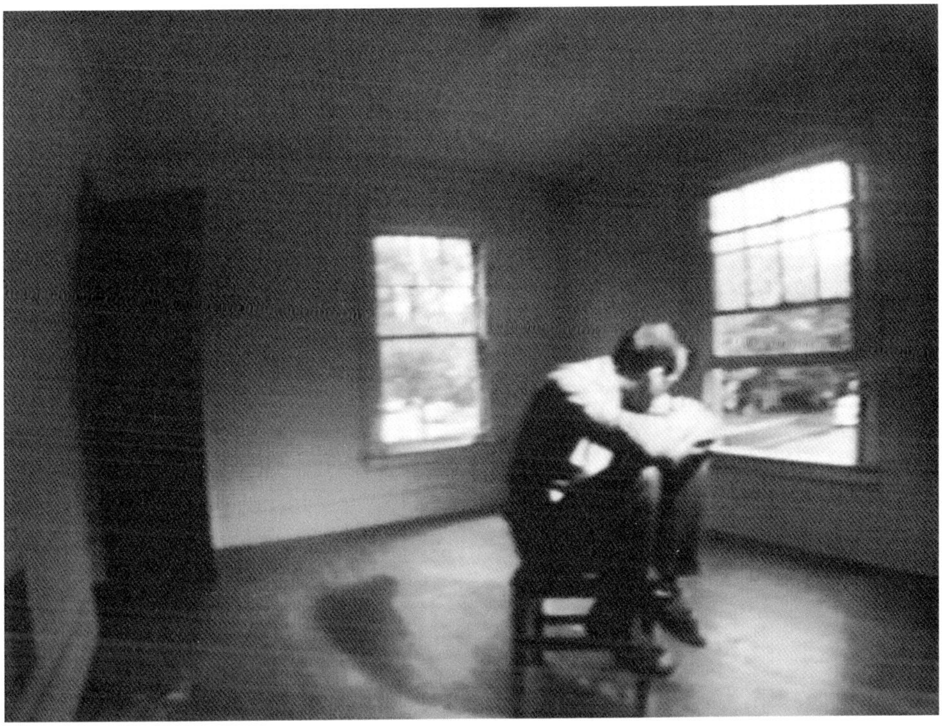

Fig. 3: Bill Viola, Reasons for Knocking at an Empty House, video still, 1983.

"Boredom is a warm, gray cloth laid out with the most glowing, colorful silk lining. We wrap ourselves within this lining when we dream, and are home in its arabesques. But the sleeper appears gray and bored beneath its covering, and when he awakes and is ready to describe his dreams, he usually conveys only this dreary ennui. For who is able to turn the lining of time inside out with one single movement? The telling of dreams is nothing other than this."[27]

Bill Viola's video works can be understood much in the same way as Walter Benjamin's *image* of dreams as a two-sided cloth, whose interior and exterior are closely interwoven and inseparable; as a sounding-out of the complex fabric of relationships.

Interior and exterior congeal in the representation and governing of spatial references which thus is explicitly understood – in the *representation of mental image production*, not in the mental image itself – is explicitly understood as a

26 Viola: *Reasons for Knocking at an Empty House*, p. 150.
27 Benjamin: *Collected Writings*, p. 1054.

linkage of activity or non-activity, bodily experience and habitat and of sensual experience as perceptual patterns. Bill Viola describes this process: "In my work, I have most strongly been aware of the camera as representation of point of view – point of consciousness. Point of view, perceptual location in a space, can be point of consciousness. But I have been interested in how we can move this point of consciousness over and through our bodies."[28]

The real space is the basis for the video "Reasons for Knocking at an Empty House"[29] from 1983.[30]

To understand this video work as an example of cognitive research that establishes itself from a comprehension of the arts reveals many things. I would like to analyze some of them in terms of their image-theoretic aspects.

Bill Viola himself can be seen in different positions in this room, close to the camera as well as – according to the measurement of the room – far from it, sitting on a chair, on the floor, leaning against a wall, standing freely in the room; sometimes one can hear him breathe and sigh. His positions and his relation to

28 Viola: *Reasons for Knocking at an Empty House*, p. 148.

29 The idea of 'Reasons for Knocking at an Empty House' already in 1982 served Bill Viola for an installation. The beholder must assume a peculiar sitting position, in which she faces an unusual spatiality. She finds herself vis-à-vis a monitor showing the image of Viola, who – after days without sleep and fathoming out the limits of consciousness – struggles with keeping himself awake. Via headphones, the beholder hears the noises produced by Viola himself, putting her in a state of felt permanence and duration. Viola and the beholder are notoriously literally beaten out of this non-state or limbo, whenever Viola receives a beat on his head, which can be heard on the headphones as an acoustic shock. Unexpectedly the instantaneous 'now' erupts into the state of duration. By means of this immediate bodily sensation, the beholder can immerge into the experience of this work. Bill Viola described this effect: "The notion of the voyeur (viewer) is very important. The inner space one experiences when sitting in the chair is an obvious metaphor for the space inside our skins, the ultimate inside/outside perimeter, but getting into the chair is like getting inside someone else's skin." The installation is a reminiscence of the worker Phineas P. Gage, who, while working for the Vermont railways in 1848, became the victim of an accident. While he was working, a demolition charge exploded prematurely, an iron rod darted into Gages left cheek and penetrated his forehead. Gage survived, but the peace-loving and gentle fellow had turned into an aggressive and unpredictable man.

30 While working on this art piece, Bill Viola spent three days and nights in an unspecified, barely furnished room. Besides a table and a chair, the beholder of the video tape can see a door at the left side of the chamber. In the background and on the right wall two windows are located. Both of them can be opened by pushing them up. The light coming in from the windows figures as the only option to understand whether it is night or day. The noise from the streets penetrates through them, and from time to time, the beholder can see a car passing by. For the whole duration of the video tape, the beholder watches this scene from a slightly elevated position on the left side of the room, so that only the wall on which the camera is placed, and some parts of the right and the left wall escape his vision. The chair is located in different positions during the course of the art piece – sometimes Viola sits down on it. The little table, on which a jar is placed, does not seem to be permanently located in the room (unless one could suppose that it might sometimes be placed in the wall, where the camera is located, and thus cannot be seen); on some of the video stills it is not present.

the room are relative to the chair that changes with Viola's positions; the chair becomes his counterpart. The slight changes of location which modify the room in a minimal sense by the three mobile "objects" – the table, the chair and Bill Viola himself – return the attention to the emptiness of the space structured only by the changes of light. The emptiness of the action thus is equivalent to the emptiness of the space.[31] This emptiness acquires a density in the perception which is effected by the lack of events that structure time. The space which is experienced is then filled with the density of duration. "Existence for existence's sake. Beyond waiting. There is nothing to wait for except to live in the next moment. Just living. Isolating time. The effects of duration. Boredom. Fatigue. Disorientation. Upset cycles. The psychology of isolation and sleep deprivation here is presented in two ways: first, the extreme wide angle cover shot of the room which never changes. A fixed frame. A constant container, both prison and security. Only the motion of the figure and his physical manipulations are visible as change. It becomes a claustrophobic viewing situation. Second – the common hallucinatory properties of sound in these situations is presented by lavalier miking – bringing the audio up close to the person in the room, often times in relation to the visual image, way out of proportion and in opposition to a normal auditory situation. In situations without sleep, even the ticking of a clock can seem deafening.[32] "The idea was to stay awake for three days, confined in an empty room of a desert house, a fixed camera observing what would happen as time became an aggressive, destructive force of this person, me."[33]

The passage of time is experienced only through changes of positions in the room, these markings are the only way to interrupt the duration, and the attention of the recipient is enhanced due to this lack of action and focuses on the minimal changes of location of the objects that become *basic* perceptual sentiments and *bodily* experience. Perceiving thus becomes a process tied to the passive body in Viola's sense, a constant and fixed constellation of events in which a perceptual process oriented along the production of differences turns into a non-linear, unanchored minimal scansion and subliminal pulse. Reflection is radically refused, seemingly without differentiation; differentiation is abolished instead of produced. With the lack of differentiation as exhibited in this video, Viola shows how identity is massively threatened by a seemingly ever-returning situation. In

31 Considering the formal disposition of this tape, Viola comes close to minimalist conceptions of spatiality. Robert Morris describes the relation of object and space: "Denn der Raum eines Zimmers ist selbst ein strukturierender Faktor, und zwar sowohl durch seine kubische Form wie auch im Sinne der verschiedenartigen Verdichtung, mit der sich unterschiedlich große und unterschiedlich proportionierte Räume auf das Subjekt-Objekt-Verhältnis auswirken können." ("The space of a room is, indeed, itself a structuring factor, which is due to both its cubic form and in the sense of divergent aggregation, by which differently sized and differently proportioned spaces can influence the relation of subject and object." – Robert Morris quoted in: Stemmrich: *Minimal Art*, p. 344.)

32 Viola: *Reasons for Knocking at an Empty House*, p. 97.

33 Ibid. p. 245.

"Reasons for Knocking at an Empty House", Viola lets the circumstances of a spatial experience become an experiment of an extreme temporal experience. This permanently unchanging state of duration is defined by the lack of events; absence is the state presented in this work. The process of differentiation that not only creates an orientation in the spatial environment but also creates perception of temporal intervals and passage of time is deconstructed in this work.

Viola's oeuvre is characterized by this subtlety in treating the physiological and subjective conditions of perception on the one hand and the material perceptual objects on the other. This virtuous treatment simultaneously shows that consciousness develops just like objects: namely through relationships.[34] One can then understand Viola's works as the attempt to return something of the Latin origin *perceptio* to seeing and perceiving, which denotes not only the seeing but rather the *taking hold* of the subject in the sense of *grasping* or *capturing.*[35] Event fields are produced, zones and passages, in which nothing objective is created but in which conditions are made visible, possibilities and options that allow for a zone hovering on the borders of virtual experiences; visionary experiences.

## IV Mental excercises – Please pay attention please

"One only gains an awareness of self identity by a certain amount of activity and not by mediating upon oneself" was Bruce Nauman's reply to Willoughby Sharp's question in a 1970 interview on the motivation for those videotapes in which massive physical movement is set into motion.[36]

In the video series "Raw Materials" and "Clown Torture", Bruce Nauman shows physical activity in virtually hysterical repetition. The soundtrack accompanying these works, which makes the obsessive repetition even more striking to the viewer, must be ignored here but not first without mentioning the verbalism, or better said, the acoustic phonetics and strength of sound.

The scansion of single words or phrases is brought into an exact choreography with eruptive body movements, just the same as a drawn-out tone – as for example in Raw Material BRRRRRR – and staged together with the movement, which transports the body into a plethora of vibration.

34 Stafford in Interventionen, p. 44.

35 Crary: *Aufmerksamkeit*, p. 15 and Flach: *Realfiktionen*.

36 Bruce Nauman: "Bewegen und Begegnen".

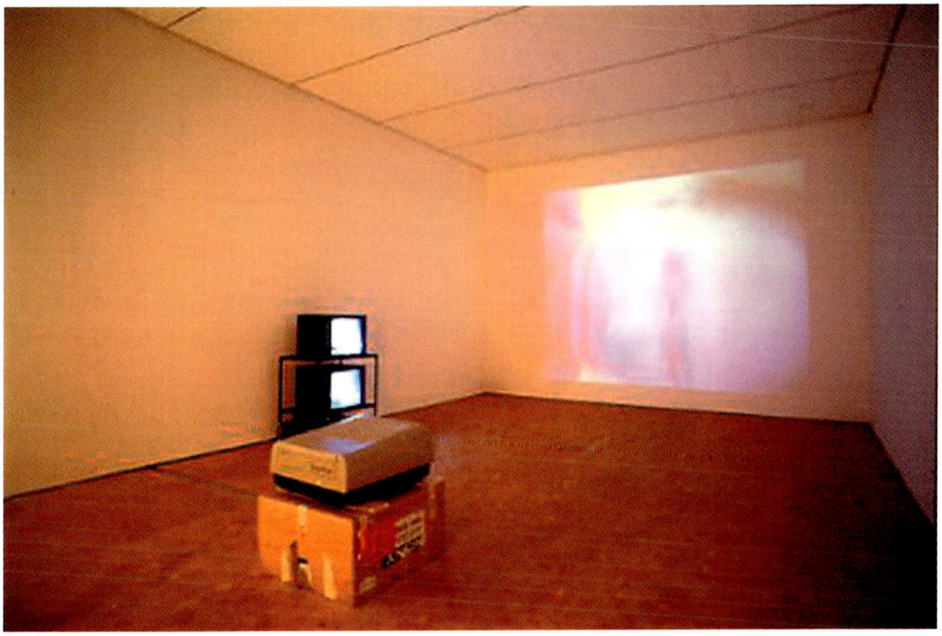

Fig. 4: Bruce Nauman, Raw Material BRRR, view on the installation, 1990.

In these "self performance pieces", claustrophobic situations are also presented and communicated to the viewer by permanent agitation which seems to be oddly stationary in its execution. An *undermining* of the strict external/internal schema arises in that it becomes obvious that an interior status determines an external one and vice versa. This manifests in penetrating, stereotypical rhythms of action and monotonous repetitions.

A tension is unleashed by the display of "compulsive repetition" which measures the room between work and recipient. By accentuation of a synchronic structure of event, it becomes obvious that it is not an individualized body represented here but rather the extracted relation, a – in Plessner's terms – "intermediate- or status sphere"[37] – which is the focus. The intensity of that presented communicates exactly this: artificiality is not only strongly systematized by the repetition, but the conceptual structure, inferior to the work, allows Nauman to also control the recipient's reaction, as he describes himself: "it is a kind of body-response, they feel (…) that tension."[38] Knowledge about the mind should not be communicated but evoked.

Thus, "enhanced gestures"[39] are shown in which the body is *in no way* considered simply an external instrument of an interior. But if such a movement – as a rhythmic structure – has always been representational activity, it will be, con-

37 Plessner: *Ausdruck und menschliche Natur*, p. 87.
38 Bruce Nauman quoted in: Korot and Schneider: *Video Art*.
39 Freud *Collected Writings* I, p. 152.

sciously or unconsciously, reproduced exactly where *no* goal-orientated action can be recognized but where something is insinuated. Rather, this "behavior" – using Plessner's term – is "psychophysically neutral", so that the "descriptively sensual" with "the descriptive data" is always ascribed as "non-objective non-objectively".[40]

Its goal is not beyond itself but has its own meaning. It wants to "be accepted as a picture and is sufficient in and to itself."[41]

When it is not the represented gesture which communicates a certain expression but rather – in the full sense of classical art theory the gestures (for example the lines in painting or drawing, the use of the camera and the room organisation in video art, etc.), which is recognized as expressive.

And when an affect is *not* exactly expressed by body posture but rather the expression's modality generates and presents a habitus, and this presenting refers to its double meaning, namely to (re)present and to present, then this habitus refers to a potential expression or, as Warburg formulates it, the expression of the art on *its style.*

Images are also to be understood as "Ereignisbilder" – 'images of an event' or even better: as "Erregungsbilder"[42] – images of an *agitation*, in which aesthetics and kinesis cannot be thought of separately; as such, kinesthesia would not simply be a perception of movement but more a perception in movement.[43]

What is relevant to an iconic episteme's concept is also equally addressed: the internal proximity between imagination and imago, between imaginativeness and image. In this sense, it is the imagination itself that uses the internal image sense to create external images.[44] The mental image and l'image objet are two aspects of one and the same phenomenon; the difference, if there is one at all, is that one picture is ephemeral and the other can be of an indeterminate duration. Or, as Jacques Derrida and Bernhard Stiegler describe it in the Échographies: "L'image en général n'existe pas. Ce que l'on appelle l'image mentale et ce que j'appellerai ici l'image-objet, [...] sont deux faces d'un seul et même phénomène qui ne peuvent pas plus être séparées [...]. La différence qui s'impose le plus immédiatement est que l'objective dure, tandis que la mentale est éphémère."[45]

40 Plessner: *Ausdruck und menschliche Natur*, pp. 83, 86.
41 Ibid., p. 90.
42 Waldenfels, Bernhard: "Von der Wirkmacht und Wirkkraft der Bilder", p. 57.
43 Ibid. p. 57.
44 Boehm: "Das Paradigma 'Bild'", p. 80.
45 Derrida and Stiegler: *Échographies*.

## V Epilogue

> All vivid reactivity is bound to differentiation, whose most prominent instrument is the body. This destiny has to be recognized as essential. The body as an instrument of differentiation of vital reactions; and only the body, is comprehensible according to its psychic vividness. The body finds one of the most important determinations of differentiation in perception.[46]

This is what Walter Benjamin writes in his essay on the "psycho-physical problem" in 1922. To see oneself seeing, to make the invisible visible, all this is conditional on tying the act of seeing to conceptions of perception, for which not only the "seeing, but the sentiment of structures"[47] is important – as Walter Benjamin further writes. The act of seeing is thus detached from the classic regime of visual sight and is tied to a model of perception and subjectivity. This model *frees* the seeing from its reduction to a purely retinal reproduction of an external visual impression and *ties* it to a notion of embodiment. With this linking of seeing to the body, seeing is just one layer of the body and the subject that sees is not determined solely and in one sense through the constructs of seeing, but through a concert of *all* senses that shape the modality of seeing in the first place. Or rather, it is about a subject that is aware of the inextricably mixed modalities and contingencies of perceiving.

## References

Arnheim, Rudolf: *Kunst und Sehen. Eine Psychologie des schöpferischen Auges.* Berlin / New York (de Gruyter) 2000.

Benjamin, Walter: "Strenge Kunstwissenschaft. Zum ersten Band der 'Kunstwissenschaftlichen Forschungen'", in: *Schriften* Vol. 3, ed. by Rolf Tiedemann und Hermann Schweppenhäuser, Frankfurt am Main (Suhrkamp) 1972, pp. 363–369.

Boehm, Gottfried: "Augenmaß. Zur Genese ikonischer Differenz", in: Gottfried Boehm, Birgit Mersmann and Christian Spieß (eds.): *Movens Bild. Zwischen Evidenz und Affekt*, Munich (Fink) 2008, pp. 14–43.

Boehm, Gottfried: "Das Paradigma 'Bild': die Tragweite der ikonischen Episteme", in: Hans Belting (ed.): *Bilderfragen. Die Bildwissenschaft im Aufbruch*, Munich (Fink) 2007, pp. 77–82.

46 Cf. also Walter Benjamin: "Schemata zum psycho-physischen Problem" (ca. 1922), here quoted in Sigrid Weigel: "Passagen und Spuren des Leib- und Bildraumes", p. 61.

47 Benjamin: "Strenge Kunstwissenschaft", p. 368.

Boehm, Gottfried: "Die Wiederkehr der Bilder", in: Gottfried Boehm: *Was ist ein Bild?*, Munich (Fink) 1994, pp. 11–38.

Dagognet, François: *Philosophie de l'image*, Paris (Vrin) 1984.

Didi-Huberman, Georges: *Vor einem Bild*, Munich (Hanser) 2000.

Flach, Sabine: '*Körper-Szenarien*' *Zum Verhältnis von Bild und Körper in Videoinstallationen*, Munich (Fink) 2003.

Flach, Sabine: On Lament, in: Sabine Flach, Daniel Margulies and Jan Söffner (eds.): *Habitus in Habitat I. Emotion and Motion*, Bern, New York, u.a. (Peter Lang) 2010

Flach, Sabine: "Realfiktionen. Versuchsanordnungen von Olafur Eliasson", in: Matthias Bruhn/Kai-Uwe Hemken (eds.): *Modernisierung des Sehens. Sehweisen zwischen Künsten und Medien*, Bielefeld (transcript) 2008, S. 287–299.

Flach, Sabine and Jan Söffner: *Emotionaler Habitus. Verkörperte Sinnlichkeit zwischen Subjektivität und Umweltrelation,* München (Fink) 2011.

James, William: *The Principles of Psychology* (1890), Vol. 1, New York (Dover) 1950.

Korot, Beryl and Ira Schneider (ed.): *Video Art. An Anthology*, New York (Harcourt) 1976.

Macho, Thomas: "Ist mir bekannt, daß ich sehe? Wittgensteins Frage nach dem inneren Sehen", in: Hans Belting and Dietmar Kamper: *Der zweite Blick. Bildgeschichte und Bildreflexion*. Munich (Fink) 2000, pp. 211–229.

Nauman, Bruce: "Bewegen und Begegnen", in: Christine Hoffmann (ed.): *Bruce Nauman. Interviews 1967–1988*, Dresden (Philo Verlagsgesellschaft) 1996, pp. 85–86.

Plessner, Helmuth: *Ausdruck und menschliche Natur* (= GS, Vol. VII), Frankfurt am Main (Suhrkamp) 1982.

Roth, Gerhard: *Das Gehirn und seine Wirklichkeit. Kognitive Neurobiologie und ihre philosophischen Konsequenzen*, Frankfurt am Main (Suhrkamp) 1996.

Stafford, Barbara: "Die kombinatorische Ästhetik der Neurobiologie", in: Jörg Huber (ed.): *Darstellung: Korrespondenz* (= *Interventionen* 9), Zürich Wien New York (Springer) 2000, p.43–61.

Spielmann, Yvonne: "Schichtung und Verdichtung im elektronischen Bild", in: Yvonne Spielmann and Gundolf Winter (eds.): *Bild – Medium – Kunst*, Munich (Fink) 1999, pp. 59–77.

Stemmrich, Gregor (ed.): *Minimal Art. Eine kritische Retrospektive*. Dresden / Basel (Verlag der Kunst) 1995.

Viola, Bill: *Reasons for Knocking at an Empty House. Writings 1973–1994*, Cambridge, MA (MIT Press) 1995.

Waldenfels, Bernhard: "Von der Wirkmacht und Wirkkraft der Bilder", in: Gottfried Boehm, Birgit Mersmann and Christian Spieß (eds.): *Movens Bild. Zwischen Evidenz und Affekt*, Munich (Fink) 2008, pp. 47–63.

Weigel, Sigrid: "Passagen und Spuren des Leib- und Bildraumes in Benjamins Schriften", in: Sigrid Weigel (ed.): *Leib- und Bildraum. Lektüren nach Benjamin.* Köln / Weimar (Böhlau) 1992.

Wiesing, Lambert: "Vom Cogito zum Video. Die bewußtseinstheoretische Bedeutung des Sehens nach René Descartes", in: Olaf Breidbach, Karl Clausberg (eds.): *Video Ergo Sum. Repräsentationen nach innen und außen zwischen Kunst- und Neurowissenschaft*, Hamburg (Verlag Hans-Bredow-Institut) 1999, p. 134–147.

Wittgenstein, Ludwig: *Vermischte Bemerkungen. Eine Auswahl aus dem Nachlaß*, ed. by Georg Henrik von Wright in collaboration with Alois Pichler, Frankfurt am Main (Suhrkamp) 1994.

Wittgenstein, Ludwig: *Zettel*, ed. by G.E.M. Anscombe and Georg Henrik von Wright (= *Werkausgabe*, Vol. 8), Frankfurt am Main (Suhrkamp) 1984.

## List of Illustrations

# The Subject 'at Rest'
# Cognitive Neuroscience's Struggle with the Dark Side of Cognition

FELICITY CALLARD / DANIEL S. MARGULIES

## 1. Introduction

If the human being is, today, specified by the property of *brainhood* – "the property of quality of *being*, rather than simply *having* a brain"[1] – what sort of brain is it that underpins her personhood? In this chapter, we are interested in the qualities and dynamic features of this brain, and how the neurosciences currently conceptualize its development, possibilities and constraints. How, in particular, is its articulation with the environment modelled? To what extent are its contours inflected by earlier models and frameworks – neurological, psychological, and philosophical – that have been used to explore the brain, and to what extent do they depart from them? What implications, moreover, might these conceptualizations of the brain have for accounts of subjectivity in the multi-disciplinary spaces of research on brain-self-environment relations?

Over the course of the first decade of the twenty-first century, discussions regarding the brain – both within and beyond the neurosciences – have arguably been most preoccupied with three poles of research:

(i) on *neuroplasticity* and *neurogenesis*, which describe the brain's capacity to reorganise itself by forming new neural connections throughout life, and the formation of new neurons in the mature brain;[2]
(ii) a renewed focus on *emotion/affect* – as a remedy for the excision of these phenomena from earlier, overly cognitive models of brain and hence of self;[3] and
(iii) on *mirror neurons* and, more generally, *social neuroscience* – the neural mechanisms of shared understanding and communications.[4]

1 Vidal: "Brainhood".
2 Malabou: *What Should We Do With Our Brain?*; Rubin: "Changing Brains".
3 See the research of Jaak Panksepp (*Affective Neuroscience*), Antonio Damasio (*Descartes' Error*, *The Feeling of What Happens*), and Joseph LeDoux *The Emotional Brain*.

Alongside these tectonic shifts within the neurosciences, and in complex articulation with them, the social sciences and humanities have been experiencing an efflorescence of theoretical and empirical research on the self and subjectivity that engages many of the same terms – for example, affect, empathy, and embodiment – that are currently common currency within the neurosciences. Indeed, some of this research in the humanities and social sciences includes the creative use, translation and reworking of research findings, as well as more general concepts, from the neurosciences.[5] The brain – as it is being conceptualised and modelled by the neurosciences, as well as disseminated beyond them – is in the process of being reframed by a fourth potent arm of research, that on the brain's *resting state* and its *default mode* of function.

* * * * *

In 2009, the *Journal of Neuroscience* commemorated the 40th anniversary of the Society for Neuroscience by asking a number of prominent neuroscientists to reflect on the changes within the field over the past 40 years. Marcus Raichle, in his paper, announced that there had recently been nothing less than a paradigm shift in functional neuroimaging.[6] Raichle contrasted two perspectives on brain function, each of which, he contended, has had a long and complex history. According to one perspective, the brain "is primarily reflexive, driven by the momentary demands of the environment"; according to the other, "the brain's operations are mainly intrinsic involving the maintenance of information for interpreting, responding to and even predicting environmental demands."[7] It is the former perspective that has characterised much of the corpus of experimental and theoretical research within the neurosciences. And it is the latter that has, accordingly, been for much of the last century the neuroscientific underdog. For this perspective explicitly departs from existing models of the brain that characterise cognitive neuroscience – and of the attendant self that that brain is said to subtend.

This emergent field is little more than a decade old. It comprises research on the brain in the absence of any explicit task, termed the 'resting state,' or 'default mode,' which has given rise to interest in the 'default mode network' (DMN), a set of brain regions that effectively underlie a novel core of cognitive function. In this paper, we map and analyse this emergent research field. In so doing, we attend specifically to the potential implications that research on the resting state

4 For a review of mirror neuron research see: Rizzolatti and Craighero: "The Mirror-Neuron System", and for social neuroscience see: Lieberman: "Social Cognitive Neuroscience".

5 E.g. Connolly: *Neuropolitics*; Massumi: *Parables for the Virtual*; Hansen: *New Philosophy*. For a consideration of the potential as well as the difficulties associated with these interdisciplinary engagements see: Cromby: "Integrating Social Science with Neuroscience" and Papoulias and Callard: *Biology's Gift*.

6 Raichle: "A Paradigm Shift".

7 Ibid.

and on the default mode of the brain have for conceptualisations of subjectivity that extend beyond the perimeter of the neurosciences. Our intention is twofold. First, we trace the emergence of 'rest' and 'the resting state' as objects of scientific enquiry, and, in so doing, indicate how such scientific constructs challenge – as well as pay certain debts to – existing psychological models used within cognitive neuroscience. Second, we reflect on potential implications of such research for conceptualisations of subjectivity that coalesce in fields adjacent as well as distal to the neurosciences. Our paper comprises a cross-disciplinary collaboration between a neuroscientist within the field of resting state functional magnetic resonance imaging (fMRI) research and a cultural theorist with expertise in the history and living present of psychiatry. Our positions within and to one side of the scientific field of resting state research allow us, we believe, to offer insights, cautionary as well as enthusiastic, regarding the potential that this field holds for reorienting some of the existing models through which subjectivity and brain-self-environment relations have been understood.

## 2. Revolutions of a restless neuroscience

The claims now being made on behalf of resting state research – as Raichle's announcement of a Kuhnian paradigm shift[8] makes clear – wish to underline its historically revolutionary status. But, notably, the claims for newness and the excitement surrounding this field are conjoined with an emphasis on its revivification of a hitherto submerged perspective on brain function. Indeed, Raichle, in proclaiming the impending paradigm shift, dwells on how "surprising discoveries"[9] in imaging research have opened up a new chapter in what has actually been an historically long-standing interest in exploring the behavioural relevance of intrinsic brain activity. He leans, here, on the genealogy presented by the eminent neuroscientist and physiologist Rodolfo Llinás.[10] Llinás contrasts the work of William James and the famous neurophysiologist Charles Sherrington with that of Sherrington's disciple, T. Graham Brown. James and Sherrington conceptualised the central nervous system as fundamentally reflexological, in which "the brain is essentially a complex input/output system driven by the momentary demands of the environment."[11] In contrast, Brown argued that the spinal cord ought not to be understood as reflexological, and indeed that movement could be intrinsically generated in the absence of sensory input:

8 Ibid.
9 Ibid.
10 Llinás: *I of the Vortex.*
11 Ibid. p. 6.

> It is therefore possible to look upon the neuraxial unit as the efferent neurone and not as the reflex arc, and *to regard as the primitive activity not the reflex but that rhythmic phenomenon* of which there still remain examples in the acts of progression and respiration.[12]

Brown's prime focus was on the rhythmic and intrinsic organisation of gait: he argued that his research demonstrated that the conditioning of rhythmic activity is largely self-generated, such that sensory input modulates but does not determine it. He thus refocuses our conceptual lenses away from the phenomenon of the reflex arc and towards that of rhythmic intrinsic organisation. Llinás argues that Brown's insights on spinal cord function may be extrapolated to the operations of the brainstem and areas of higher brain function. On this view of the brain, sensory input "modulates rather than informs"[13] the intrinsic system of nervous system function. Such a view runs counter to many theoretical frameworks employed by various disciplines in the course of the twentieth century to understand and model the human brain and cognition, not least behaviourism, orthodox cognitive psychology, and later cognitive neuroscience. Indeed, such a view entails a potential reconfiguring of the articulation between brain, self and environment – or between internal and external world – from the one familiar to us from cognitive science.

Resting state research, in explicitly allying itself with Brown over Sherrington, positions itself on one side of a long running duel, one whose axis centres on the opposition between the reflexive and the intrinsic. But how did rest and 'the resting state' emerge as topics of explicit scientific enquiry within neuroscience? In this section, we present a brief genealogy, paying particular attention to some of the manoeuvring of different neuroscientific sub-disciplines, and to the moments at which initially distinct constructs and terms coalesced. Of particular interest are two distinct paths – with distinct methodologies, techniques and fields of expertise – out of which the field as we know it today has been constituted: cognitive psychology and neurophysiology. We contend that, over the course of the last decade, the terminology employed within this field has been transformed – in the process moving to vocabulary that is less contentious, arguably more tightly bounded, and primed for a neuroscientific reframing of inner mental life.

### *2.1 Lineage I – 'default mode'*

A cross with arms of equal length (Figure 1) is an ancient ideogram and also semiotically complex: for mathematicians, it indicates addition, or two perpendicular bisecting line segments; for art historians, the crucifix; perhaps it also sug-

12 Brown: "On the Nature of the Fundamental Activity of the Nervous System", p. 45 [italics added].

13 Llinás: *I of the Vortex*, p. 7.

gests a target – for those in the business of aiming at things. For cognitive psychologists and neuroscientists, this cross signifies a classic condition for the control state during an experiment. It is the state of rest, a neutral state, baseline, the moment of 'crosshair fixation.' For cognitive neuroscience, this state has long been on the opposing side of the cognition it aimed to study.

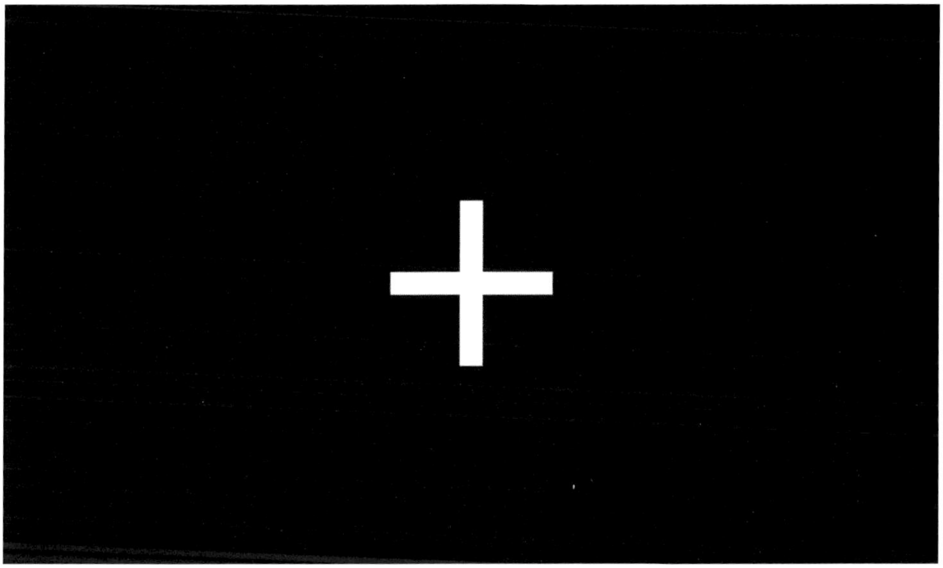

Fig. 1: An example of a standard cross-hair used for baseline fixation during psychological task paradigms.

Most categories of study in cognitive neuroscience emerged from a century-old lineage of experimental psychology.[14] The traditional approach in neuroimaging studies, both in positron emission tomography (PET) and continuing with fMRI, was the contrast of a specific state (e.g. visual stimulus, sustained attention, memory retrieval) with a state in which subjects were simply asked to rest. Depending on the experimental condition, this 'resting-state' could be with eyes closed, eyes open, or fixation on a crosshair. Rest was implicitly considered a cognitive baseline against which task demands elevated brain activity in function-specific regions.

14 Although the tools of non-invasive neuroimaging with high spatial resolution were developed in fields such as physics, chemistry and medicine, their application to mapping cognitive function was the product of their union with concepts and task paradigms predominantly drawn from experimental psychology. Bringing cognitive psychology's tools into the neuroimaging environment thus enabled the rapid growth in the field of cognitive neuroscience in the 1980s. Many of the tools of cognitive psychology are, in turn, highly indebted to research by the pioneers of late nineteenth- and early twentieth-century experimental psychology on basic cognitive processes such as sensation, perception, attention and memory (see: George Mandler: *A History of Modern Experimental Psychology*; Kurt Danzinger: *Constructing the Subject*).

Gordon Shulman and colleagues at Washington University in St. Louis (one of the foremost institutions in the field of cognitive neuroscience) noted some regions of the brain appeared to *decrease* in activity during the task condition. In 1997, they published their findings in the *Journal of Cognitive Neuroscience* showing that a distribution of regions including the medial prefrontal, posterior cingulate/precuneus, and lateral parietal cortex were more active when subjects were resting.[15] This paper also argued that while a passive control condition in the experimental design might for some appear to be "too underspecified" to act as a reliable control, their analysis indicated that "passive conditions" across a wide variety of experiments produced a "consistent set of blood flow changes" and could thereby serve as a control state.[16] Notably, this paper also ruminated on the blood flow decreases caused by ongoing processes in the passive mental state, suggesting the possibility of unconstrained verbal thought processes, monitoring of the external environment, and monitoring of the body image. (Such constructs would, notably, return in later attempts to theorize what is happening cognitively when the brain is 'at rest.') They explicitly considered that processes in the 'passive condition' might have an 'antithetical relationship' to active task processes (as sleep is antithetical to an alert state, a 'general exploratory/monitoring state' might be antithetical to a task-focused state). This shift – which we shall term 'The Flipping of Contrasts' – presented cognitive neuroscience with the problem of how to make sense of the data. If a large swath of cortex is more active during a state of rest, what is happening *psychologically* during rest that is driving this increased activity?

The term 'default mode' entered the cognitive neuroscience vocabulary to describe the functional state of rest, in the contemporary sense, with Marcus Raichle's and colleagues' publication of three papers in 2001.[17] Many of these task-induced decreases in brain activity appeared to be "largely task independent, varying little in their location across a wide range of tasks." Such consistency made them consider whether there might be "an organized mode of brain function that is present as a baseline or default state and is suspended during specific goal-directed behaviors."[18] Through a semiotic linking of functional neuroanatomy to the regions found to be more active during rest, several hypotheses were proposed regarding the psychological content of the resting state. Debra Gusnard and colleagues postulated that the observed medial prefrontal cortex activity reflected the predominance of self-referential mental activity (also observed to implicate the medial prefrontal cortex) that occurs in the absence of environmen-

15 Shulman et al.: "Common Blood Flow".

16 Ibid.

17 See: Gusnard et al.: "Medial Prefrontal Cortex"; Gusnard and Raichle: "Searching for a Baseline"; Raichle: "A Default Mode". Buckner and colleagues note that references to 'default mode' are first found in the literature on cognition, in other words prior to the term's appearance in explanations of neural and metabolic phenomena (Buckner et al.: The Brain's Default Network).

18 Gusnard et al.: "Medial Prefrontal Cortex".

tal demands. They furthermore tentatively proposed that such activity was involved in the "processing of such representations that *embody aspects of self*,"[19] and linked such processing to the concept of the autobiographical self proposed by Damasio and that of the narrative self proposed by the philosopher Shaun Gallagher.[20] Gusnard and Raichle's review in *Nature Reviews Neuroscience* elaborated their theory of a default mode of brain function based in neurophysiological, as well as psychological questions, thus invigorating long neglected research questions regarding internally-driven mental states.[21] These three papers were central – and not solely in terms of their inauguration of a new research field. For they indicated that one "useful way" to address the "important concept" of the self was "to further explore the nature of default state activity"[22]: in so doing, these authors established an enduring and intimate tie between the resting state and investigation of the neural architecture of the self.

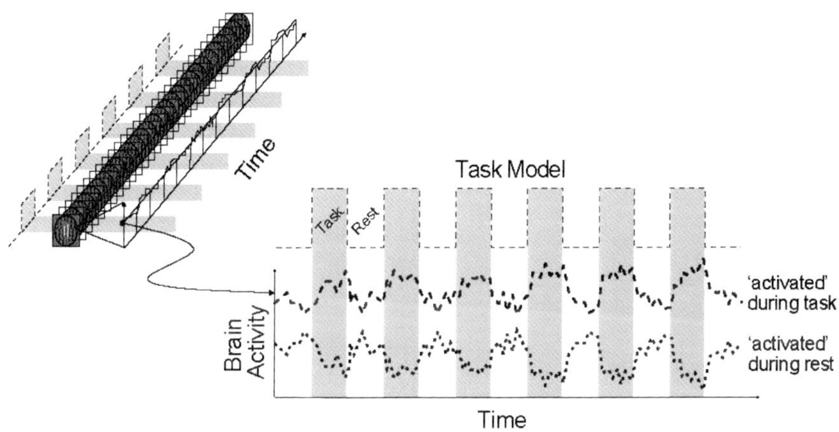


Fig. 2: Traditionally, cognitive neuroscience studies focus on the brain regions which covary in activity with a task. 'The Flipping of Contrasts' by Shulman and colleagues[23] involved inverting the traditional contrast of 'task-over-baseline' in order to assess regions that were more active during the resting condition.

It would take us too far afield from the central concerns of this paper adequately to address the numerous research findings and debates regarding the default mode since 2001.[24] What follows is a schematic outline of some of those that are most critical to the arguments of this paper.

19 Ibid. [italics added].
20 Damasio: *The Feeling of What Happens*; Gallagher: "Philosophical Conceptions of the Self".
21 Gusnard and Raichle: "Searching for a Baseline".
22 Gusnard et al.: "Medial Prefrontal Cortex".
23 Shulman et al.: "Common Blood Flow".
24 Two significant and growing bodies of research that we do not discuss in this paper comprise: (i) The clinical psychiatric literature, which has expanded rapidly to touch on all major diag-

### *(i) Goal-directedness*

While activity during the default mode was initially set in opposition to "goal-directed behaviour,"[25] it was subsequently reconceptualised as involved in long-term, goal-directed planning, as numerous studies hypothesized its role in prospection, or future-oriented thinking.[26]

### *(ii) Quantification of stimulus-independent thoughts and the invigoration of research on mind-wandering*

More recently, we have witnessed the coalescence of research on the default mode network with other cross-disciplinary areas of research. Most notably, previously dispersed research on stimulus-independent thoughts, task-unrelated thoughts and 'zone outs' has been gathered together under the umbrella term of 'mind-wandering'.[27] Through such research, phenomena such as mind-wandering, which have previously been marginal to the theorisations of brain and self undertaken by cognitive science, have been installed as far more fundamental. Mason and colleagues' study in *Science*, for example, contended that mind-wandering constitutes "a psychological baseline that emerges when the brain is otherwise unoccupied" and that is underpinned by activity in a default network of cortical regions.[28] (That the dissemination of such research into the public sphere is undertaken via the use of such statements as "Daydreaming seems to be the default setting of the human mind" underlines how such research is effecting a shift away from a model of the self oriented towards external goals so beloved by orthodox cognitive psychology.)

nostic categories. (For a review see: Greicius: "Resting-State Functional Connectivity.") (ii) Cross-species resting state research, which provides a means of studying the physiology underlying spontaneous low-frequency fluctuations (for example: Biswal and Kannurpatti "Resting-State Functional Connectivity"), and to facilitate cross-species comparative studies of functional neuroanatomy (see: Margulies et al.: "Precuneus"; Vincent et al.: "Intrinsic Functional Architecture").

25 Shulman et al.: "Common Blood Flow".

26 Spreng et al.: "The Common Neural Basis".

27 Christoff et al.: "Experience Sampling"; Gilbert et al.: "Comment"; Mason et al.: "Wandering Minds"; Smallwood et al: "Going AWOL in the Brain". A paper by Smallwood and Schooler – entitled, interestingly, "The Restless Mind" – helped to bring about the current scientific popularity of the term 'mind wandering.' The authors, noting precisely the fact that research was proceeding using a variety of "disparate constructs", called for the phenomenon to be referred to as 'mind wandering': because this term is familiar to the lay person, its use would, they believed, aid the elevation of such research into mainstream psychological thinking (see: Smallwood and Schooler: "The Restless Mind").

28 Mason et al.: "Wandering Minds".

### *(iii) Self-related processing, episodic memory, social cognition and sense of agency*

Topics of inner rumination, reflection and motivation have been subsumed under the heading of default mode function, with task-based studies used to support the specialized roles of the implicated regions.[29] Much support has been drawn from the rationale that the content of mind-wandering is composed of episodic memory, prospection, and the consideration of social relationships. Given the diversity of roles attributed to the default mode network (DMN), more recent work has attempted a network-based rendition of the modular theory of brain function (which postulates that each functional area of the brain has a singular role), thus subdividing the DMN in order to accommodate such diverse theories of function.[30]

Regardless, however, of the cohesiveness of the cognitive constructs under development, or of the precise spatial distribution of the responsible network, a cognitive neuroscience theory of unquantifiable inner experience was taking form through the linking functional roles of brain regions that are more activated during the state of rest with the psychology of unconstrained mental activity.

## *2.2 Lineage II – spontaneous brain activity*

We have thus far focused on cognitive neuropsychology as it established the foundations and terminology for studying the brain's function in the psychological state of rest. However, interest in 'resting' brain activity, albeit of a different sort, preceded Shulman's 1997 'The Flipping of Contrasts'. Bharat Biswal and other physicist colleagues, who were then based at the University of Wisconsin in Milwaukee, were working under the guidance of James Hyde (a major innovator in the development of fMRI technologies). Rather than asking the *neuropsychological* question posed by Shulman and colleagues, they posed a parallel question about the role of the spontaneous activity that was discarded as noise in analytic models.[31] Instead of inquiring about a functionally relevant psychological baseline condition, Biswal and colleagues explored the possibility that baseline physiological activity might be functionally significant for maintaining neural organization.

29 Goldberg et al.: "Neural Correlates"; Moll et al.: "The Self"; Schilbach et al.: "Minds at Rest?"; Spreng et al.: "The Common Neural Basis".

30 Andrews-Hanna et al.: "Functional-Anatomic Fractionation".

31 For a visual example of the temporal dynamics in an fMRI dataset, see: http://vimeo.com/9871689, which presents real-time fMRI data of a single individual listening to music. Similar fluctuations are also present in the absence of any overt sensory or behavioural activity.

That spontaneous neurophysiological activity was functionally relevant was not a new idea,[32] but it had fallen behind the hypothesis of the input-output model driving behavioural psychology. If the brain were instead primarily driven by the requirement to maintain its own dynamics, with environmental input only modulating, rather than driving its function, the spontaneous endogenous dynamics would be meaningful and not simply unconstrained noise. Biswal and colleagues addressed this question in 1995 with a remarkably simple paradigm.[33] They began with a standard finger-tapping task in a boxcar design, and expectedly, the motor cortex was activated more during tapping than during the resting-condition. Their innovation was to then take data collected from the same subjects during a rest-only condition and to analyse the correlation between the spontaneous fluctuations occurring in a small portion of the motor cortex and the rest of the brain. They found that the same distribution of motor cortex activated during the tapping-task was correlated in its spontaneous fluctuations. Here, the title of their seminal article: "Functional connectivity in the motor cortex of resting human brain using echo-planar MRI," reflects the union of fields that was to follow almost a decade later. Thus, it appeared that the brain was functionally coordinated into spatially consistent areas *even in a task-independent state of rest.*

### *2.3 Consolidating the 'resting-state' field of research*

The links between the field of dynamic physiological properties in the resting human brain with the field of dynamic psychological properties in the resting human brain were not as obvious as they perhaps might now seem. Biswal's findings were not initially popular within the imaging community, and cognitive neuroscience did not know how to integrate Raichle's work. One may conjecture that the two groups were unaware of each other's work, as no cross citations exist prior to 2003.[34]

32 E.g. David Ingvar's research on high resting blood flow in the prefrontal cortex, which he attributed to spontaneous self-generated mental activity of the resting human brain (Ingvar: "Memory of the Future").

33 Biswal et al.: "Functional Connectivity".

34 The assertion that the research communities were independent from one another prior to 2003 can be justified by the lack of any prior cross citations. This claim is supported by the consistency with which Raichle cites Biswal as the seminal researcher in the field in articles and lectures appearing after 2003 (for example: *video.google.com/videoplay?docid=7393045011 768458913*). From the perspective of the surrounding research community, personal correspondence with numerous neuroimaging researchers supports the early general neglect of the 'task-induced deactivations' Raichle was describing. Likewise, Biswal's findings ran so contrary to the popular assumptions in the field that his findings were attacked (personal communication). Another example comes from the closing discussion of the first international conference on resting state research in December 2008, where a participant commended Biswal's perseverance by quoting Ghandi: "First they ignore you, then they ridicule you, then

A young researcher named Michael Greicius who was working in the laboratory of Vinod Menon at Stanford University made the connection. His article, published in *Proceedings of the National Academy of Sciences* and edited by Raichle, was entitled "Functional connectivity in the resting brain [*note the Biswal reference*]: a network analysis of the default mode hypothesis [*note the Raichle reference*]."[35] The unification of these two approaches, one psychological, the other physiological, and both essentially a break with the dominant model of input-output brain function, marked the beginning of what we now know as 'resting-state fMRI'. It was here that Greicius and colleagues coined the functional-anatomical term that has become almost synonymous with the name of the field itself: the 'default-mode *network*'. It was this network, they argued, that "account[ed], in large part, for the phenomenon of task-related decreases in brain activity."[36] The blending of the two fields is most exemplified by a statement by Raichle and Snyder from a response paper published in 2007 in the journal *NeuroImage*: "The important distinction is not between "rest" and "task" but rather between intrinsic and evoked activity."[37] The yoking of the physiological and the psychological approaches to one another has meant that, even as the 'resting state' research field now appears to be a unitary one, it retains within it distinct theoretical foundations and terminologies. This theoretical fecundity has been advantageous in terms of sparking wide-ranging empirical research as well as giving extra impetus to model building. But it has also meant that the 'resting state' and the mapping of the cognitive function of the default mode network are frequently conflated. The creative semiotic terrain produced through the mixing of these terminologies has aided and will, we suggest, continue to aid the transmission of this research into other disciplinary arenas and into the public sphere.

## 3. Implications of a revised rest

The previous sections have attempted to depict the complexity of the field of transformations produced through the emergence of the resting state research field and its self-proclaimed inauguration of a new paradigm in functional neuroimaging. These transformations have been not only technical and methodological, but have been accompanied by disciplinary disturbances as well as ontological and epistemological shifts in how the brain is conceptualized and scientifically interrogated. In the remainder, we analyse in greater detail some of

they fight you, then you win." To which Biswal responded: "... and we all know what happened to Ghandi. ... They shot him."

35 Greicius et al.: "Functional Connectivity".

36 Ibid. p. 256.

37 Raichle et al.: "A Default Mode".

the potential implications of these transformations for models of brain, self and subjectivity.

The methods and objects of resting state research potentially catalyse a new model of brain and self. The intrigue with and focus on non-observable and unconstrained mental activity, for example, contributes to the emergence of an account of the self grounded as much through mind-wandering and introspection as through deliberate, goal-focused activity; the focus on the rhythm of the intrinsic and spontaneous dynamics of the brain contributes to the emergence of an account of the self specified through and anchored by those dynamics rather than through her responses to the environment and the exteroceptive stimuli that impinge upon her. As resting state and DMN findings begin to be disseminated, it is possible to discern already how they are being used to ground particular visions both of the self and of the intimate tie between brain and self. The neuroscientists Susan Whitfield-Gabrieli and John Gabrieli, for example, in an online article for *Scientific American* have suggested that the:

> exciting discoveries about the resting human brain raise the question of whether we are gaining the novel capacity to measure quantitatively our most intimate and unique inner selves. Are you most "you" when you're racing through work? Or when you're simply sitting in a chair, mind adrift, just being?[38]

And Raichle, himself, in a recent cover feature for the *Scientific American*, writes:

> The brain's default mode of function serves as a master organizer of its dark energy. Over time neural dark energy may ultimately be revealed as the very essence of what makes us tick.[39]

If, as Nikolas Rose has argued, the spaces of contemporary biomedicine and biopolitics are opening up "new ideas of what human beings are,"[40] then there appear already to be indications that the resting state and the DMN might be installed as a new foundation for the self. In these two quotations, it is the subject 'at rest' that – by dint of her default mode brain activity – potentially holds the key to subjectivity *tout court*. We can see the ease with which the analytical distance between resting state data, models of DMN activity, and claims about the nature of subjectivity can be flattened.

The explosive growth of resting state research has, then, started to make its mark felt beyond the laboratory. In the process, 'rest' has been rewritten to comprise various active, internal psychological states. The past century of experimental psychology was built upon those aspects of cognition that it could modulate and measure externally. The emergence of the concept of a default mode of neur-

38 Whitfield-Gabrieli and Gabrieli: "Idle Minds".
39 Raichle: "The Brain's Dark Energy", p. 49.
40 Rose: *The Politics of Life Itself*, p. 6.

al and psychological activity has impinged on the inner territory of the subject, and, in the process, rendered it tangible to experimental neuroscientific paradigms. In little more than a decade, the 'task induced deactivations' noticed by Shulman and colleagues have moved from being a complete mystery, to being configured as a coherent network that has been described in *ScienceNews* as "one of the hardest-working systems in the brain" – "despite its laid-back name."[41] Rest – to follow Raichle in his frequent use of a quotation from Seneca – has in this formulation certainly become "far from restful."[42]

We wish to comment on one particularly noticeable consequence of this reconfiguration of 'rest', not least because it returns us to the problematics we considered in the introduction to this chapter. It also significantly reorients some of the previous assumptions and guiding models used within the humanities and social sciences to describe and conceptualize a self who is not engaged in deliberate and purposive activity. It is our contention that through the reconfiguration of rest, the resting brain has been territorialized: it is conceptualized and materialized as a matrix that is constituted as perpetually productive, as intrinsically creative, and as thrown towards the future. Most notably, the increased focus on the importance of mind-wandering and daydreaming in no way gainsays the brain's industriousness. Buckner and colleagues, for example, in describing resting state activity, speculate that: "Rather than let the moments pass with idle brain activity, we capitalize on them to consolidate past experience in ways that are adaptive for our future needs."[43] Raichle and Snyder make no bones about the fact that, for them, study of the default mode of the brain enhances investigation of "the real reason we have a brain": "not to reminisce about the past nor react in the moment but, rather, to envision the future."[44] The brain, on Raichle's account, functions as a kind of "Bayesian inference engine" through which it is able to generate predictions of the future, and to link these predictions with its reflections on the past. Such abilities are, moreover, central to "the development of unique human attributes such as imagination and creativity."[45] Unsurprisingly, then, as this research travels through non-peer reviewed publications, the use of tropes of productivity to characterize states of only apparent idleness, multiply. As Saey puts it: "It may be off when you're on, but the brain network behind daydreams and a sense of self is no slacker."[46]

41 Saey: "You Are Who You Are By Default", p. 16.

42 Raichle is quoting from Seneca: "The fact that the body is lying down is no reason for supposing that the mind is at peace. Rest is … far from restful" (Seneca: *Epistulae morales*). Interestingly, Seneca is describing the state of individual who has not found serenity because his emotions are in turmoil and hence his sleep is "far from restful"; Raichle, in contrast, quotes Seneca in the service of embedding the restlessness of rest as a generic rather than phenomenologically (and ethically) specific condition.

43 Buckner et al.: "The Brain's Default Network", p. 31.

44 Raichle et al.: "A Default Mode", p. 1089.

45 Raichle: "The Brain's Dark Energy", p. 1250.

46 Saey: "You Are Who You Are By Default", p. 16.

The model of mind-wandering as industriousness is in distinct contrast to those accounts of day-dreaming and mind wandering that dominated late nineteenth and twentieth-century philosophy and social theory. For Freud, for example, the key conceptual term in his famous essay "Writers and Day-Dreaming" is *play*; this is "serious play", certainly, but play nonetheless.[47] Freud's mind is one in which "hardly anything is harder for a man than to give up a pleasure which he has once experienced." Indeed, the subject does not give something up but exchanges one thing for another, such that as the child grows, he "builds castles in the air" rather than castles made out of bricks. The contrast between Freud's formulation (in which subjectivity is weighted by the pull of the past) and that of Raichle and Buckner (with the subject's adaptive orientation to the future) could not be more marked.

The territorialization of rest is also reframing older, analytical frameworks and constructs that functioned in a binary manner. One way in which William James, for example, divided the field of consciousness was to oppose attention to the state of absentmindedness conjured up by the French term *distraction* and the German *Zerstreutheit*. For James, it was the abolition of the state of distraction that signalled the awakening of the attention.[48] In contrast, the model of attention being developed in the DMN literature reformulates absentmindedness or mind-wandering as a form of introspective attention. Here, network brain activity 'at rest' is mapped on to the psychological category of attention, such that attention's opposite no longer exists. Instead, we have two types of attention – the intro- and the extrospective. The neuroscientist Peter Fransson, in a similar manoeuvre, argues that activity during the default mode disallows the possibility that one might, metaphorically speaking, "lose track of oneself." While he acknowledges that there is still uncertainty as regards the "exact function of this core of intrinsic activity", he speculates that:

> it represents unconscious and continuously on-going processes that are necessary to maintain a coherent neuronal representation of the "self." We believe that irrespective of how focused we are on a specific task [such task-based focus implies lower levels of DMN activity] and no matter how computationally demanding that task is, we cannot, metaphorically speaking, "lose track of ourselves". At all times, the brain needs to have a coherent mental model of the self. Cognitive faculties that might be administered by this model include having a sense of who we are and where in space we are and the passage of time.[49]

47 Freud: "Writers and Day-Dreaming".

48 James: *Principles of Psychology*. It is fascinating that James notes that the "curious state of inhibition" that he is describing can be "produced at will by fixing the eyes on vacancy", and that some individuals are able "voluntarily [to] empty their minds and 'think of nothing.'" James here almost exactly describes the instructions commonly given to research subjects in resting state studies.

49 Fransson: "How Default Is the Default Mode", p. 2844.

Fransson is here talking at the level of the brain rather than about the phenomenological self. Nonetheless, his claim that the brain's unceasing and coherent mental model of the self might administer cognitive functions that include such fundamental subjective categories as the 'sense of who we are', conjures up a conception of the self that is unable to lose its moorings or, in short, to unfix itself from its self. If the resting state and DMN literature present a brain and a self preoccupied with daydreaming and fantasy, and characterised by unconstrained mental activity, such activities should, in fact, be regarded as tethered and directed rather than formless and indeterminate.

## 4. Rest moves

We have described how resting state research is in the process of reconceptualising models of brain and self within – and potentially outside of – the neurosciences. While such transformations are in certain ways building on – and committed to expanding – already established cognitivist frameworks (e.g. note the use and extension of standard psychological constructs such as attention), they are, we suggest, simultaneously delineating a rather different account of the self, one which is ripe for movement into other fields.

The polysemy and complexity of the two terms at the heart of this new research field – *rest* and *default* – are, we consider, likely to continue to be central to the interest in, debates over, and dissemination of findings within this neuroscientific research field. *Default:* The current meaning of default – a condition that obtains in the absence of active intervention – is etymologically very recent: the *Oxford English Dictionary* traces its use to 1966: to define a preselected option adopted by a computer when no alternative is specified by the user or programmer.[50] Here, the 'default' is something that is specifically programmed into a system, rather than being immanent to it. But the artificiality of the system disappears once the term travels beyond the realm of programming, such that the 'default' connotes the neutral state of the system – how it might act in the absence of interventions/stimuli. Such a 'neutral state' easily slides towards connoting the core, functional state of the system; from there, to what the system most 'naturally' returns to; and from there, perhaps, to connoting the 'core' of the self. (Let us recall, for example, how this research field is re-positioning the subject as a default daydreamer. Or how Whitfield Gabrieli and Gabrieli pose their rhetorical question in relation to the default mode: "Are you most 'you' when you're racing through work? Or when you're simply sitting in a chair, mind adrift, just being?"[51]

50 Weinberg: *PL/I.*
51 Whitfield-Gabrieli and Gabrieli: "Idle Minds".

*Rest:* This term has, of course, a rich philosophical, anthropological, religious and sociological – as well as biological and physiological – history. It is therefore metaphorically and metonymically very rich, a characteristic that has, as we have seen, been exploited to the full by scientists, external commentators and critics when discussing research on the resting state. (Those of us who are social scientists ought not to imagine that the term 'rest' has lain uninterrogated by scientists. Indeed, resting state scientists – along with their interlocutors – have done much conceptual ground-clearing vis-à-vis the difficulties of the term.) The etymology of 'rest', as described by the *Oxford English Dictionary*, indicates that uses of the word have included: a natural repose or relief from activity; the intermission of labour or exertion (hence the Sabbath as the day of rest); freedom from distress or trouble; quiet or tranquillity of mind; an interval of silence or a pause (in music); the cessation of motion; and continuance in the same position or place. In this sense, rest can variously be regarded as the opposite of: activity, busyness, labour, movement, restlessness and agitation. We have indicated how the resting state research field has reworked most of these axes such that the resting brain is now characterized by ceaseless activity, exertion, industriousness and movement. (The only axis that has not obviously been reworked is the affectively freighted axis that opposes rest to agitation, distress or trouble.) We have also seen the ease with which the focus can move between analysing a 'resting' state metabolically, physiologically and psychologically. Resting state researchers' characterizations of the 'resting brain' are, indeed, largely intended to be characterizations of *the brain* (whether at a metabolic, physiological or psychological level). Nonetheless, neuroscientific styles of thought are frequently underpinned by what Vidal has described as a "brain-self-consubstantiality,"[52] such that the 'self' quickly becomes co-terminous with those attributes of the brain.

What is noticeable in the rise to visibility of resting state research is the language used to describe and conceptualize the new scientific object. Both the peer-reviewed and non-peer-reviewed literature frequently employ tropes connoting wildness or an underside when describing the resting state and the DMN. Raichle's two papers (one peer-reviewed, one not) entitled "The Brain's Dark Energy"[53] point to a fundamental and mysterious property of the brain; Jarrett (in a non-peer-reviewed article), comments, in a similar vein, that "Perhaps resting brain activity, and the mind-wandering it gives rise to, is psychology's very own *dark matter.*"[54] Others invoke the well-worn trope of exploration: leading neuroscientist Giulio Tononi describes "the discovery of a major system within the brain, an organ within an organ, that hid for decades right before our eyes," and comments that "It's like finding a new continent."[55] Buckner and Vincent explain

52 Vidal: "Brainhood", p. 7.
53 Raichle: "The Brain's Dark Energy".
54 Jarrett: "The Restless Brain".
55 Glausiusz: "Devoted to Distraction".

that "we are in uncharted territory."[56] But the very moment at which this mysterious new object comes into view is also the moment in which there is a drive either to rebut its strangeness (e.g. Morcom and Fletcher's unease that 'mysterious functions' might be attributed to the resting brain),[57] or to render the new object co-terminous with other, more familiar constructs.

* * * * *

How is the brain that is said to underpin our personhood being conceptualised within and beyond the neuroscientific laboratories? Brains that are emotional, brains that are neuroplastic, and brains that are characterised by mirror neurons are arguably beginning to make significant inroads into public discourse, and to be themselves subjected to critical interrogation.[58] But while the emergent field of resting state research is, as we have demonstrated, already making a significant impact both empirically and conceptually within the neurosciences, it has as yet not been subject to any sustained critical analysis from a perspective external to or to one side of the neurosciences.

That has been the task we have set ourselves in this chapter, through offering a schematic outline of the field's genealogy and an initial assessment of how it is reconfiguring models of brain-environment relations and of the self. The impact and extent of such reorderings within as well as beyond the neurosciences is not yet clear. What is clear is that this nascent field is both deeply engaged with and raising to greater visibility many problematics – mind-wandering and day-dreaming, somatic rhythms, introspection, memory and the anticipation of the future, the consolidation and experiencing of the self – that are also topics of live debate and enquiry within the social sciences and the humanities. Both these latter disciplinary domains are, moreover, currently preoccupied with how to use and respond to insights from other fields of expertise when conducting conceptual and empirical explorations of self and subjectivity. 'Resting state' research, we believe, is at the cusp of being taken up and put to use by social scientists and humanities scholars.

We write at a moment in which articles with such titles as "The Restless Brain",[59] "Devoted to Distraction",[60] "Daydream Achiever",[61] "Perchance to Daydream ... and Degenerate"[62] and "You Are Who You Are By Default"[63] are beginning to disseminate research concerning the resting state and the default mode network to various publics. It is precisely because processes of diffusion,

56 Buckner and Vincent: "Unrest at Rest".
57 Morcom and Fletcher: "Does the Brain Have a Baseline?".
58 Rees: "Being Neurologically Human"; Rubin: "Changing Brains".
59 Jarrett: "The Restless Brain".
60 Glausiusz: "Devoted to Distraction".
61 Lehrer: "Daydream Achiever".
62 Valeo: "Perchance to Daydream".
63 Saey: "You Are Who You Are By Default".

dissemination and translation have only recently begun – and hence that the paths that such diffusion and translation will take are as yet underdetermined – that we consider it important to delineate some of the directions of travel, the consolidation of constructs, and the openings, as well as the potential perils, that such a field offers to those beyond its borders. The rapidity of dissemination and translation of research on mirror neurons is instructive in this regard. That the experimental corpus on mirror neurons was both small and specific did not slow the speed with which mirror neurons were taken up to add weight to hypotheses and models being developed in other neuroscientific fields. And it was certainly no block to the excitement with which 'mirror neurons' were greeted and set to work by diverse researchers within the social sciences and humanities.[64]

In the course of the paper, we have argued that the 'new continent' of the default mode network is – as it is ushered into the light – being mapped, filled in, and hence reconceptualised as positivity. In the process, many of the previous characteristics and connotations of 'rest', and the constructs associated with it, are being reframed and/or overturned. In the eagerness with which 'rest' is being redescribed as the brain's industriousness, the moment of uncovering the mystery of the resting state is also, perhaps, the moment in which its mystery is colonised. Resting state research has opened up to neuroscience what was hitherto unquantifiable inner experience, and, in so doing, has destabilised many of the assumptions built into the models of cognitive science. For the social sciences and humanities to engage with resting state research, then, holds open the possibility of engaging with, and contributing to the building of, a different model of the self and of subjectivity from that one familiar to us by dint of the dominance of orthodox cognitive psychology. But we have also argued that the resting state field is simultaneously engaged in a reworking of cognitive constructs such as attention and of memory. Such reworking is, we have suggested, incorporating – and territorialising – resting state activity. In this reworking, the openings beyond cognitivism are arguably being closed. We write at a moment in which to borrow from resting state research enables the possibility of borrowing in a currency different from that of cognitive – and cognitivist – science. Whether those exchanges will take place in a different currency or, as both the resting state field and the exchanges grow, return to the same currency, remains to be seen.

64 E.g. Orbach: *Bodies*; Stafford: *Echo Objects*; Thrift: "Pass It On".

## Acknowledgements:

Felicity Callard acknowledges the financial support of the NIHR Biomedical Research Centre for Mental Health, South London and Maudsley NHS Foundation Trust/Institute of Psychiatry (King's College London). Daniel Margulies acknowledges the financial support of the Max Planck Institute for Human Cognitive and Brain Sciences, Leipzig and The Neuro Bureau of Berlin. The authors also acknowledge the support of the European Neuroscience and Society Network (funded by the European Science Foundation [ESF]) for providing the opportunity to initiate this collaboration.

Parts of this chapter appear in an earlier article, which is appearing in a special issue of the journal *Subjectivity*, published by Palgrave, entitled *Neuroscience and Subjectivity* (Felicity Callard and Daniel S. Margulies "The Subject at Rest: Novel Conceptualisations of Self and Brain from Neuroscience's Study of the 'Resting State'").

## References

Andrews-Hanna, J. R., J. S. Reidler, J. Sepulcre, R. Poulin, and R.L. Buckner: "Functional-Anatomic Fractionation of the Brain's Default Network", in: *Neuron* 65 (2010) 4, pp. 550–62.

Biswal, B. and S. S. Kannurpatti: "Resting-State Functional Connectivity in Animal Models: Modulations by Exsanguination", in: *Methods in Molecular Biology* 489 (2009), pp. 255–74.

Biswal, B., F.Z. Yetkin, V.M. Haughton, and J. S. Hyde: "Functional Connectivity in the Motor Cortex of Resting Human Brain Using Echo-Planar MRI", in: *Magnetic Resonance in Medicine* 34 (1995) 4, pp. 537–41.

Brown, T. G.: "On the Nature of the Fundamental Activity of the Nervous Centres. Together with an Analysis of the Conditioning of Rhythmic Activity in Progression, and a Theory of the Evolution of Function in the Nervous System", in: *The Journal of Physiology* 48 (1914), pp. 18–46.

Buckner, R. L. and J. L. Vincent: "Unrest at Rest: Default Activity and Spontaneous Network Correlations", in: *NeuroImage* 37 (2007), pp. 1091–1096.

Buckner, R. L., J. R. Andrews-Hanna and D. L. Schacter: "The Brain's Default Network: Anatomy, Function, and Relevance to Disease", in: *Annuals of the New York Academy of Sciences* 1124 (2008), pp. 1–38.

Christoff, K., A. M. Gordon, J. Smallwood, R. Smith, and J. W. Schooler: "Experience Sampling During Fmri Reveals Default Network and Executive Sys-

tem Contributions to Mind Wandering", in: *Proceedings of the National Academy of Sciences* 106 (2009) 21, pp. 8719–8724.
Connolly, W. E.: *Neuropolitics: Thinking – Culture – Speed*, Minneapolis (Minnesota Press) 2002.
Cromby, J.: "Integrating Social Science with Neuroscience: Potentials and Problems", in: *BioSocieties* 2 (2007), pp. 149–169.
Damasio, A.: Descartes' Error: Emotion, Reason, and the Human Brain, New York (Avon) 1994.
Danzinger, K.: *Constructing the Subject: Historical Origins of Psychological Research*, Cambridge (Cambridge University Press) 1990.
Fransson, P.: "How Default Is the Default Mode of Brain Function?: Further Evidence from Intrinsic Bold Signal Fluctuations", in: *Neuropsychologia* 44 (2006) 14, pp. 2836–2845.
Freud, S.: "Writers and Day-Dreaming", in: *The Standard Edition of the Complete Psychological Works of Sigmund Freud*, Vol. 9, ed. by James Stratchey, London (Hogarth Press and the Institute of Psycho-Analysis) 1908.
Gallagher, S.: "Philosophical Conceptions of the Self: Implications for Cognitive Science", in: *Trends in Cognitive Sciences* 4 (2000) 1, pp. 14–21.
Gilbert, S.J. et al.: "Comment On 'Wandering Minds: The Default Network and Stimulus-Independent Thought'", in: *Science* 317 (2007) 5834, p. 43.
Glausiusz, J.: "Devoted to Distraction", in: *Psychology Today* (March / April 2009), pp. 84–91.
Goldberg, I., S. Ullman, and R. Malach: "Neuronal Correlates Of 'Free Will': Are Associated with Regional Specialization in the Human Intrinsic/Default Network", in: *Consciousness and Cognition* 17 (2008) 3, pp. 587–601.
Greicius, M.D., B. Krasnow, A.L. Reiss, and V. Menon: "Functional Connectivity in the Resting Brain: A Network Analysis of the Default Mode Hypothesis", in: *Proceedings of the National Academy of Sciences of the United States of America* 100 (2003) 1, pp. 253–258.
Greicius, M. D.: "Resting-State Functional Connectivity in Neuropsychiatric Disorders", in: *Current Opinion in Neurobiology* 21 (2008), pp. 424–430.
Gusnard, D. A. and M.E. Raichle: "Searching for a Baseline: Functional Imaging and the Resting Human Brain", in: *Nature Reviews Neuroscience* 2 (2001), pp. 685–694.
Gusnard, D. A., E. Akbudak, G.L. Shulman, and Marcus E. Raichle: "Medial Prefrontal Cortex and Self-Referential Mental Activity: Relation to a Default Mode of Brain Function", in: *Proceedings of the National Academy of Sciences of the United States of America* 98 (2001) 7, pp. 4259–4264.
Hansen, M. B. N.: *New Philosophy for New Media*, Cambridge MA (MIT Press) 2004.
Ingvar, D. H.: "'Memory of the Future': An Essay on the Temporal Organization of Conscious Awareness", in: *Human Neurobiology* 4 (1985), pp. 127–136.
James, W.: *The Principles of Psychology*, New York (Dover Publications) 1890.

Jarrett, C.: "The Restless Brain", in: *The Psychologist* 22 (2009), pp. 836–839.
LeDoux, J. E.: *The Emotional Brain: The Mysterious Underpinnings of Emotional Life*, New York (Simon & Schuster) 1996.
Lehrer, J.: "Daydream Achiever", in: *Boston Globe* (31 August 2008).
Lieberman, M. D.: "Social Cognitive Neuroscience: A Review of Core Processes", in: *Annual Review of Psychology* 58 (2007), pp. 259–289.
Llinás, R.R.: *I of the Vortex: From neurons to self*, Cambridge, MA (MIT Press) 2001.
Malabou, C.: *What Should We Do with Our Brain?*, New York (Fordham University Press) 2008.
Mandler, G.: *A History of Modern Experimental Psychology: From James and Wundt to Cognitive Science*, Cambridge, MA (MIT Press) 2007.
Margulies, D. S., J. L. Vincent, C. Kelly, G. Lohmann, L. Q. Uddin, B. B. Biswal, A. Villringer, F. X. Castellanos, M. P. Milham, and M. Petrides: "Precuneus Shares Intrinsic Functional Architecture in Humans and Monkeys", in: *Proceedings of the National Academy of Sciences of the United States of America* 106 (2009) 47, pp. 20069–20074.
Mason, M. F., M. I. Norton, J. D. Van Horn, D. M. Wegner, S. T. Grafton, and C. Neil Macrae: "Wandering Minds: The Default Network and Stimulus-Independent Thought", in: *Science* 315 (2007) 5810, pp. 393–395.
Massumi, B.: *Parables for the Virtual: Movement, Affect, Sensation*, Durham and London (Duke University Press) 2002.
Moll, J., R. de Oliveira-Souza, G. J. Garrido, I. E. Bramati, E. M. A. Caparelli-Daquer, M. L. M. F. Paiva, R. Zahn, and J. Grafman: "The Self as a Moral Agent: Linking the Neural Bases of Social Agency and Moral Sensitivity", in: *Social Neuroscience* 2 (2007) 3, pp. 336–52.
Morcom, A. M., and P. C. Fletcher: "Does the Brain Have a Baseline? Why We Should Be Resisting a Rest", in: *Neuroimage* 37 (2007) 4, pp. 1073–1082.
Orbach, S.: *Bodies*. New York (Picador) 2009.
Panksepp, J.: *Affective Neuroscience: The Foundations of Human and Animal Emotions*, New York & Oxford (Oxford University Press) 1998.
Papoulias, C. and F. Callard: "Biology's Gift: Interrogating the Turn to Affect", in: *Body & Society* 16 (2010) 1, pp. 29–56.
Raichle, M. E. et al.: "A Default Mode of Brain Function", in: *Proceedings of the National Academy of Sciences of the United States of America* 98, (2001) 2, pp. 676–682.
Raichle, M. E., and Abraham Z. Snyder: "A Default Mode of Brain Function: A Brief History of an Evolving Idea", in: *NeuroImage* 37 (2007), pp. 1083–1090.
Raichle, M. E.: "A Paradigm Shift in Functional Brain Imaging", in: *The Journal of Neurosciences* 29 (2009), pp. 12729–12734.
Raichle, M. E.: "The Brain's Dark Energy", in: *Science* 314 (2006) 5803, pp. 1249–1250.

Raichle, M. E.: "The Brain's Dark Energy", in: *Scientific American* 302 (2010), pp. 44–49.

Rees, T.: "Being Neurologically Human Today: Life and Science and Adult Cerebral Plasticity (an Ethical Analysis)", in: *American Ethnologist* 37 (2010), pp. 150–166.

Rizzolatti, G. and L. Craighero: "The Mirror-Neuron System", in: *Annual Review of Neuroscience* 27 (2004), pp. 169–192.

Rose, N.: *The Politics of Life Itself: Biomedicine, Power, and Subjectivity in the Twenty-First Century*. Princeton, NJ (Princeton University Press) 2007.

Rubin, B. P.: "Changing Brains: The Emergence of the Field of Adult Neurogenesis", in: *BioSocieties* 4 (2009), pp. 407–424.

Saey, T.H.: "You Are Who You Are By Default", in: *ScienceNews* (19 July 2009).

Schilbach, L., S. B. Eickhoff, A. Rotarska-Jagiela, G. R. Fink, and K. Vogeley: "Minds at Rest? Social Cognition as the Default Mode of Cognizing and Its Putative Relationship to The 'Default System' Of the Brain", in: *Consciousness and Cognition* 17 (2008) 2, pp. 457–467.

Seneca, L. D.: *Letters from a Stoic: Epistulae morales ad Lucilium*, New York (Penguin Books) 1969.

Shulman, G. L., J. A. Fiez, M. Corbetta, R. L. Buckner, F. M. Miezin, M. E. Raichle, and S. E. Petersen: "Common Blood Flow Changes across Visual Tasks: II. Decreases in Cerebral Cortex", in: *Journal of Cognitive Neuroscience* 9 (1997) 5, pp. 648–663.

Smallwood, J., and J. W. Schooler: "The Restless Mind", in: *Psychological Bulletin* 132 (2006) 6, pp. 946–958.

Smallwood, J., E. Beach, J.W. Schooler, and T.C. Handy: "Going AWOL in the Brain: Mind Wandering Redues Cortical Analysis of External Events", in: *Journal of Cognitive Neuroscience* 20 (2008) 3, pp. 458–469.

Spreng, R.N., R.A. Mar, and A.S.N. Kim: "The Common Neural Basis of Autobiographical Memory, Prospection, Navigation, Theory of Mind, and the Default Mode: A Quantitative Meta-Analysis", in: *Journal of Cognitive Neuroscience* 21 (2009) 3, pp. 489–510.

Stafford, B. M.: *Echo Objects: The Cognitive Work of Images*, Chicago, IL (Chicago University Press) 2007.

Thompson, E.: "Embodied Self-Awareness and the 'Resting state': A Neurophenomenological Approach", talk at the *International Conference: Interdisciplinary Perspectives on Coherence and Disorders of the Embodied Self*, Heidelberg 2008.

Thrift, N.: "Pass It On: Towards a Political Economy of Propensity", in: *Emotion, Space and Society* 1 (2008) 2, pp. 83–96.

Valeo, T.: "Perchance to Daydream ... and Degenerate. The Brain's Default Network May Help Make Us Human, But at a Cost", in: *Dana Foundation* 2008 (http://www.dana.org/news/brainwork/detail.aspx?id=13180).

Vidal, F.: "Brainhood, Anthropological Figure of Modernity", in: *History of the Human Sciences* 22 (2009), pp. 5–36.

Vincent, J. L., G.H Patel, M.D. Fox, A.Z. Snyder, J.T. Baker, D.C. Van Essen, J.M. Zempel, L.H. Snyder, M. Corbetta, M.E. Raichle: "Intrinsic Functional Architecture in the Anaesthetized Monkey Brain", in: *Nature* 447 (2007) 7140, pp. 83–86.

Weinberg, G. M.: *PL/I Programming Primer*, New York (McGraw-Hill) 1966.

Whitfield-Gabrieli, S. and J. Gabrieli: "Idle Minds and What They May Say About Intelligence", in: *Scientific American* (January 5th 2010).

# *Attention and Boredom*

# We Were Never Being Boring
# Between Concentration and Inattention

NICOLAS DE OLIVEIRA AND NICOLA OXLEY

This text focuses on notions of disengagement, boredom and vacuity as strategies employed by artists and audiences. These ideas have become ubiquitous in contemporary art. Informed by mass communication and telematics, today's art competes with the rampant spread of technological innovation and the spatio-temporal shrinking of our environment. This is characterised by the rise of two interlinked phenomena: the special effect, a symptom of the spectacle, and the ability to 'pay attention'.

In a commodified culture, art is progressively construed as part of the entertainment industry. During the experience of a spectacle, the audience seesaws between utter captivity, when paying attention to an event, and dejection or boredom, when there is nothing to be seen. The spectacle, as the name suggests, relies largely on the scopic, and has, according to the American art historian Jonathan Crary, been a major driving force of culture for at least 150 years. It follows that sight must be located somewhere the audience can focus upon and, the narrower the field of scrutiny, the more absorbed we become. Contrariwise, the opening up of vision might suggest a loss of attention, and a gain in autonomous experience. Terms such as immersion and participation have become closely linked with current art practice, partly devised – it would appear – to draw the spectator into the work itself by way of a personal experience. Attention is then devolved from the object to the subject, to the self; consequently, the spectator might be said to be looking at something which returns the gaze from whence it came, establishing a circular vision and in short, a relationship between the individual and the world.

This process of passing across the threshold between inner and outer underlines the importance of liminality in the present that takes us beyond the experience of entertainment, activated through persuasion and attraction.

In the Contemporary, artists have developed corresponding and countering strategies that often invoke the boundaries of perception; accordingly, artists often place audiences at the threshold of different states of consciousness, between remembrance and oblivion, between light and dark (twilight), between waking and sleeping (daydreaming), between concentration and inattention (boredom).

These apparent strategies of disengagement, however, are not what they appear to be. Neither a form of refuge or entrenchment on the part of the artist, nor a refusal to connect with the work by the audience, rather, they represent different forms of 'circumspect sensing', other ways of engaging and sharpening our faculties and sensitivities. The discussion will revolve around the work of key artists, including Marit Folstad (Norway), Hans Op de Beeck (Belgium) Patrick Jolley (Ireland), and Stefan Bruggemann (Mexico), artists whose reception by audiences is neither immersive nor participatory but empathetic. Their works strip what appears before our eyes to the bare essentials, and at times to even less; their depiction of reduction, emptiness and boredom could be understood as representing the symptomatic loss of cohesive meaning in contemporary Western culture, yet their work also asks us to examine these terms as productive strategies.

Boredom is at once an effect of a culture in which expectations are set so high that only a constant delivery of stimuli can stave it off, as well as a technique of switching into a state of neutrality, or, to fall headlong into a present-day cliché, "going on screensaver." "If boredom increases" writes Lars Svendson, "it means that there is a serious fault in society or culture as a conveyor of meaning."[1] However, radical thinking often derives from a period of boredom, and it is this kind of critical action that we demand of art today. According to Martin Heidegger, boredom and disengagement are connected to the passage of time. The German term 'Langeweile', meaning to suffer from an extension of time, suggests both a fear of time and an attunement to it. He suggests not going out of one's way to make oneself bored, but rather learn "*not to resist straightaway* but *to let resonate...* only by not being opposed to it, but letting it approach us and tell us what it wants, what is going on with it."

Patricia Meyer Spacks asserts that one of the key reasons for boredom is "the intensification of concern with individual rights,"[2] including the right to happiness and the spurious need to be endlessly pleasured by commodities. Today, as confidence in sexuality wanes, the best available, if temporary, cures for boredom are drugs, glamour and shopping. Furthermore, she argues that we have an evolving focus on "inner experience", on the growing sense that people have complex worlds – filled with feelings, wishes, thoughts, desires, prejudices – that are located somewhere inside them. As we become more psychically discriminating, we become more sensitive to our sense of vacuity and more obsessed by what we lack. Countering such an internalised experience necessitates a functioning link to a productive exterior. The aptitude to connect with the world and to reach out relies upon empathy, or the possibility of conceiving the *Other*, be it in the form of an individual, a place, or an object. Jacques Lacan tells his famous anecdote on the occasion of a fishing trip: a sardine tin, bobbing in the sea,

1 Svendson: *A Philosophy of Boredom*, p.22.
2 Meyer Spacks: *Boredom*.

catches a glint of sunlight and is seen by another fisherman, who shouts out to Lacan: "You see that can? Do you see it? Well, it doesn't see you!" He was, of course wrong, since the thing receives the look, and by an act of mirroring, returns the gaze.

Identification provides one of the most direct forms of generating empathy; this is especially so in film, where the viewer engages with the characters in the narrative, firstly, because they are there as a focal point, and secondly, because they drive the narrative. By contrast, if the characters are uninteresting, or even boring to the point where they actively refuse to perform, the audience may fail to empathise. However, this form of disengagement may also be seen as a technique of another form of localisation, whereby the stripping down of the depicted individual demands that the viewer take his/her place, an empathy that would appear to be more engaged. The video work of the Norwegian artist Marit Folstad takes the idea of perceived emptiness, a laconic refusal of identification, and turns it into nothing but a shimmering, diaphorological surface. "With the Lights Out" (2008) depicts slowed-down footage of a man smoking, or rather, exhaling smoke. The smoke is, at times, wispy and insubstantial, while at others it masks the face in a shroud. The smoke tarries and subsides, making curlicued figures and patterns in the air. Smoke is not an object, but a *thing*, insubstantial, without body, yet infinitely lingering and persistent, a marker of waiting, of time ungainfully spent, an embodiment of a nameless epic. Without purpose or punctum, the smoke signifies a liminal state of becoming that refutes fixity or boundary.

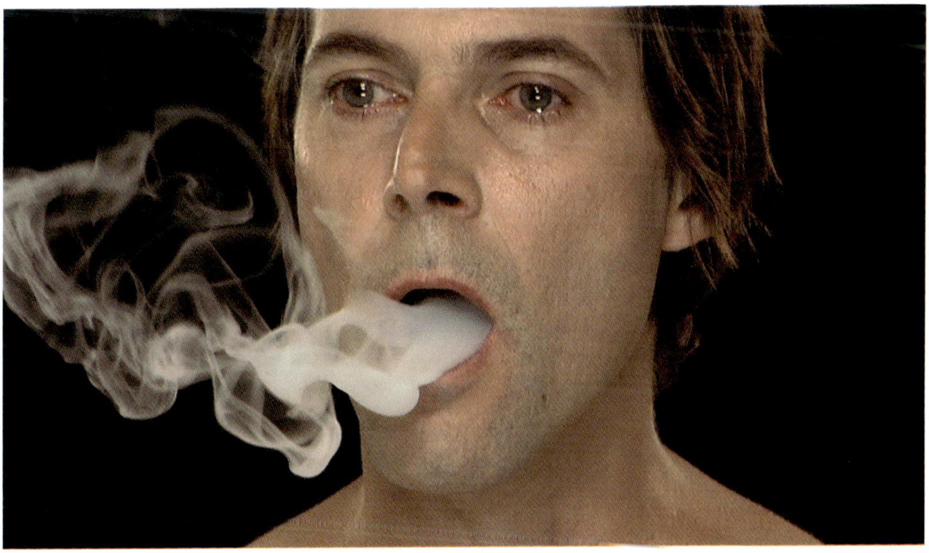

Fig. 1 :Marit Følstad, video still from: With the Lights Out, 2008.

Folstad's images return us to the body. This is not a spectacular body though, immersing the audience in ever greater sensory expectation, but rather a body that experiences slowly, empirically. Qualities of stillness and slowness pervade the works, and are manifested in the oppositional motifs of expansion and reduction. The audience is made to anticipate the work's narrative; we are always one step ahead. Slowness allows us to perceive the world with Heidegger's term "Umsicht," a pre-reflective, circumspect vision, also termed "aletheic." Sight is then embedded within a visual field, not outside of it: "Letting something be encountered is primarily circumspective; it is not just sensing something, or staring at it. It implies circumspective concern."[3]

Therefore, the body becomes a kind of 'material' that gives shape and presence to actions, ideas and emotions located elsewhere; one might say that the body quite literally *endures*: it does not control the flow of time but instead submits to a state of waiting. Folstad's increasingly elegiac videos tend towards stillness. These pin-sharp, high-definition recordings show actions undertaken with immense deliberation, over and over again. The clarity of these images is deceptive, since the video is more than lifelike: it is, in fact, 'hyperreal', as its oversize scale and high-definition picture quality is not naturalistic and brooks no intimacy. Indeed, this 'overdefinition' of the human figure is welcomed by the viewer's eye because vision is greedy, always wanting more; however, our understanding, which is empathetic, leaves us uncertain about the image's overdetermined sharpness. We are fascinated and seduced by the surface but are unable to empathise with it. Thus the body in the work is perceived as a simulacrum, recognizable and familiar, though essentially unknowable.

Ultimately, the ability to withstand or endure confers greater control than to *do*, as stillness triumphs over motion.

The closer and over-defined the world becomes, the greater the amount of mediation that takes place, the further we travel to escape. London, New York and Beijing are no longer sufficient. Our increasingly sedentary lifestyles have turned us into armchair travellers, making us yearn for the Great Arctic wastes, for parched deserts, and for inaccessible mountains. The very hostility of these places becomes attractive since there is no need to actually be there. Furthermore, since these places only exist in our mind's eye, they become rooted as metaphors, as placeholders *for* our powers of imagination.

The vast scope of the Belgian artist Hans Op de Beeck's ambitious work, "Location [6]" belies its remarkably simple ambition: to show the viewer little or nothing they have not already experienced, albeit transposed into a spectacular setting. Where the panorama of the 19th Century presented the promise of exotic locations and undreamed of places, Op de Beeck shows us an infinite white world punctuated with wispy, careworn trees without shadows that display a kind of wordless sorrow. The central chamber from which the panorama unfolds is an idealised space for a single viewer, suggesting the artist's preference for solitary, contemplative viewing. At a time when most of our activities are designated as collective, here individual experience is emphasized.

3 Heidegger: *Being and Time*, p. 176.

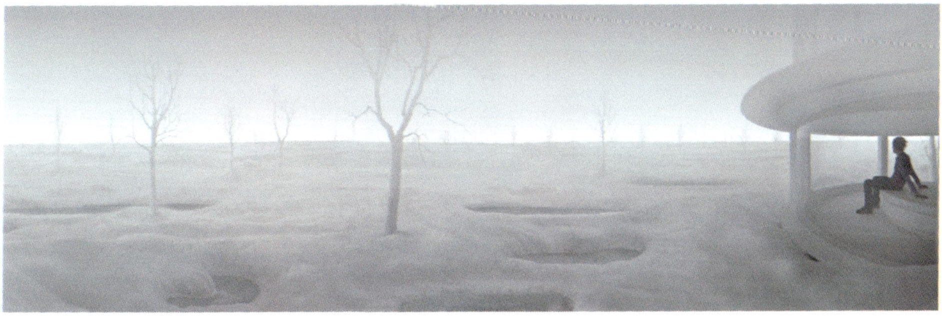

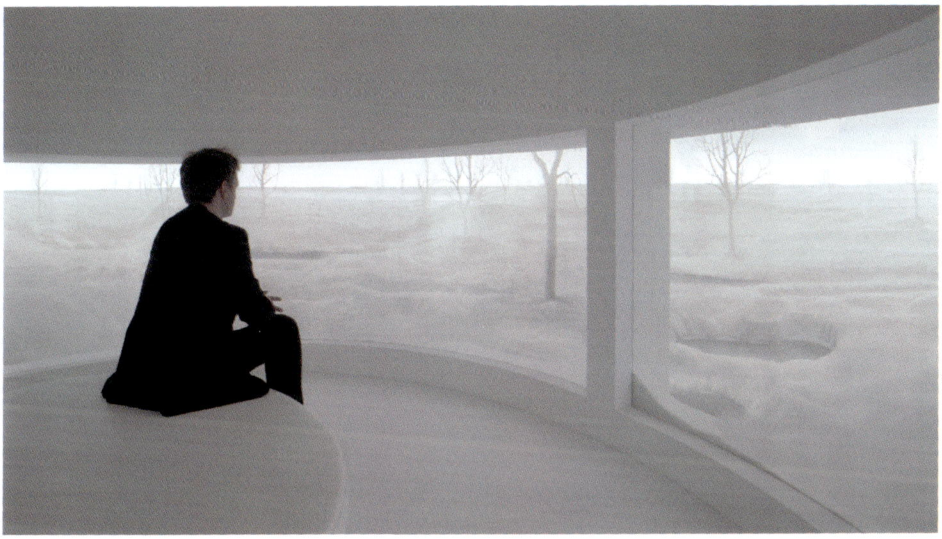

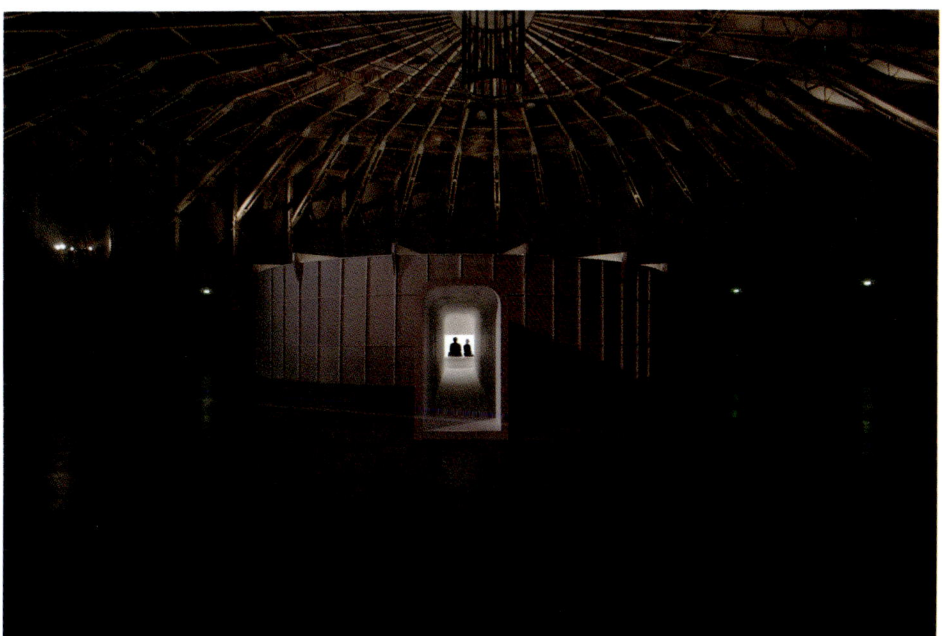

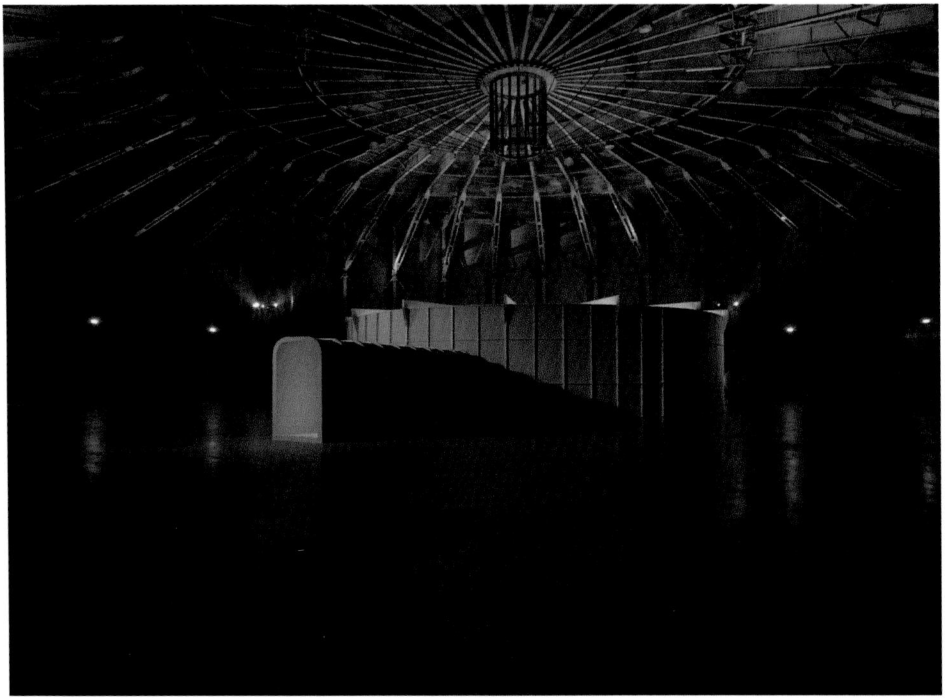

Fig. 2–5: Hans op de Beek, Location (6), 2008.

Telematic and virtual technologies have succeeded in substituting reality with the signs of the real, whereby sensation and excitement can be fabricated; individual experience is replaced with collective sensation through the wonders of artifice.

Op de Beeck's panorama, however, does not transport us to an exotic location; instead it emphasises a stripped-down, everyday experience, which is both diminished and heightened by the display, the landscape appearing at once reduced and augmented.

Such mutability in its physical perception serves only to stress its metaphorical presence: this is not any particular snowy landscape, and yet it represents *every* such place, moving us from the verbal dimension of enumerating and *telling* to that of *showing*. This notion of a 'summative' view bears a direct relationship to the idea of the "age of the world [as] picture".[4] By locating the perception of space in human sight, "the world is re-staged [...] and space becomes an effect of the human look"[5] with the eye at the centre. Op de Beeck's staged world is laid out with the eye in mind; the eye explores the landscape right up to its boundary, the horizon, and makes contact with the object that transcends sight. Maurice Blanchot points towards such an expanded notion of visual perception by asking "What happens when what you see, even though from a dis-

4 Heidegger: "The Age of the World Picture".
5 Osborne: *Travelling light*, p. 6.

tance, seems to touch you with a grasping contact, when the matter of seeing is a sort of touch, when seeing is a contact at a distance?"[6] Thus sight evolves from a purely scopic function that *emanates* from the body to one that *receives* stimuli, as in the event of touch. Tactility invokes slowness in a world dominated by the speed of pure vision, inviting an intimacy based on reciprocity absent from the simple exchange of glances.

The set appears lifelike, not because of the weight of detailed evidence it provides, but due to what it does not. Memory, after all, is based on observation, at best an inexact activity. If our initial observations are partial, they are further compounded by an inability to recall exactly, thus calling for a continuous checking or circling between an event and its remembrance. Op de Beeck's works accentuate the ordinary by generic reenactment; the mundane ceases to be a verifiable occurrence, but instead stands in for every instance of the banal. The ordinary, endlessly reprised, lacks features, perhaps because repetition has worn experience smooth. Yet no matter how simple or sumptuous the thing looked upon, the viewer can only grasp the most fragmentary information. Indeed, an abundance of detail may be detrimental to the object's ability to transgress its own physicality; a surfeit of information allows the viewer to become trapped in the tangible aspects of the illusion, while the mind actually searches for a means of transcending its physical and thus reductive nature.

But it is the very artifice of the illusion that makes it arresting. The spectacle is, in fact, always connected to the audience's ability to suspend disbelief. The closer we come to melding artifice and reality, the more the 'gap' of belief is reduced; in other words, the audience begins to conflate the real with the fake. Today, the profusion of virtual technologies sees a drastic reduction of this gap and conspires to rob the audience of the need to visualize, imagine and 'fill in' what is presented, to transform it into a personal experience.

Artifice can be a means of obfuscation, of rendering the viewer 'unconscious', and, conversely, it may be employed to return the viewer to a waking, creative state; the resulting condition of reverie induces the viewer to be immersed *and* conscious of his/her own state. Accordingly, daydreaming is actually inseparable from attentive behaviour.

Gaston Bachelard invokes the state of daydreaming as an important element within our creative lives: "In point of fact, daydreaming, from the very first second, is an entirely constituted state. We do not see it start, and yet it always starts the same way, that is to flee the object nearby and right away it is far off, elsewhere, in the space of elsewhere. When this elsewhere is in natural surroundings...when it is not lodged in the houses of the past, it is immense. And one might say that daydream is original contemplation."[7] Bachelard argues that we rely on what is nearby to quickly take us elsewhere: "As soon as we become

6 Blanchot: *The Gaze of Orpheus*, p. 71.
7 Bachelard: *The Poetics of Space*, p. 184.

motionless, we are elsewhere; we are dreaming in a world that is immense. Indeed, immensity is the movement of motionless man. It is one of the dynamic characteristics of quiet daydreaming."[8]

This fluid relationship between temporal modes is vertiginous as we slingshot in a perpetual motion to and from the past. Gilles Deleuze argues that in this fluid movement resides what he calls difference, a state of being that is radical and promotes real change. Furthermore, if time is thus *out of joint* it induces a kind of vertigo, experienced when events rush toward one another, inducing a sensation of falling in the subject. Though physical experience is felt to belong in the present, memory returns us by revealing *shreds* of the past. The constant movement of memory thus induces the G-forces of vertiginous descent and exposes the individual to an infinite weariness.

Walter Benjamin, writing about Franz Kafka's characters, asks:

> Why do they vegetate? Could they be the descendents of the figures of Atlas that support globes with their shoulders? [...] But it is not the globe they are carrying; it is just that even the most commonplace things have their weight…[9]

The Irish artist Patrick Jolley's installations and films showcase the dilapidated and careworn appearance of the constructed locations: derelict buildings, threadbare furnishings, the air choked in languid clouds of dust. This apparent lack of care, this state of abandon is shared by the protagonists that dwell in these surroundings whose laconic resignation signals not only complete detachment and alienation from the world, but perhaps also a separation from the self. They refute our desire for identification since they barely acknowledge their own humanity. We do not wonder who they might be since our presence does not register; they are akin to *monads*, or empty shells, who are utterly unmoved by external forces yet have an unknowable internal motivation that compels them to act as they do.

The durational aspect of Jolly's films is a clear indication of the individual's impotence when faced with time that cannot be measured, but must be lived or felt. Jolly points us toward knowledge, not as an *a priori* state, but one that results from the burden of experience. His characters refuse to *tell* of their sense of being, leaving the audience to reflect on the experience offered by the work. The limbo-like state in which his characters are held, in turn, engulfs the audience, asking us to suspend our usual sense of time: we cannot measure and thus *know* this experience. "The time that is felt and consciously endured seems slow, thick, opaque",[10] writes Harold Schweizer, arguing that, according to Henri Bergson, if it cannot be protracted or contracted at will, it ceases to be a "transparent medium

8 Ibid., p. 184.
9 Benjamin: *Illuminations*, p. 109.
10 Schweizer: *On Waiting*, p. 16.

or instrument".[11] In this way, duration and the waiter who endures it cannot be separated, they become one. Thus, the silent figures in Jolley's work are waiting, enduring; they become identified with a state of resignation and are unable to control their own time, their duration. It is they who wait in the viewer's stead; as placeholders, they endure for us.

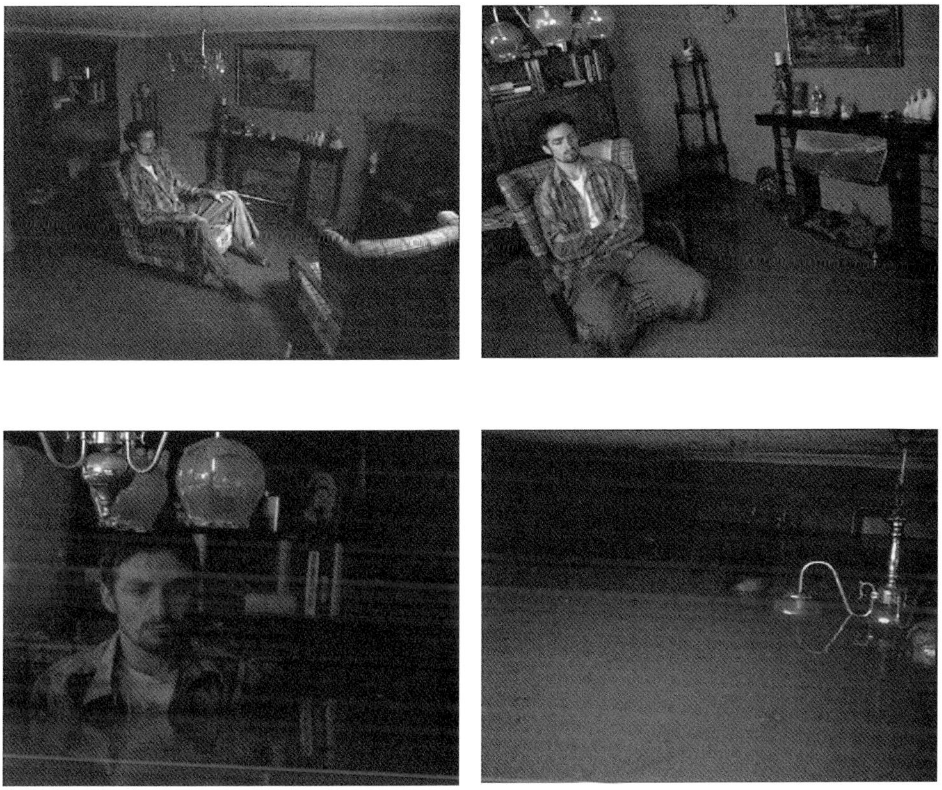

Fig. 6–9: Patrick Jolley, sequential images from Sinking Room, 2009.

Human traits, according to Benjamin, are transferred to the spaces themselves, turning them into vagabonds in their own right.[12] Thus, we might argue that it is the spaces that *roam*, rather than the empty protagonists that fill them. Their silence is absorbed by the space they inhabit and the building comes to life. Stooped by the burden of their shared predicament, figures, furniture, objects and surrounding architecture begin to resemble one another. The film 'Untitled' (2009) depicts a male character sitting in an armchair in a room that is slowly flooded with water; the protagonist, like the room, simply waits and submits to the inevitability of drowning.

11 Ibid, p. 17.
12 Benjamin, quoted in: Vidler: *Warped Space*, p. 116.

The condition of waiting, writes Laura Tanner, "is frequently experienced as a collapse into the powerlessness of pure object status."[13] Similarly, in much of Samuel Beckett's work, waiting and the trap of duration forms an essential key to the understanding of what motivates the characters; the visible world is reduced to a stratum of utensils as in an emergency refuge where everything awaits evacuation. The body is no longer at the centre of a world of objects that are subservient to his/her wishes and can be directed or employed to perform some useful function. This loss of control over duration then also leads to a collapse into objecthood: as we wait, we cease to *become*, a state reserved for human beings, and turn into objects. The lack of strategy regarding objects weakens and fragments the individual's subjectivity and he/she comes to resemble them as "gratuitous, accidental, enduring".[14] We therefore become separated from ourselves, condemned, like Vladimir and Estragon in 'Waiting for Godot' to wait as strangers to ourselves – always held by the knowledge of the 'not yet'. According to Blanchot, this affliction of separation from the sensible and meaningful world compels us to "endure 'pure' time, time without event, without project and without possibility; a kind of empty perpetuity that must be borne infinitely…'"[15]

> While the flow of images at 24 frames per second tends to assert a "now-ness" to the picture, stillness allows access to the time of the film's registration, its "then-ness". This is the point of, essentially located in the single frame, where the cinema meets the still photograph, both registering a moment of time frozen and thus fossilized.[16]

It is the artist's often imperceptible switching between temporal modalities, between real-time and slow motion or "time-out-of-joint" that reveals the artifice most clearly. "Duration", writes Pamela M. Lee "is dialectically conditioned by that which interrupts it," before going on to assert that "slowness reveals the fissures and gaps within duration that may otherwise appear without incident [and] is as much linked to mobility as immobility – and the extent to which the existence of immobility interrupts the apparently seamless flow of things."[17] It follows that time is neither a monolith nor a monument fixed in perpetuity or rolling on inexorably. Instead, its body is formed by Bachelard's "micro-events",[18] infinitesimal accretions of moments. Bachelard disputed Bergson's notion of uninterrupted and homogeneous duration, describing it instead as heterogeneous and interrupted; lived time, in short, is not successive but fragmented and highly subjective.

13 Tanner: *Lost Bodies*, p. 120–121.
14 Schweizer: *On Waiting*, p. 31.
15 Blanchot: *The Infinite Conversation*, p. 121
16 Mulvey: *Death 24x a Second*, p. 102.
17 Lee: *Chronophobia*, p. 121.
18 Bachelard: *The Dialectic of Duration*.

Roland Barthes assesses the idea of endurance differently, describing it as a dissimilar state, and going as far as to argue that the "Neutral" undoes the binary paradigmatic oppositions that structure Western thought:

> The Neutral doesn't refer to " impressions" of grayness, of "Neutrality", of indifference. The Neutral – my Neutral – can refer to intense, strong, unprecedented states. "To out play the paradigm" is an ardent, burning activity.[19]

In this way, Barthes contends that this state is neither active nor passive, but a creative position on its own where the subject disappears. "That means not sleeping but putting oneself in a process [...] of progressive degradation, of extenuation: " to will" – " to think" – " to dream" – " to daydream" – to be sitting doing nothing at all,' 'to be slowed down all the way to [one's] thinking."[20] Blanchot picks up on the neutral subject's inactivity by linking it to the condition of weariness:

> Weariness is the most modest of misfortunes, the most neutral of neutrals; an experience that, if one could choose, no one would choose out of vanity. O neutral, free me from my weariness, lead me to that which, though preoccupying me to the point of occupying everything, does not concern me,– But this is what weariness is, a state that is not possessive, that absorbs without putting into question.[21]

Neutrality, waiting and weariness are terms that, in their own particular ways, point toward states of absence. The loss of a goal, the weariness of waiting for something that never arrives are states that are inextricably linked to the idea of Modernism, promulgated by rapid change in material, spatial and temporal conditions. It is unsurprising that this kind of *lack* be closely associated with much creative endeavour from the early twentieth century to the present. Thus, far from being seen solely as a detrimental state, the notion of absence becomes a productive space.

> Now the Sirens have a still more fatal weapon than their song, namely their silence. [...] it is conceivable that someone might possibly have escaped from their singing; but from their silence certainly never.[22]

Franz Kafka's paradox refers to the power of absence, of nothingness. We struggle with the concept of nothing, since absence is difficult to grasp. By relating it only to our sensory perception, the question is difficult to address. The idea of nothing is often equated with the perception of darkness, a state in which nothing is visible. Blindness can then be equated with absence. According to Maurice

19 Barthes: *The Neutral*, p. 7.
20 Ibid., p. 185.
21 Blanchot: *The Infinite Conversation.*, p.xx
22 Kafka: *The Complete Stories and Parables.*

Merleau-Ponty, the world is revealed as strange and paradoxical and can only be *seen* through the intellect, through reflection. Seeing, then, becomes a form of 'writing the world', through blindness and oblivion.

In his essay "Walking in the City", Michel de Certeau argues that walkers in the city are akin to writers but not readers, they are inscribing the streets and neighbourhoods through the movement of their limbs and eyes, and, in so doing, are written upon by the gaze of others. Yet they are not readers since their view is utterly partial and they remain blind to their predicament, unaware of the larger picture.

In the film "A Production of Nothing" (2005) by the Mexican artist Stefan Bruggemann, a female protagonist is shown moving through the industrial quarter of an unnamed city. Her journey is accompanied by a female voice-over narrating a philosophical endgame. The film, unable to depict absence, functions as an accompaniment to the spoken text, which addresses "nothing" as a linguistic construct. His use of visual seduction masks the impossibility of the depiction of absence. We are made aware that "*nothing*" does not rely on sensory input. An object, no matter how small, on the other hand, does. As such, "*nothing*" cannot be seen; it cannot be perceived with the senses. The very act of perception is based on particular hard-wired and learnt principles that structure, among other senses, our vision. The world, then, is not simply 'out there' but is constructed in the process of perception. The perceptual codes are responsible for constructing a 'Weltbild', an all-encompassing idea of the world that surrounds us. Faced with nothing, no image is produced to slot into this 'picture'. We are left with an absence, a void. This inability to describe disturbs our picture, and we seek recourse in images that may circumscribe it.

The lack of visual pathos in much post-conceptual work might be related to the understanding that images simply fulfill the role of the placeholder, a stand-in for the unpresentable. And, according to Jean-François Lyotard, the task of postmodern art is encapsulated in the attempt to present the unpresentable. But since it cannot be represented as *itself*, something else is brought in as a substitution. What is told or presented is often something quite different in appearance or in meaning of what cannot be shown. However, what is put in its place does not replace it; instead, it underdetermines what cannot be represented. It is arguable that something is unrepresentable if it cannot be brought before our eyes, or if an adequate material form of presentation cannot be found. More accurately though, argues Jacques Ranciére, "a thing cannot be represented by artistic means on account of the very nature of those very means",[23] due to a surplus of presence. He refers to art as a vehicle that carries meaning, whereby the material and the form produce a surplus that "overstates" what it attempts to represent.

Perhaps we might understand the artists' favouring an aesthetics of disengagement as caused by the concern with such a surplus. And yet, concealed with-

23 Rancière: *The Future of the Image*, p. 110.

in this reductivism, this affected boredom, this laconism and darkness, lurks its inverse: a desire for abundance and plenty. The next time we leave the lights on at home when we are not there we might reflect that this is because "the margin of surplus itself feels like life."[24]

## References

Benjamin, Walter: *Illuminations,* translated by Harry Zohn, ed. by Hanna Arendt, New York (Schocken Books) 1968.

Bachelard, Gaston: *The Poetics of Space* (1958), Boston (Beacon Press) 1969.

Bachelard, Gaston: *The Dialectic of Duration*, Mary McAllester Jones (trans.) Clinamen Press (Manchester), 2000.

Barthes, Roland: *The Neutral*, Rosalind E. Krauss and Dennis Hollier (trans.), New York (Columbia University Press) 2005.

Blanchot, Maurice: *The Gaze of Orpheus and other Literary Essays*, translated by Lydia Davis, New York (Station Hill) 1981.

Blanchot, Maurice: *The Infinite Conversation*, translated by Susan Hanson, Minneapolis (University of Minnesota Press) 1993.

Heidegger, Martin: *Being and Time* (1927), translated by John Macquarrie and Edward Robinson, New York (Harper & Row) 1962.

Heidegger, Martin: "The Age of the World Picture" (1938), in: *The Question concerning Technology and other Essays*, New York (Harper) 1982, pp. 128–30.

Kafka, Franz: *The Complete Stories and Parables* 3–4, ed. by Nahum N. Glatzer, translated by Willa & Edwin Muir, New York (Quality Paperback Book Club) 1971.

Lee, Pamela M.: *Chronophobia: On Time in the art of the 1960s*, Cambridge MA (MIT Press) 2004

Meyer Spacks, Patricia: *Boredom: The Literary History of a State of Mind*, Chicago (University of Chicago Press) 1995.

Mulvey, Laura: *Death 24x a Second: Stillness and the Moving Image*, London (Reaktion Books Ltd) 2006

Osborne, Peter D.: *Travelling light: Photography, Travel and Visual Culture*, Manchester and New York (Manchester University Press) 2000.

Rancière, Jacques: *The Future of the Image*, London and New York (Verso) 2007.

Schweizer, Harold: *On Waiting*, Abingdon, Oxon (Routledge) 2008.

Svendson, Lars: *A Philosophy of Boredom*, London (Reaktion Books) 2005.

24 Wood: *How Fiction Works*, p. 69.

Tanner, Laura: *Lost Bodies: Inhabiting the Borders of Life and Death,* Ithaca (Cornell University Press) 2006.
Vidler, Anthony: *Warped Space: Art, Architecture, and Anxiety in Modern Culture*, Cambridge MA and London (MIT Press) 2001.
Wood, James: *How Fiction Works*, London (Jonathan Cape) 2008.

## List of Illustrations

Fig. 1 Marit Følstad, Video With the Lights Out, 2008 HD video, duration: 17'13" Soundtrack: Lasse Marhaug, Courtesy of the Artist and Gallery Riis.
Fig. 2–5 Hans op de Beeck, Location (6), 2008, sculptural installation, mixed media, mist and artificial light, 18 metres diameter x 4 metres high (cylinder), Courtesy Galleria Continua, San Gimignano – Beijing – Le Moulin, Coproduced by Holland Festival.
Fig. 6–9: Patrick Jolley, sequential images from Sinking Room, 2009, 32 millimeter film stock.

# The Generativity of Boredom
# Morton Feldman, Aphex Twin and Einstürzende Neubauten

HOLGER SCHULZE

Imagine yourself, sitting in a concert hall, highly attentive, tense and full of expectation. You carefully prepared your appearance in the public milieu of an opera house or a concert hall; you expect some social encounters and sensual experience with emotions and turmoil (music is for the emotions, they all say) – and then: the orchestra plays a piece of – one might say – repetitive, sleepy and for some listeners even annoying, screeching and scratching noises.

Fig. 1: Morton Feldman, Coptic Light, 1985.

You might imagine then that this late avant-garde piece by Morton Feldman by the title of *Coptic Light*, released in 1985, fuelled even in the mid-1990s a fairly outdated anti-avant-garde aggression in concert halls in the U.S. and in Europe. People screamed and shouted; they left the concert hall, slamming the doors loudly. And after the piece ended the listeners who liked it gave even more engaged shouts of approval and respect for this (in my opinion) great musical piece. But why all this?

If you had the opportunity to listen to this piece, just for, let's say five minutes – you could now (while reading this article) recall your own, fairly transitional and tiny experience with this piece, I assume that even this tiny excerpt provoked – let me put it this way – *not exclusively* positive and cheering emotions in all of you. Even I, listening to this piece a lot in the last few weeks, had some moments when I truly did not want to listen to it: I was not in an appropriate state of mind then, or did not have the sensibility to enjoy this piece.

At other times, though, I did not want the piece to *stop*. I had to listen to it over and over again, as if I had become addicted to hearing it. And again: Why?

Some of you might say: There really is a bluntly repetitive and absolutely mono-tonous and not at all varying quality in this piece. But isn't this true for almost every composition coined as *minimal music*? And we all know there are and have been fairly successful minimalist composers (such as Philip Glass or Steve Reich), whose operas and movies attracted and still do attract big and broad audiences worldwide.

So: What is it that can hinder you and me merely enjoying this piece? Are we really too bound to old European codes of consonances and dissonances, of *musical development* (a truly questionable term), of variation and counterpoint?

Do they keep us from simply diving and immersing ourselves trustfully into such a truly minimalist repetitive auditory structure?

*

Imagine – just for a second, if you will – what it would be like if you were not reading this text right now (at home, at your desk or on your way somewhere, sitting in public transport maybe); but if you could relax; if you could even give in to a kind of tiredness, of letting loose, of closing your eyes; roll over in your bed – or just drift away into a dreamy state of half-consciousness.

Imagine yourself diving into a twilight zone of your own consciousness. Maybe you don't want that to happen. Maybe you hear sounds then, and murmurs; noises from far away. And you feel a warm blanket around you. And you simply like it.

In this article I do not *want* to and *do* not speak from the position of a musicologist; I do not dive into musical analysis of compositional structures or the traditions of musical aesthetics, of musical development or tonality or dynamics. But I will analyze the effects of this auditory event from the standpoint of a *hearing perspective* (Sam Auinger).

This research position is best described in a research field that evolved recently, in the last decade, under the names of *Auditory* or *Sound Studies*. My specific approach is that of Historical Anthropology: a field of research which focuses on human beings under changing and highly diverse cultural and historical circumstances, of different ages, sexes and ethnicities: how those human beings experience and live with sonic and auditory events in their world. Media Anthropology and Sensory Studies come into play here.

So I pose the question: How can it be possible that human beings perceive an auditory artefact (like the before-mentioned piece by Morton Feldman) as boring – and what could be the generative, the even productive quality of such an experience?

Can boredom be a good thing?

# I. Sensory Anthropology of Alertness and Sleepiness

In contrast to common aesthetic and cognitive postulations of a fully alert, present and self-reflexive individual, auto-nomous and self-sufficient under all circumstances, there is another side to cognition. A side of cognition that needs and deserves a kind of tiredness, a sleepiness; a dizzy and sometimes even cliché-like dreamy state of consciousness.

After all: Most of the time you and I are definitely not fully present and highly alert – which is a good thing!

We *are* distracted all of the time. The cultural form or *dispositif* of human beings being able and forced to sit still and non-moving in a closed architectural box for about forty-five minutes (like in school) or for ninety minutes (in university or theatres) or for up to eight or even fourteen hours in assembly lines or other capitalist and even post-Fordist workspaces, this cultural form is – according to common studies on alertness and its structure – merely ridiculous; anthropologically analyzed.

Human beings drift and imagine, think and resonate, perceive bodily reactions and sensations; they react to possibly any events outside (or just at the fringe) of those eminent events we *should* be paying attention to – all the time. Luckily, we are not concentrating all the time. And luckily, human beings do *not* immediately follow all the outside forces in their environment that demand their attention. If we *did* so, we would be truly distracted all the time from everything. Alertness is luckily highly selective and involuntary, and – depending on the individual character – it takes erratic jumps and saltations, back and forth, zooming in and zooming out.

So, the body as a whole is a listening organ of wandering foci of perception and of changing timespans of increased or decreased alertness. It is *a receptive organ of supramodality*: the modes of perception and cognition are not separated as such; culture demands such strange separations into different senses. But human beings do not *necessarily* need this separation; and different cultures as well as different historical eras establish different sensory regimes and hierarchies.

A sensory anthropology now tries to formulate the framework into a theory or even an art form of this non-linear, non-determined receptivity or alertness; the starting point for this was vigorously postulated by science historian and mathematician *Michel Serres*, in the year 1985:

> Transmission trumps listening, we know how to project a sound and how it spreads, we know how to relay it, we are not good at receiving.[1]

1 Michel Serres: *The Five Senses*.

Michel Serres' work *Les Cinq Sens* (i.e.: *The Five Senses*) is a groundwork for sensory anthropology. Though this volume has just recently been published in the English language, 24 years after it was originally published in French; it will, I am very sure, change the way the English-speaking world of academia thinks and writes and undertakes research on the senses.

I predict: It will question deeply the paradigm of signal or data processing as a dominant model of sensory perception; and theories of embodiment and immersion, of the individual, experiential and highly narrative side of sensory experience will gain more acknowledgement than ever before.

## II. Tension and Aggression

So, coming back to my initial piece by Morton Feldman, what you can perceive here is a kind of *auditory ennui.* This *auditory proprioceptive event* is first of all a physiological event – not a mere isolated mental or neural state.

We like to think of music as only being constructed and understood in the mind or in the emotional realm of our personality, which is obviously only *partially* true.

We like to forget a fact that *Auditory Studies* emphatically remind us of: Any auditory experience (I do not say: *listening to a musical piece*) is at first a holistic bodily state which you and I enter. Through any sound event (be it noises or musical performances or electro-acoustic amplified or even generated sound art), our bodies are dipped into changing spheres of resonating and basically vibrating material substances. Gases and solid substances that surround us transmit the auditory disruption to us. Or, as the seminal definition in the *Encyclopedia Britannica* puts it: Sound is a

> Mechanical disturbance from a state of equilibrium that propagates through an elastic material medium.

Via this disturbance in the material continuum around us, we acquire this tension, this specific cohesion that emerges spherically from sonic events.

Our bodies and we – as merely listening and receptive individuals – cannot help but swing and resonate and repeat those auditory events in our own bodies: Vibrations are transmitted to us. And areas in our corpus that are able to resonate – *do* resonate. This is physiologically speaking *banal* – but for a theory of receptivity it is of high interest.

If we dislike or like an auditory and physically perceptible tension, this fact might be irrelevant for a *receptive* body – as almost every non-pathologically disturbed body is; but: as social beings, thinking of ourselves as being autonomous and individual, as being characters and maybe even logic-driven creatures, we do not like being *forced* to perceive, feel or think something. We like the idea of being able to freely decide what we do or have done with us and our bodies.

So we like to stop noises or sounds we do not like immediately and with *tense aggression*. Just as we defend ourselves from being forced to an involuntarily auditory experience.

I would like to give you another example of this; another three minutes. If you have any access to this example you should listen to the piece by Richard D. James alias Aphex Twin, Selected Ambient Works, Volume II, Warp Records Sheffield 1994, CD 1, Track 11, 0:00-3:00.

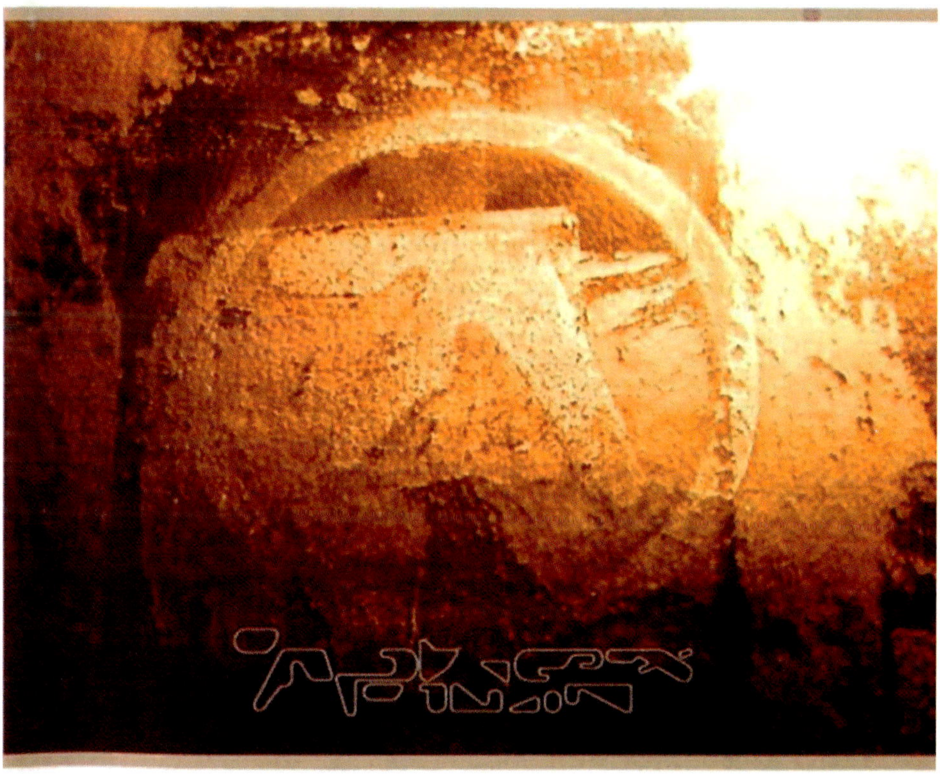

Fig. 2: Aphex Twin, Selected Ambient Works, Vol. 2, 1994.

Is there? Are we not bored by repetition? Do we not demand diversity and development, variation and nuances, differentiations and distinctions? Is it not *this* that constitutes culture and thought?

At this point I could sidetrack and divert attention towards the arguments for a fruitful merging of the qualities of any *difference* in any *repetition* – as for instance elaborated by Gilles Deleuze in his seminal study from 1968; but this would entail fleeing from the question: *Why do we hate such moments of repetitive comfort?* Do we miss the opportunity to find any hint or insinuation of a sign that we could interpret and understand as *intentional*, swimming in a stream of repetitiveness? Do we miss a language-like structure that we could take as "*speaking to us*"?

But there might be something else. Something granted by the aforementioned *rapport* – a bodily experience? Although and because we do feel lost in a dead end – without signs and signifiers.

## III. A Generative Theory of the Body and the Signs

What connection could we find in experiences of boredom between semiotics – and a corporeal and sensory, even material perspective?

It is often stated there must be a clear line between a perspective on signs and meanings, arguments and interpretation on the one hand; and on the other hand a perspective on the physical and physiological substances, the sensory impressions, the dense synaesthetic web or even knot our sensory experience is made of. But can this be true? Doesn't this permeate the age-old and recurrently deconstructed mind-body division?

Is this truly implicated in traditional writings of semiotics by – just to name them – Charles Sanders Peirce, Ferdinand Saussure, Max Bense or even Umberto Eco? All of these (not seldom monist!) authors stressed the material and the physical quality of sign processes. *Semiosis*, the process of generating and thus using and understanding signs, has been defined by all these famous thinkers of semiotics as a process in *material* substances.

Bluntly said: There is no *immaterial* way of transmitting meaning – as well as there might well be no really meaningless use of physical, material substances.

So, besides meaning we have materials; besides semiotics we have mediology; and beside the category of *coherence* we have the category of *cohesion* (a term from textual linguistics to describe non-semantic relations in texts) – or tension, as Jean-Luc Nancy put it:

> Un corps, c'est donc une tension. Et l'origine grecque du mot est « tonus », le ton. Un corps est un ton. Et je ne dis rien là qu'un anatomiste ne puisse approuver: un corps, c'est un tonus.[2]

This basic tension and its background emotions are now fundamental in a theory of generativity and semiogenesis formulated by American philosopher, phenomenologist and psychologist Eugene T. Gendlin. *Generativity* is used here as a fruitful and more general alternative to terms we often use such as *action, productivity, creativity* or even *work;* concepts so deeply rooted in 19th century capitalist thinking and ideology of industrial production that we could be witnessing their disappearance as key concepts in the next few decades.[3]

Eugene T. Gendlin now uses a concept of generativity in a term for embodied, but not yet explicated meaning called: *bodily felt sense.*

*Bodily felt sense* means the grounding and proprioceptive sensory events we perceive all the time. We feel ourselves in our bodies, in situations, among other people and with certain constellations of expectations, obsessions and fears. And we do not *interpret* this all the time; but in certain instances we suddenly do. An example from Eugene Gendlin:

> For example, suppose you were at a party and felt you were bored and needed to go home. But suppose that instead of going home, you opened up the boredom and found anger. And suppose that in finding the anger you found also that you needed to stay and say something directly about the anger to someone. In a similar way as we pursue a goal, the goal seems to change. But later we say the new goal is the one we really wanted all along but we didn't know it.[4]

So, as in this example, boredom can have a generative quality. It draws us back from routines of perception, interpretation and even feeling, and it draws us back from a prefabricated set of emotions we are almost *demanded* to feel in a cliché-like manner in a certain situation. The Italian philosopher *Mario Perniola* calls these coined emotions in his book *Del Sentire* (About Feeling) from 1991 *Ready-Felts.* An effect, he argues (obviously deeply impressed by the neo-feudalist regime of Silvio Berlusconi), of a highly mediatized society he calls: *sensology* – a parallel to the *Ready-Thoughts* of the *ideologies* in the last century.

Boredom can now bring us back to our specific and individual felt senses – pertaining exclusively to a particular situation; it can open us up for the intrinsic and specific qualities of a situation and of the practices around us; as Gendlin puts it:

2 Nancy: *Corpus*, p. 124. In English: "A body is therefore a tension. And the Greek root of the word is *tonos*, tone. A body is a tone. And here I am saying nothing which an anatomist could not agree with: a body is an energy."

3 Terms such as *action*, *productivity*, *creativity* or even *work* tend to cover the fact that *work* in our understanding is still today a rather minor concept – looked at globally; concepts of *slavery*, on the other hand, and of non-productive and unsalaried occupations and practices still *do* dominate the lives of most of the human beings living on this planet right now.

4 Gendlin: *The Wider Role of Bodily Sense*, p. 203.

> Any situation, any bit of practice, implies much more than has **ever** been said.[5]

We often do not sense these intricate implications. We need something to grant us time and space and openness – and sometimes even the non-intentionality, the drifting and non-intentional proprioceptivity to realize the potential of semiogenesis that lies in a situation. Or a moment.

Boredom is thus – not surprisingly – often related to play and even childlike, infantile, non-adult, sometimes pathological concepts of experience and generativity; final example of auditory boredom by the German post-punk and experimental noise-group Einstürzende Neubauten from the year 1983 called *Hospitalistische Kinder – Engel der Vernichtung (Hospitalish Children/Exterminating Angel),* first released on their Album *Zeichnungen des Patienten O.T.*

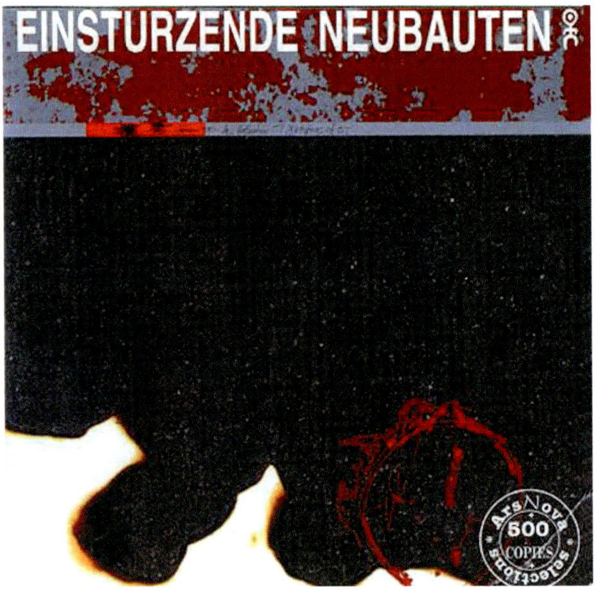


Fig. 3: Einstürzende Neubauten, Zeichnungen des Patienten O.T., 1983.

They articulate the following lines:

> Ja – warum?… Spurenabdrücke… Ja… Wovon sollte das sein? … Komm! … Du sammelst alles auf was du siehst… Gut… So... Vielleicht war das Ungeheuer das... Ja, das kann sein... Vielleicht auch nicht... Der Nächste bitte![6]

Boredom – which can seem either *lethal* or eternally *joyful* to children, as in this example – seems to grant us a non-linear, non-intentional and non-directive time

5 Ibid., p. 201.

6 Einstürzende Neubauten: "Hospitalistische Kinder – Engel der Vernichtung". English translation: "Yes – why?… Forensic traces… Yes… what's that supposed to be?… Come on… you pick up everything you see… good… right… maybe it was the monster which… yes, maybe… but maybe not… Next, please!"

bracket. This is a valuable gem in societies and cultures of never-ending entertainment, of *Infinite Jest* (D. F. Wallace).

> Keine Hemmungen mehr bis zur Sintflut
> Na und, dann nagel doch
> Hört ihr Leute laßt euch sagen:
> einen Engel als Beute werden wir erschlagen
> Hab meinen Verstand begraben
> wie meine Seele im Wüstenboden
> ... und ich will nicht länger warten
> Bis Gottes unendlicher Hoden
> Endlich in Flammen aufgeht
> Engel der Vernichtung
> Engel der Vernichtung
> Engel der Vernichtung
> Engel der Vernichtung[7]

A timespan in which we are not hastily forced to *do* something – but in which we can allow ourselves to let something come. Or as Eugene T. Gendlin puts it:

> This coming is characteristic of the body. What else comes like that? Sleep comes like that, and appetites. If they don't come, you just have to wait. We all know that. Tears come like that, and orgasm. Emotions come like that, and so also this felt sense, which is wider and at first not clear, comes like that.[8]

> You can feign joy or anger but to have them, they must come. So also does the muse come, when she is willing and not otherwise. And new ideas, the lines of a new design, and steps of therapy come this way.[9]

I would like to end this brief digression on the joys of boredom with a sentence by Austrian writer Peter Handke; at a press conference after the world premiere of his play *Das Spiel vom Fragen / The Art of Asking*, he was asked by a journalist why he wrote the play.

Handke paused for a moment, seemed to search for the true reason – and answered with a kind of exhibitionist's sincerity:

> Mir war langweilig.
>
> I was bored.

7 Einstürzende Neubauten: "Hospitalistische Kinder – Engel der Vernichtung". English translation: "No more inhibitions before the deluge / so what – nail it then! / Hear ye people, let us tell you: / we will slay an angel as our prey / I have buried my brain / like my soul in desert terrain / … and I no longer want to wait / until God's infinite scrotum / finally goes up in flames / Exterminating angel / Exterminating angel / Exterminating angel / Exterminating angel"

8 Gendlin: *The Wider Role of Bodily Sense*, p. 194.

9 Ibid., p. 202.

## References

Gendlin, Eugene T.: "The Wider Role of Bodily Sense in Thought and Language", in: Maxine Sheets-Johnstone (ed.), *Giving the Body its Due*, Albany (SUNY Press) 1992, pp. 192–207.

Howes, David (ed.): *Empire of the Senses. The Sensual Culture Reader*, London (Berg Publishers) 2005.

Nancy, Jean-Luc: *Corpus*, Paris (Metailié) 1992/2000.

Perniola, Mario: *Del Sentire*, Turin (Einaudi) 1991.

Schulze, Holger (ed.), *Sound Studies: Traditionen – Methoden – Desiderate. Eine Einführung* (Sound Studies Volume 1), Bielefeld (transcript Verlag) 2008.

Schulze, Holger: "Berührung. Touched by Sound", in: *Open Space Magazine* 8/9, 2007.

Schulze, Holger: "Bewegung Berührung Übertragung. Einführung in eine historische Anthropologie des Klangs", in: Holger Schulze (ed.), *Sound Studies. Traditionen – Methoden – Desiderate*, Sound Studies Volume 1, Bielefeld (transcript Verlag) 2008, pp. 137–159.

Schulze, Holger: "Der Raumkörperklang. Eine Anthropologie des Mit", in: Carsten Seiffarth & Martin Sturm (eds.): *Sam Auinger. Katalog*, Wien-Bozen (Folio Verlag) 2007, pp. 33–46 (Engl.: "Spatial Body Sound. An Anthropology of With", in: ibid., pp. 75–87).

Schulze, Holger: "Hypercorporealismus. Eine Wissenschaftsgeschichte des körperlichen Schalls", in: Peter Wicke (ed.), *Das Sonische – Sounds zwischen Akustik und Ästhetik* (= *Popscriptum* 16 [2008] 10).

Schulze, Holger: "Wissensformen des Klangs. Zum Erfahrungswissen in einer historischen Anthropologie des Klangs", in: *Musiktheorie – Zeitschrift für Musikwissenschaft*, 22 (2007) 4, Laaber (Laaber Verlag) 2007, pp. 347–355.

Seitter, Walter: *Physik der Medien. Materialien, Apparate, Präsentierungen*, Weimar (Verlag und Datenbank für Geisteswissenschaften) 2002.

Seitter, Walter: *Physik des Daseins. Bausteine zu einer Philosophie der Erscheinungen*, Wien (Sonderzahl Verlagsgesellschaft) 1997.

Serres, Michel: The Five Senses. A Philosophy of Mingled Bodies, trans. Margaret Sankey and Peter Cowley, London / New York (Continuum International Publishing Group) 2009.

Wallace, David: *Infinite Jest*, London (Little, Brown Book Group) 1997.

Wulf, Christoph & Holger Schulze (eds.): *Klanganthropologie: Performativität – Imagination – Narration. Paragrana 16* (2007) H. 2, Berlin (Akademie Verlag) 2007.

## Pieces of music

Aphex Twin, *Selected Ambient Works*, Volume II, Sheffield (Warp Records) 1994.

Einstürzende Neubauten, "Hospitalistische Kinder – Engel der Vernichtung", in: Einstürzende Neubauten, *Zeichnungen des Patienten O.T.*, London (Rough Trade Records) 1983.

Einstürzende Neubauten, *Zeichnungen des Patienten O.T.*, London (Rough Trade Records) 1983.

Morton Feldman, *Coptic Light* (1985), Symphonieorchester des Bayerischen Rundfunks, cond. by Peter Rundel, Bayerischer Rundfunk Munich 2002.

Prince, "Joy In Repetition", in: Prince, *Graffiti Bridge*, Chanhassen (Paisley Park/Warner Bros) 1990, Track 8.

## List of Illustrations

Fig. 1 Morton Feldman, Cover of: *Coptic Light* (1985), Symphonieorchester des Bayerischen Rundfunks, cond. by Peter Rundel Bayerischer Rundfunk München 2002.

Fig. 2 Aphex Twin, Cover of: *Selected Ambient Works*, Volume II, Warp Records Sheffield 1994.

Fig. 3 Einstürzende Neubauten, Cover of: Zeichnungen des Patienten O.T., Rough Trade Records, 1983.

# The Other Side of Existence
## Heidegger on Boredom

JAN SLABY

> Tedium is not the disease of being bored because there's nothing to do, but the more serious disease of feeling that there's nothing worth doing. This means that the more there is to do, the more tedium one will feel.
>
> Fernando Pessoa[1]

Emotions and moods are the other side of cognition: all-important elements in our relatedness to the world and indispensable ingredients of thought, judgement and evaluation; still, they have both long been neglected and, what is in some ways worse, misclassified as antagonists of reason (while what they in fact are is invaluable ingredients of our rational perspective on the world). In a time where the overall perspective that the sciences and the humanities adopt towards affective phenomena has changed dramatically to the better, we are still far away from an adequate understanding of the emotional spectrum. In fact, it is not even clear that an adequate descriptive approach to affective phenomena in humans has been found and established. The purpose of the present chapter is to make some progress in this direction. Since it is always more effective to work from a single case to a more general conclusion, I will focus exclusively on one particular kind of feeling: On boredom.[2]

## 1. Introduction

Boredom, if looked at in the right way, can reveal elements of the predicament of human existence, although the restlessness and consequent urge to engage in diverting activities that usually come along with the advent of boredom easily prevent insight into this structure. In boredom, the significance of the world and the self drain away, motivation ceases, and even the temporality of our existence is altered in a strange way: Nothing seems to happen and thus time seems to stand still, and can thereby become strangely obtrusive. In his 1929/1930 lectures

1 Pessoa: *The Book of Disquiet*, fragment 445, p. 365.
2 We will soon see that it is not quite correct to call boredom a 'feeling'.

on *The Fundamental Concepts of Metaphysics*, Heidegger offers a remarkable existential interpretation of three varieties of boredom: "becoming bored by something", "being bored with something", and "profound boredom" as expressed in the phrase *it is boring for one*. According to Heidegger, these three varieties of boredom reveal a skein of relations between the temporality of human existence and what one could call 'existential significance' (*mattering*, 'meaning of life'). The temporality of human existence, the temporal constitution of our very being, and existential meaning – the significance that intrinsically orients a human life – hang together inextricably: The draining away of existential significance *is identical to* the strange slowing or even halting of time in boredom. Heidegger then goes on to claim that the experience of profound boredom, understood in its full existential depth, makes manifest that a human being is the free and responsible creator of whatever meaning there is in one's life. Not only that, but profound boredom moreover amounts to a *call* to actively take charge of one's existence so as *to endow* it with meaning, and thereby effect a fundamental change in existential temporality.

Heidegger's discussion of boredom is an exercise in the existential interpretation of human affectivity, and as such it can serve as a source of inspiration for attempts to understand human emotion and feeling. The aim of this article is to begin illustrating this by means of a reconstruction of Heidegger's analysis. I will show that Heidegger operates with an understanding of human affectivity as a passive sense of possibility, so that feelings are understood on the one hand as passive, involuntary reactions, but on the other hand also as proto-conceptually shaped ways of 'being open towards the world' – they manifest what Heidegger calls 'disclosedness' or 'understanding of being', at any time mediated by language understood in an inclusive way as 'articulated intelligibility'. In our feelings, we are oriented in a certain way towards possibilities of conduct, of existence, of being, and equally away from other possibilities of this kind. The possibilities in question are existential possibilities – *ways of being*, encompassing modes of conduct, of leading one's life. Manifested in our affectivity, the world presents itself as a space of possibilities. Our sense of possibilities is at the same time a way of being open to (or its privation: being closed off from) the world. Talking about this openness to the world is to talk about a general dimension of human feelings, their directedness towards something, what I have elsewhere called *affective intentionality*.[3] The study of affective intentionality has to be at the centre of the philosophy of affective phenomena in humans – philosophy of emotion, in short.

My main aim in the following is to characterize this key strand of reflection upon human feeling through a discussion of Heidegger's interpretation of boredom. In the concluding section I will cast some doubt upon the final stage of Heidegger's interpretation, suggesting that it too aggressively forces quite a spe-

3 See Slaby: *Gefühl und Weltbezug*; Slaby and Stephan: "Affective Intentionality".

cific understanding of existence upon the most profound variety of boredom. A brief glance at Fernando Pessoa's *Book of Disquiet* will support this critical line of thought. This final move, however, will not change my overall assessment that Heidegger can serve as a valuable guide in our efforts to shed light upon the hitherto underexplored 'other sides of cognition'.

I prepare the grounds for my subsequent analysis by outlining some general contours of the broader theoretical orientation that one might adopt in order to come to grips with Heidegger's interpretation of boredom. What will become particularly clear from this initial clarification is the widening of the analytical perspective from single states of experience to the whole of a person's perspective on the world – what I choose to call 'human existence'. This broadened perspective can help improve our thinking about human feelings and other human capacities, as it avoids a narrowing of one's focus on artificially isolated elements. Working back and forth from the broad existential perspective to its various constituent elements is the best way to proceed. In this way, the other sides of cognition become the 'other sides of existence'.

## 2. From states of consciousness to existential orientations

According to Heidegger, moods are not subjective states of feeling, but rather something we might call *existential orientations*. As such they concern the entirety of a person's situated existence and thereby also the textures of the situations in which the person finds herself. Boredom is a good example of this re-orientation. From a distance, we might think of boredom as an affective state, a kind of feeling, a certain type of mood. But boredom seems quite unlike many paradigm cases of feeling. We are not gripped by boredom in the same way than we are gripped by other kinds of feeling. That is why we are better off understanding boredom as an *existential orientation*.[4] Existential orientations are background structures of experience, ways of being situated in the world as well as more active adoptions of stances towards oneself and the world. Existential orientations encompass experience, thought, volition, action and other forms of demeanour. In an existential orientation, all of these comportments are modified and shaped in specific ways depending on the kind of existential orientation in question.

Existential orientations overlap to some extent with conscious states, but they importantly include more than these. Existential orientations are, most fun-

4 The notion of an existential orientation was recently introduced into the philosophical debate about human emotions by Matthew Ratcliffe (see Ratcliffe: "Feeling of Being" and Ratcliffe: *Feelings of Being*).

damentally, the basic structures of our *ways of being*, the ways in which we *are*. They comprise all the meaningful ways in which a person relates to the world, herself and other people in action, experience, thought, feeling, posture and demeanour – existential orientations prepare and configure all our ways of relating to the world (where both 'world' and 'relating to' have to be understood in an inclusive way). Existential orientations form a background framework of intentionality, insofar as they pre-configure foreground intentional states. Examples of existential orientations include fearfulness, self-confidence, motivatedness, alertness and vigilance, hostility, cheerfulness, open-mindedness, resoluteness and determination, boredom, anxiety, depression, etc. Not all manifestations of the conditions that go under the names just listed are existential orientations, though. Some instances of fearfulness, open-mindedness, hostility etc. are more appropriately thought of as character traits, while other instances rather qualify as 'foreground intentional states', concretely directed at something specific. Existential orientations are the middle ground between dispositional character traits and the common foreground intentional states. They are manifest in experience in a certain sense, but are not (usually) in the foreground of awareness. Rather, they figure in experience as background structures. It is *from* existential orientations that attention, emotion, experience and action are directed to the world – that is why it is often so hard to 'notice' existential orientations. For the most part, attention is focused not on one's existential orientations but rather *through them* onto something else. Their experiential aspects concern the ways of one's attending (and not attending) to something. However, there are indirect ways of 'getting hold' of existential orientations. For once, existential orientations can change, sometimes even quite abruptly, thus changing our ways of relating to the world. Insofar as they are transparent experiential structures, these changes in our relatedness to the world change the way the world appears to us. Sometimes, the way we orient ourselves towards the world changes quite subtly, as when our background state changes from contentment to slight irritation, so that some of what happens around us suddenly appears slightly annoying, offensive, or threatening. Our overall condition has changed, and we might become aware of this by noticing the subtle change in how the world appears first.

Existential orientations are neither restricted to what happens to us, nor to what we bring about intentionally. Instead, they combine elements of both, to varying degrees. Thus, many existential orientations are clearly a matter of *feeling* a certain way – to borrow another useful term from Matthew Ratcliffe: in these cases they are *existential feelings* or "feelings of being".[5] Your existential orientation could be a *feeling* of being unwelcome, of being at home, being in control, unloved, stared at, offended, comfortable, etc. As feelings, these are passive occurrences rather than activities. On the other hand, existential orientations could also be, to some extent at least, actively adopted. This is the case when you

5 See Ratcliffe: *Feelings of Being*.

choose to adopt a certain stance or attitude towards things in general, towards aspects of your life, your projects, your friends, loved ones or fellow humans in general. Thus, you could try (and succeed) to motivate yourself, to make yourself live in a more open-minded, more attentive way, to try to be less irritable, to have a warmer, more friendly attitude towards others, etc.[6] If you succeed, you *actively orient* yourself (towards something), as opposed to merely *being* (passively) *oriented.* Usually, active and passive elements are mixed together inextricably, and it is not easy to determine to what extent one has a say in shaping one's existential orientations. Often, mood-like existential orientations simply assail us – however, most affective states allow for *some* voluntary control or regulation. This activity of '*holding oneself*' in an existential orientation comes quite close to what Aristotle called 'hexis', and something like this is crucially involved in character formation, in personal development, and in virtue.[7]

The exploration of possible ways to *orient oneself existentially* is one of the many fascinating themes in the writings of the early Heidegger, and it of course plays an important role in his analysis of boredom.

This preliminary discussion brings us in a good position to understand some of the things Heidegger says in his analysis of mood. An understanding of existential orientations, for instance, might help us to understand Heidegger's claims about moods not being psychological states, their not being something 'internal'. Instead, he famously claims that a mood is a way of being – "the fundamental way in which Dasein *is* as Dasein" (p. 101/67 – my emphasis),[8] "the way of our being-there with one another" (p. 100/66), and moreover "the 'presupposition for' and 'medium' for our thinking and acting" (p. 102/68). Heidegger takes moods to be existential orientations. This is in accord with his concept of *Befindlichkeit,* which can be translated as *attunement.* Looked at superficially, *Befindlichkeit* is Heidegger's generic term for affective phenomena. However, given the way in which he introduces it as a technical term, it seems to correspond more to the concept of an existential orientation as described above than to a generic term for affective states. What one has to take into account is that Heidegger construes attunement to be inextricably joined together with *understanding.* And as he understands the latter, it amounts exactly to an active holding oneself in an existential possibility – for instance, in *Being and Time* he explains

6 These attempts often involve affectivity, at least to some degree – often, you need to bring yourself in the right kind of emotional state in order to genuinely succeed in adopting a certain attitude. Attitudinal and affective modulation go hand-in-hand. See Slaby: *Gefühl und Weltbezug*, chapter 7.

7 In German, the appropriate translation of 'hexis' is *Haltung* – a term that nicely captures the idea that one often has to actively *hold oneself* in an existential orientation. The English terms that come the closest to the German *Haltung* are 'stance' and 'posture'.

8 All quotations in the text that are marked by page numbers only refer to Heidegger: *Grundbegriffe der Metaphysik*, in such a way that the first number always refers to the page number in the German edition, while the second number refers to the corresponding page number of the English translation by McNeill and Walker from which I have taken all quotations.

that understanding "is not a having-discovered a fact, but rather a holding-oneself in an existential possibility", (p. 336 – *my translation*). Since, according to Heidegger, each attunement "is understanding" and each understanding has its attunement (*Being and Time* p. 335, see also p. 142), I take it that we should not exclusively reserve the notion of existential orientation to the passive aspects of human existence (i.e., to affectivity), but rather allow it to include active elements that belong to understanding.[9]

The most important point for present purposes, in any case, is that, according to Heidegger, our attunements reach deeper into our very being than anything else – it is "in them that we first meet ourselves" (p. 101/68). It is here, in studying existential orientations, that we enter the dimension that we can call our being – our existence. So let us follow Heidegger's lead and try to meet ourselves – *in boredom.*

## 3. Heidegger on Boredom

With his detailed interpretation of different varieties of boredom, Heidegger wants to prepare the grounds for his metaphysical questioning concerning the world, finitude and solitude – these three being his "fundamental concepts of metaphysics". Remarkably, he wants to do this by *awakening the fundamental attunement*, the *Grundstimmung*, for 'our' philosophizing. As this fundamental attunement he identifies "profound boredom". The reason why a state of boredom, of all things, is the ultimate precondition for metaphysical philosophizing is briefly hinted at, in the form of a vague foreshadowing only, in § 20. Boredom, as the experience of *Lange-weile* – of a time that becomes long – points towards *time* as that which the fundamental questions of metaphysics are intimately tied up with.

From this it is already clear that Heidegger does not want to merely provide *descriptions* of varieties of boredom. He wants to *stimulate* boredom in his listeners. His goal is to create a specific readiness *for* certain experiences, and a kind of attentiveness or wakefulness *in* experience. This approach is based in part on the observation that although we are always in some existential orientation or other, we are for the most part not *attentively* in it. Dasein – being-*there* – as the kind of being proper to us as humans – is constitutively correlated to being-*away*, which means existing in any of a variety of non-attentive, absent-minded, unfo-

9 In the German original, the relevant passages read as follows: "Die Befindlichkeit ist *eine* der existenzialen Strukturen, in denen sich das Sein des "Da" hält. Gleichursprünglich mit ihr konstituiert dieses Sein das *Verstehen*. Befindlichkeit hat je ihr Verständnis, wenn auch nur so, daß sie es niederhält. Verstehen ist immer gestimmtes" (p. 142). And: "Jedes Verstehen has seine Stimmung. Jede Befindlichkeit ist verstehend" (p. 335).

cused modes of being (cf. p. 95/63). According to Heidegger, these various modes of being-away are in fact our default ways of being, only rarely (if ever) interrupted by spells of lucid attentiveness, of wakefulness and awareness, which then truly deserve to be called being-*there*. This is why, according to Heidegger, we do not initially have a clear idea of what boredom and other existential orientations really are, what they do to us or make manifest to us, even despite the fact that they structure experience in pervasive ways and are thus continuously 'there' in a certain way. This is also why, in order to gain an understanding of boredom, we need to *wake up to it*, attend to it, *live it* in some lucid sort of way. No amount of amassing factual knowledge can replace this *event* of waking up in and to the attunement of boredom. Thus, methodologically, Heidegger's work on boredom is an exercise in what could be called *performative* and *transformative* phenomenology, in that it has an active purpose instead of merely providing theoretical insight. This approach significantly diverges from many descriptive approaches.

In boredom, the default tendency of Dasein towards being-away seems to be particularly powerful. There is an active tendency to turn away from it. In boredom, just as in anxiety, the default tendency is not to be inattentively bored, but to actively seek distractions in order *not* to be bored. For this reason, a person on the verge of becoming bored constantly engages in activities that serve the sole purpose of 'passing time'. This makes it particularly difficult to get a hold of boredom. Most of the time, it seems to most people that they are in fact *not* bored.

So in order to perform the phenomenological act of waking us up to boredom, there is no need to create a state of boredom in the first place. Instead, one has to inhibit the activities and distractions that routinely fill most of one's regular life. Once these shallow surface activities are halted, boredom is revealed to be already there, lurking beneath the surface of diverting activities. Expect this procedure to be quite painful though, once all routine distractions are disallowed. Only then, in the resulting state of withholding all distractions and lofty engagements, do we have a chance of getting hold of our boredom, probably in a state of ever-increasing unrest, in a conspicuous and oppressive *felt emptiness* that threatens to drive us crazy.

### *3.1 Becoming bored by something*

The first variety, *becoming bored by something*, is the most common one and has a fairly simple structure – there is something (an object, a person etc.) that is boring. Thus, one is bored because of the "boringness" of this item. The second variety is more difficult, Heidegger calls it *sich langweilen bei etwas* ('being bored with something'), where it is not easy to determine what it is that is boring. The third variety is the strangest, as there is nothing in particular that is boring here – it is a profound, unconditioned boredom expressible in the puzzling phrase "one is bored" (*Es ist einem langweilig*).

The basic phenomenological characterization that Heidegger provides of the first variety of boredom is that one is *held in limbo* and *left empty* by it. In the most clear-cut cases, this is because the item in question does not grant us a fulfilment that we expect from it. For example, a railway station is boring if it occasions an overly long wait for a train to arrive. It leaves us empty by not offering us occasion for fulfilling activities, and it holds us in limbo by stubbornly postponing the activity proper to our being at the station, namely boarding a train. A book we read is boring insofar as it is uninspiring and uninteresting, thus it leaves us empty; and in reading it, we are "held in limbo" by the book since, though occupying our attention, it keeps providing uninspiring material and thus constantly postpones the fulfilment we are seeking in reading it. It makes us wait for what would be a proper result of reading: e.g., being moved or enthralled by a good story. Thus, what is boring is such that we are *held in limbo* and *left empty*. Boring is what *postpones* (probably indefinitely) an expected fulfilment.

And while we are thus held in limbo and left empty, what we eagerly and nervously strive to do is to 'fill up' the dead time by engaging in diverting activities that present themselves to us in the given situation. We nervously strive to make time pass. Heidegger nicely describes our wait at the village train station: What we might do is draw circles in the sand, count the trees in the alley, and glance repeatedly at our watch in increasingly shorter intervals, eager to check how much time we have made pass already. Thus diverting ourselves, we inadvertently make sure that the boredom doesn't reach a deeper level – that the boredom doesn't grip us more fully, and so we prevent ourselves from gaining a deeper insight into what goes on.

### *3.2 Being bored with something*

The first variety of boredom is an existential orientation that is dominated by some clearly identifiable intentional object – an external item, a structure or situation, such as the deserted train station in the first example, a book or an uninspiring interlocutor. The thing or person bores us because, although we are somehow bound to that item in expecting a specific fulfilment, the item withholds that fulfilment and thus leaves us empty – what is boring in this sense enchains us, keeps us fixated upon it without granting us what we want. The second variety – being bored with something – is not focused on some item or other in such a straightforward way. Heidegger's example is an evening invitation to which he decides to go after a good day's work:

> We have been invited out somewhere for the evening. We do not need to go along. Still, we have been tense all day, and we have time in the evening. So we go along. There we find the usual food and the usual table conversation, everything is not only very tasty, but tasteful as well. Afterward, people sit together having a lively discussion, as they say, perhaps listening to music, having a chat, and things are witty and amusing. And already it is time to leave. The

> ladies assure us, not merely when leaving, but downstairs and outside too as we gather to leave, that it was really nice, or that it was terribly charming. Indeed. There is nothing at all to be found that might have been boring about this evening, neither the conversation, nor the people, nor the rooms. Thus we come home quite satisfied. We cast a quick glance at the work we interrupted that evening, make a rough assessment of things and look ahead to the next day – and then it comes: I was bored after all this evening, on the occasion of this invitation.(p. 165/109)

Poor Martin. What happened? As opposed to the train delay at the uninspiring village station, the evening invitation is an event that he had freely chosen to attend, and of which he knew exactly what to expect – all of the usual things proper to a dinner party did in fact take place. We were bored nonetheless.

Heidegger analyses the situation by again trying to identify the characteristic 'passing of time' and the two structural features that were so striking in the first variety: being left empty (*Leergelassenheit*) and being held in limbo (*Hingehaltenheit*). At first sight, neither the 'passing of time' nor the two features seem present. But, as Heidegger goes on to demonstrate, on closer inspection they in fact do present themselves.

The first observation is that the routine passing of time is actually much more pervasive, and it is for this reason that we can easily overlook the fact that it takes place. This time, the entirety of the situation – *everything* that one does while engaging in the dinner party activities – qualifies as a kind of *Zeitvertreib* ('passing of time'). What we are bored with is not in fact distinct from our killing time:

> The evening is that with which we are bored, and *simultaneously*, *what* we are bored *with* here is *passing the time*. In this boring situation, *boredom and passing the time become intertwined* in a peculiar way. Passing the time creeps into our becoming bored and, diffused throughout the whole situation, achieves peculiar proportions that it is never able to assume in the first form in our discontinued and restless attempts. We find nothing boring, and yet passing the time takes on such proportions that it lays claim to the whole situation for itself. Strange! (p. 113/170)[10]

This strange entangling of the boring with our passing time is taken by Heidegger to indicate that boredom of the second variety is 'more profound' than the first variety, because in it the entirety of one's situation is infected by it, as opposed to merely one specific aspect. The boredom is increasingly focused on ourselves, while details of the situation don't matter so much.

10 The argument here is not so easy to discern. What I take to be the grounds for the claim that indeed *all* our dinner party activities qualify as 'Zeitvertreib' is the fact that we were bored while engaging in them. This is a typical Heideggerian argument in that it has a circular structure: The fact that we were bored manifests itself in that all activities we engaged in are revealed as mere attempts to kill time – i.e., they were not genuinely based in authentic care. This is simply the phenomenological profile of the second variety of boredom. I hope this will become clearer in the remainder of the present section.

What about the two phenomenal features characteristic of the first variety of boredom – being held in limbo and being left empty? At first sight, both seem to be missing in the second variety. Heidegger undertakes to show that these features do in fact appear in the second form, but that they also have taken on a different appearance. The feature of 'being left empty' has changed in line with the overall structure of the second variety into something that is not caused by something in our environment (as was the case in the first variety). Instead, the emptiness in question is of our own making. By letting ourselves be casually swept away and taken along by the usual dinner party activities, by freely submitting to whatever it is that happens at the dinner, we create a peculiar emptiness in ourselves. It is this *casualness* ('Lässigkeit' in German) in which we submit, unthinkingly, to whatever goes on at the party, that gives the decisive hint as to what goes on here:

> In this chatting along with whatever is happening we have, not wrongly or to our detriment, but legitimately, left our proper self behind in a certain way. In this seeking nothing further here, which is self-evident for us, we *slip away* from ourselves in a certain manner. [...] In this casualness of leaving ourselves behind in abandoning ourselves to whatever there is going on, *an emptiness can form*. Becoming bored or being bored is determined by this emptiness forming itself in our apparently satisfied going along with whatever there is going on. [...] This emptiness is a being left behind of our proper self. (p. 180/119–20)

This is what is what is at the root of the emptiness: A casual dinner party is not something that would fulfil us, not something crucial to our lives. Thus, although we seem heartily engaged in it, this engagement remains shallow. Since it originates in ourselves as our free choice – as opposed to being forced upon from something external that we do not control (like a train delay) – it makes sense to say that this emptiness is of our own making. This is why indeed *we* are bored in the sense of the German *Sichlangweilen bei* ("being bored with..." or "...at...") as opposed to *Gelangweiltwerden von...* ("becoming bored by..."). The emptiness in questions results from us *leaving behind our authentic self* ("die Zurückgelassenheit unseres eigentlichen Selbst", p. 180/120) – which in the case of the dinner party example means that this dinner is not among the things that we are looking for in our lives. The party is *existentially irrelevant* to us. That is why our involvement in it leaves us empty.

What about the temporality of the second form of boredom, the strange feature of 'being held in limbo'? As opposed to the first variety of boredom, where something specific stalls us, in the second form of boredom we have freely chosen to spend some time at the party. It therefore seems that we genuinely *have* time and thus could be quite relaxed. Nothing remotely resembles the panic-like situation at the railway station, where the delay stole us a precious amount of our time, forcing upon us a painful period of futile waiting. Heidegger points to the peculiarity of the fact that we have "*taken time*" to attend the party. He asks:

> We have *taken time* for the evening. What does it mean to take time? *What* time have we taken for ourselves here? Some span of time that is freely lying around and belongs to no one? Or does the time that we are taking *belong* to someone? *It belongs to us*. (p. 185/123)

We have taken a part of the time that is *our time* – a part of our lifetime. This period of our time we now generously spend; we use it up by attending the party. What happens in this "spending our time"? Heidegger puzzles his readers at this point by claiming that the flow of time, the constant succession of "Nows", is interrupted – that somehow, *time has come to a halt*. What results is an extended moment, a *standing Now* ("stehendes Jetzt", p. 186–9/123–26). The standing Now is such that during it we are fully engaged in the present moment, the activities offered to us at the dinner party. We are completely absorbed by the situation, immersed in the pure present of what goes on.

Why does this absorption in the present count as an instance of boredom? The crucial aspect is that this strange *standing Now* is created by our "lived present" being radically cut off both from what has been and from what will be. The temporality of our engaging in the party activities thus is an *isolated* present, with no meaningful connection to a past and no transition to a meaningful future. That is why it seems to stand still. The seamless and natural transition from a past via a mattering present to anticipated futures (possibilities) has come to a halt. Total isolation from the overall temporal framework of past and future turns the experience of present time at the dinner party into an awkward modification of existential temporality. Cut off from our past and not projected towards a relevant future, we are delivered over entirely to the present situation. Heidegger proceeds to perform a crucial identification that is in line with his analysis of primordial temporality in *Being and Time* (see § 65): The halted time at the core of our being bored with something is nothing other than our "self" – however, our self in a state of *existential abandonment*, because it is cut off from both what it had been and what it will be. The self left hanging in a temporary void of meaninglessness.

The oppressive standing Now is *us* – our very being cut off from the significance-yielding contexts of its full temporal horizons, past and future. Thus dangling in the isolated (meaningless) situation is being bored.

Let's quickly recapitulate on this complex interpretation of 'being bored with something': By taking time for the dinner party, we allow time to be transformed into a standing Now. This happens through our total immersion into the present of the ongoing party activities. The standing Now emerges as a specific emptiness that forms an odd contrast to the flurry of activities we engage in. The emerging emptiness is what captures us, fixes and thus delays us as our abandoned own self, cut off from its significance-yielding relations to past and future. In this way, we now see that and how both characteristic features of boredom – being left empty and being held in limbo – are present in the second variety of boredom. We are left empty because what goes on does not matter (enough) to us, and this fact amounts to us being held in limbo in that we have transformed a period of our lifetime into a disconnected “standing Now”. Both these features characteristic of boredom in the end come down to the same thing. Moreover, in the context of Heidegger’s conception of the being of Dasein (existence), they are revealed to be nothing other than our own ‘self’ in a state of existential abandonment:

> We said the time we take for ourselves is *our* time. This time in its standing – this is our sealed off having been and our unbound future, i.e., our whole time of our Dasein in a peculiar transformation. In this transformed form our whole time is compressed into this standing ‘now’ of the duration of the evening. This standing time – this *is we ourselves*; it is *our self* as that which *has been left behind* with respect to its *provenance* and *future*. This standing ‘now’ can, in its standing, precisely tell us that we have left it standing, which means, however, that it precisely is not releasing us, but that our being bound to it is impressing itself upon us. The standing ‘now’, the “during” of the evening in which the invitation endures, can manifest to us as such precisely this being held in limbo, being bound to our time. [...] When, letting ourselves go along with being there and part of things, we are thus set in place by the standing ‘now’ that is our own, albeit relinquished and empty self, then we are bored. (p. 189–90/125–4)

By agreeing to take time for the evening invitation, we have thrown ourselves, for a certain time, out of our existential track.[11] We linger on, existentially derailed, as mere shadows of ourselves, and it is indeed true and quite correct to say that what ultimately bores us is – *us*. When in this state, it is in a certain sense quite right to say that we have become boring to ourselves.

### *3.3 Profound Boredom*

> [W]e can see that the more profound it becomes, the more completely boredom is rooted in time – in the time that we ourselves are.
> (Heidegger: Basic Concepts, p. 201/133)

A characterization of the third and most profound form of boredom develops almost naturally out of the second variety – by means of a radicalization. Whereas in the second form we are still embedded in some specific situation or other even when it is not the situation as such that seems boring, this is not the case in the third form of boredom. Here, all one can say is that “it is boring for one”. Boredom has become total, all-encompassing, decoupled from any relatedness to specific situations. In a remarkable descriptive sequence, Heidegger claims that,

11 This ‘track’ is nothing other than what Heidegger calls ‘care’: meaningful projections (of future possibilities) from a pre-given (factive) ground in the context of which entities stand out as presently mattering to us in specific ways: Being-ahead//having-been//being-amidst (see Heidegger: *Sein und Zeit*, § 41).

in profound boredom, utter anonymity of self, wholesale meaninglessness of world, and total unrelatedness are fused together to create an existential extreme.

Who is it that suffers from deep boredom? Not you, not me, not us – but rather 'one'. The self has become an "undifferentiated no one" (p. 203/135), stripped off everything specific, stripped of its everyday personality; in fact, one is completely *de-personalized* in this state (cf. p. 207/138). Equally and correlatively, the entirety of entities – the world – not just a specific situation, has been stripped of its significance. Nothing matters any more, everything is utterly and indifferently irrelevant. A non-person, a 'no one' is facing an all-encompassing void. This, in turn, leads to a third dimension of emptiness: Non-self and insignificant world are related in a mode of 'unrelatedness'. In this respect, profound boredom is an extreme modification of intentionality: A Non-self is *negatively related* to an utterly meaningless totality of beings. This peculiar 'negative relatedness' results from the dual insignificance of both self and world. As the self in deep boredom is without concerns and interests and thus incapable of having things matter to it, its relation to the world is one of profound indifference – not more than a dumb staring at the totality of beings in utter estrangement. This is an absolute borderline case of encountering entities, a breakdown of *being-in-the-world.*

Because of this extreme character of the third variety of boredom, Heidegger holds that it cannot be discussed by means of a concrete example. There simply is no example (cf. p. 203/135). Since it is all-encompassing, this kind of boredom has only one possible manifestation – affecting *the entirety* of self and *the entirety* of beings – everything there is.[12] There also is no 'passing of time' involved in deep boredom. Once in its grip, it is out of the question that any attempt to make time pass could ever succeed. We are stuck, there is no way out – and it is a part of profound boredom that we intuitively *know* this. ('Know' is meant here not in the sense of an explicit act of reflection, but in the sense of an unreflective 'holding oneself' in this predicament.)

In fact, profound boredom is so deep that Dasein itself is transformed by it – transformed into a state that facilitates 'existential understanding'. Profound boredom offers us the possibility of getting to know how things stand with regard to our existence as such. As all Heideggerian moods have the character of making something manifest, and *disclosing* something about ourselves (cf. p. 205/136), this also applies to profound boredom. However, profound boredom is special in that it offers the possibility of understanding our existential predicament in general (this applies to only a small number of moods, anxiety of course

12 This is different from the fact that profound boredom might be *occasioned* by some specific situation or other. Heidegger suggests, in a remark that nicely exemplifies his self-assured provinciality, that 'it is boring for one' "to walk through the streets of a large city on a Sunday afternoon." (p. 203/135).

being another one).[13] This is the ontological dimension of boredom – the characteristic that makes it special.

A message is forced upon us in deep boredom. First, the extreme orientation described above – a depersonalized 'self' left hanging in a total void in a mode of utter unrelatedness – is described by Heidegger as *being delivered over to the entirety of beings withdrawing themselves in their entirety* (cf. p. 210/139). Beings in their entirety 'withdrawing themselves': worldly entities in general have ceased to offer any possibilities to Dasein. (This is the manifestation of the structural feature of *being left empty* in the third variety of boredom.)

What follows is the crucial move: Heidegger claims that this withdrawal or 'telling refusal' of possibilities is at the same time an *announcing* of these very possibilities. He plays an etymological trick here that doesn't quite work in English, by claiming that "alles *Ver*sagen ist in sich ein *Sagen*, d.h. Offenbarmachen" (p. 211/140) – which literally however un-etymologically translates to: "all withholding is a telling, i.e. a making manifest".[14] But how can a refusal be at the same time a *telling* or a *revealing*? One answer could be that, while in profound boredom everything – both self and world – have lost all significance whatsoever, it is nevertheless still boredom which is a *negative* existential quality (as opposed to the presumably neutral 'utter indifference'). This negativity of the existential orientation in the absence of anything specific to focus on or turn away from inevitably creates a state of 'responsiveness' in which the profoundly bored person is open, probably for the first time, to grasping basic truths about her existence.

However, a more important consideration is to place the 'telling' involved in profound boredom in the context of Heidegger's overall understanding of language ('Rede' and, in his later works, 'Sage'). Heidegger views language as a structural feature of Dasein, as the discursive articulation of intelligibility in general. In this context, it is not totally surprising to take worldly entities as constantly 'telling us things', i.e. calling for responses, 'laying claims upon us'. In this sense, the situation in which beings withhold themselves in their entirety has to be taken as a privation of the general ontological structure of telling, a modification in the structure of the world's intelligibility. By not offering anything, beings become conspicuous through the very fact that they 'fall silent', and this will inevitably impinge upon our conceptually articulated responsiveness to our

13 In the first variety of boredom, we "shout down" boredom's potential "message" through hyperactive killing of time; in the second variety of boredom, we don't want to listen to the message... (cf. p. 205/136) – whereas in profound boredom *we are compelled* to listen to it, there is "a peculiar compulsion in it" (p. 209/139).

14 McNeill and Walker translate the passage in question as follows: "All telling refusal [Ver-*sagen*] is in itself a telling [Sagen], i.e., a making manifest" (p. 140). It is of course a stretching of language to coin the expression "telling refusal" to capture the connotation of "telling" in the German "versagen," which would have to be translated literally as 'deny', 'refuse' or 'withhold'.

surroundings. In this way, beings 'telling refusal' can be said to force a message upon us.[15]

But what is it that is 'told to' Dasein by 'beings telling refusal in their entirety'? According to Heidegger, what is announced are the *possibilities* that Dasein has (or might have). In the worldly entities' receding, in their not offering us anything, they 'point to' the possibilities that they nevertheless *would* or *could* offer to Dasein – the beings' withholding announces these possibilities exactly by refusing, by denying them (cf. p. 212/141). As soon as the emptiness and meaningless of the world becomes aggressively conspicuous, there is a *dawning* of the possibilities that Dasein could have, but that so far lay idle in its existence. (This is what Heidegger will then identify as the third variety of boredom's manifestation of the feature of being held in limbo – the temporal character of this becomes clear in what follows.)

The crucial final piece of the explication follows suit. What is still missing is the connection between deep boredom and time. So far, nothing in the characterization of deep boredom seemed to be specifically related to time. But this is just a superficial impression. Looked at correctly, even the first main feature of deep boredom – the all-encompassing void that was created by a total refusal of beings in their entirety – is a temporal phenomenon. In this all-encompassing void, Dasein is *entranced* ('gebannt' in German) by time – by its own time, by the very time that constitutes Dasein's existence (cf. p. 221/147). Thus entranced, Dasein fails to relate to any beings – beings tellingly withhold in their entirety and all significance drains away. Being-left-empty in profound boredom is a being-entranced by the temporal horizon as such. A conspicuous feature of this is the complete disappearance of any concrete Now. As opposed to the second variety of boredom (which is centred upon a conspicuous *standing Now*), the Now is eliminated in profound boredom. What remains is an awkward merging of all three temporal dimensions – past, present, future – into an unarticulated temporal unity (cf. p. 222/148).

As this widening and fusion of the temporal dimension matches the telling refusal of beings in their entirety and their consequent meaninglessness, the second crucial temporal feature of profound boredom matches the strange announcing of possibilities in their telling refusal: The very entrancement by time amounts to a being forced into the centre of what enables Dasein as such – and this is, paradoxically, the present moment or "moment of vision" (the 'Augenblick'). Thus, just as Dasein's possibilities are announced in their very refusal, Dasein's specific *being-in-the-present* (in the *Augenblick*) is opened up in the disappearance of the present into the dimensional indifference of a unified tem-

15 This is backed by things Heidegger explains at various places in the *Zollikon Seminars*. John Haugeland in "Truth and Finitude" offers a good rationale for translating Heidegger's 'Rede' not as 'discourse' but rather as 'telling.' This is very much in line with the later Heidegger's switching from talking about 'Rede' to talking about 'Sagen' and 'Sage', which is of course much closer to the English 'telling'.

porality. From this, finally, Heidegger draws his ultimate conclusion, reporting the fusion of the temporal and the existential dimension in profound boredom:

> Yet whatever that which entrances as such, namely time, announces and tells of as something in fact refused [...] is nothing less than the *freedom of Dasein* as such. (p. 223/148–149)

This freedom, Heidegger explains, transpires only in the act of *freeing-itself* performed by Dasein. And this act of freeing-itself, in turn, happens only in the unlocking or disclosing of Dasein – in Dasein's disclosing itself as a Being-*there* (in the present), which is nothing other than *acting* in the here and now. Thus, Dasein is called upon in deep boredom to disclose-itself, i.e. to resolutely take over its particular existence in the here and now and amidst the entities of its world. This act of unlocking is the *Augenblick*, the "moment of vision":

> Only in the resolute self-disclosure of Dasein to itself, in the moment of vision, does it make use of that which properly makes it possible, namely time as the moment of vision itself. (p. 224/149)

Basic structural features of Dasein – the predicament of having to take over one's existential situation (its concrete possibilities), and one's having to perform free acts in the here and now – become conspicuous in deep boredom precisely through their vanishing, their 'telling refusal'. *Through* their very disappearance, Dasein is called upon to actively retrieve these features. The conspicuous felt absence of all possibilities takes on the character of a call to actively grasp and realize one's possibilities – and this corresponds to (or rather: is another description of) the disappearance of the present into an unarticulated temporal horizon which is at the same time a *forcing* of Dasein back into the very moment – into the present-moment of action in the here and now. That is why Heidegger can conclude that in profound boredom, bounded, finite human freedom 'announces itself' – i.e. makes a claim upon us, calls us back into resolute action. Each of us is thereby revealed to be the ultimate creator of any 'meaning in life' that there can possibly be.

## 4. Concluding remarks

> I feel like a mere void, the illusion of a soul, the locus of a being, a conscious darkness where a strange insect vainly seeks at least the warm memory of a light.
>
> Fernando Pessoa[16]

Boredom grows from the temporality of human existence. In boredom, when it is allowed to become profound and is not evaded through diversions or kept shallow in one of its more mundane varieties, our very being is modified to an extreme. In the deeper forms of the second variety of boredom ('being bored with something'), the bored person's existence literally turns into a span of 'dead time'. The 'self' (understood essentially as 'lived temporality') is abandoned by being cut off from a meaningful temporal context – from a significance-yielding history and from a constructive projection towards a meaningful future. Consequently, experience in the present is turned into a 'standing now', which is nothing less than existential futility – nothing really happens, nothing really matters. In profound boredom (the third variety), not just a short period of our life invested in a specific activity, but rather our entire existence is modified into our turning literally into a 'no one', and correspondingly, the world in its entirety ceases to offer anything of significance. In terms of temporality, profound boredom amounts to the loss of a lively present, as the three dimensions that make up existential temporality fuse into one another indifferently.

So far, so plausible. Next, Heidegger attempts to persuade us of the possibility of a 'message' being thrust upon us in profound boredom. From this point on, his interpretation can seem somewhat forced. Once at the deepest point of all-consuming boredom (rarely if ever experienced in the course of an ordinary human life), Heidegger reckons with the emergence of a quite specific possibility: The extreme transformation of existence creates a situation of heightened responsiveness in which the very features of existence that had been modified in profound boredom are made manifest to us. In this way, profound boredom is thought to facilitate our *waking up* again – what Heidegger glosses as a "waking up to ourselves". Profound boredom, according to Heidegger, calls us back into the present-moment in order to freely and responsibly take charge of our existence. Profound boredom would then have the potential to awake our freedom by forcing us back into our existential present – into the *lived presence of the "moment of vision"*.

In the last few sentences I purposely worded my phrases in order to distance myself somewhat from this interpretation. Without being explicit about this, Heidegger seems to think that failing to heed the message of profound boredom is falling short, somehow missing out on a profound existential possibility. Conse-

16 Pessoa: *Book of Disquiet*, fragment 219, p. 192.

quently, the state resulting from *not answering* the call of profound boredom – not 're-starting' resolute existence in the here and now of determined action – is implicitly construed as an inauthentic or otherwise defective mode of being. But what if someone lingered on indefinitely in profound boredom – existing, as it were, as an 'undifferentiated no one' in the wasteland of a meaningless world, relating to this world in a mode of 'utter unrelatedness'? How would this be? Maybe there is even a calm resting place that gives us peace of mind in depersonalized detachment, and in the pure, disinterested beholding of one's surroundings, unstirred by the vicissitudes of ordinary life. Viewed from this angle, it can seem like an impertinence to demand initiative and action. Why shouldn't we submit willfully to the bliss of indifference? From this (admittedly unusual) vantage point, it seems that Heidegger tends to impose an activist ideal upon human existence – inscribing a relentless demand to be oriented towards what matters, even to the point of grasping the existential truth that nothing really matters for its own sake. Even in the absence of all meaning, existence is tied slavishly to significance, by having profound boredom force a message upon us, by pulling us back into resolute being, into relentless caring, significance-yielding projections and into a way of life that, like Sisyphus, creates and sustains those projections against one's better judgment. As my choice of motto for this section indicates, I have in mind an existential orientation like the one that Bernardo Soares – anti-hero (and author's alter ego) of Fernando Pessoa's wonderful *Book of Disquiet* – is burdened (or blessed?) with. In this fictional 'autobiography without facts' we find an abundance of confessions by an assistant bookkeeper from Lisbon – confessions that testify of quite a different stance towards existential emptiness than the one offered by Heidegger. The following fragments are presented in the hope that they can kindle an idea of a way to dwell in a boredom-like existential orientation:

> Some say that without hope life is impossible, others say that with hope it's empty. For me, since I've stopped hoping or not hoping, live is simply an external picture that includes me and that I look at, like a show without a plot, made only to please the eyes – an incoherent dance, a rustling of leaves in the wind, clouds in which the sunlight changes colour, ancient streets that wind every which way around the city.[17]

> To goldenly stagnate in the sun, like a murky pond surrounded by flowers. To possess, in the shade, that nobility of spirit that makes no demands on life. To be in the whirl of the worlds like dust of flowers, sailing through the afternoon air on an unknown wind and falling, in the torpor of dusk, wherever it falls, lost among larger things. To be this with a sure understanding, neither happy nor sad, grateful to the sun for its brilliance and to the stars for their remoteness. To be no more, have no more, want no more...[18]

17 Ibid., fragment 193, p. 169.
18 Ibid., fragment 45, p. 46.

> My happiest moments are those when I think nothing, want nothing and dream nothing, being lost in a torpor like some accidental plant, like mere moss growing on life's surface. I savour without bitterness this absurd awareness of being nothing, this foretaste of death and extinction.[19]

These remarks open up a dimension that makes the final steps of Heidegger's interpretation seem questionable. There might be many more and quite different questions to ask about profound boredom. Maybe there are other ways to deal with profound boredom than being forced back into resolute existence. What vast universes of possible being are laid out before us when we let go of the fixation upon 'meaning in life'? What unexplored spaces of possibility await us when we, like Pessoa's alter ego in the *Book of Disquiet*, commit our existence to unrelenting passivity, pure beholding and literary imagination? Heidegger's interpretation of boredom, remarkable though it is, may in the end offer no more than initial glimpses of insight into the way in which temporality, selfhood, existential significance, and freedom hang together in human existence. It now seems as though the act of *freeing-oneself* in the 'moment of vision,' whereby Dasein is able to access the present situation so as to act meaningfully in it, is only one of various ways open to us in profound boredom. There might be other, quite different ways of transforming one's existential orientation from tedium into absorption in the present. The book on boredom and related orientations is far from closed. Its existential analysis has only just begun.

## References

Haugeland, John: "Truth and Finitude. Heidegger's Transcendental Existentialism", in: Mark Wrathall/Jeff Malpas (eds.): *Heidegger, Authenticity, and Modernity. Essays in Honor of Hubert L. Dreyfus, Vol. 1*, Cambridge, MA (MIT Press) 2000, pp. 43–77.

Heidegger, Martin: *Sein und Zeit* (1927), Tübingen (Max Niemeyer) 1993.

Heidegger, Martin: *Grundbegriffe der Metaphysik. Welt – Endlichkeit – Einsamkeit* (1929/30), Frankfurt (Klostermann) 2004; translated by William McNeil and Nicholas Walker: *Basic Concepts of Metaphysics. World – Finitude – Solitude*, Bloomington, Ind. (Indiana University Press) 1995.

Heidegger, Martin: *Zollikon Seminars: Protocols – Conversations – Letters*, Evanston, IL. (Northwestern University Press) 2001.

Pessoa, Fernando: *The Book of Disquiet*, edited and translated by Richard Zenith, London (Penguin Classics) 2002.

19 Ibid., fragment 461, p. 379.

Ratcliffe, Matthew: "The Feeling of Being", in: *Journal of Consciousness Studies* 12 (2005) 8–10, pp. 43–60.

Ratcliffe, Matthew: *Feelings of Being: Phenomenology, Psychiatry and the Sense of Reality*, Oxford (Oxford University Press) 2008.

Slaby, Jan: *Gefühl und Weltbezug*, Paderborn (mentis) 2008.

Slaby, Jan and Achim Stephan: "Affective Intentionality and Self-Consciousness", in: *Consciousness and Cognition* 17, 2008, pp. 506–513.

# The Other Side of the Frame
# Artistic Experience as Felt Framing: Fundamental Principles of an Artistic Theory of Relativity[1]

JULIAN KLEIN

## Prologue on the theater: Stagework

Please imagine attending a rehearsal of a theatre production: We are sitting back in the last row, observing the preparations being made for the first run-through of a Shakespeare scene. Stage technicians assemble the scenery, actors and actresses are warming up, names are being called out across the stage; someone is practicing some excerpted sentences, and someone else is testing a new position for a monologue. Finally, all the preparations wind down, and the piece begins with the first sentence.

There is nothing exceptional about all this; nearly every initial run-through of a theater production resembles this description. But some days later, we also attend the premiere. There we experience the very same procedure: the stage technicians assembling the scenery, actors and actresses running through positions, names being called out, and excerpts being practiced. The entire spectacle seems just like a rehearsal, and then the piece begins.

Had we not visited the rehearsal, we would probably consider it self-evident that all of this is just acting, and we might not be capable of believing that anyone might actually consider it real. But we did visit the rehearsal, where we experienced the very same situation. At the rehearsal, we thought that the technicians were doing for real what they seemed to be doing; for us, they were preparing a rehearsal, and not rehearsing their preparations.

Wherein lies the distinction? Why did we not 'understand' during the rehearsal that the preparations were actually staged? Were the technicians 'better' during the rehearsal because it did not occur to us at the time that they were just acting out their work? Or, conversely, were they 'not convincing enough', since their actions allowed the possibility for us to 'misunderstand' what they were doing, and take it for real? This shows that the properties of things – or, as in this

1 This article is an abridged English version of a text originally published in German, in Klein (ed.): *per.SPICE!*, pp. 104–134. I wish to thank Gratia Stryker-Haertel, Doris Kolesch, Cord Müller, Kurt Koegel, and numerous discussants for improvements of this version. Contact: julianklein@artistic-research.de

case, the behavior of the performers – are occasionally unable to make much of a contribution to how we see them and what we perceive them to be. The fact that we first saw the technicians as a stage crew and later as performers was not an effect of any sort of change in their behavior (as it did not in fact change), but rather of a change to the way in which we perceived them. In this case, the reason underlying the change is a tiny piece of paper in our hands. What changed for us was not any content but the framework – and along with it, our mode of perception.

## First Act: From Presence to Representation

Theorists have suggested various designations to describe the difference between our ways of seeing things (the stage technicians in the rehearsal, the stage appearance of the technicians in the premiere and the appearance of the actors as characters in a drama). These are all intended to subdivide the continuum between acting and non-acting to a greater or lesser degree of fine-cut precision.

Making the distinction that the stage technicians and actors in our experiment were at the center of our attention in the rehearsal situation to a greater degree than, for example, in the cafeteria before the rehearsal, provides us with a first possibility in terms of undertaking this subdivision. While in the cafeteria they were just present in a rather pure manner of existence, we could say, the stage lent them a special *presence* within our perception. Nonetheless, for us, the stage technicians (in the rehearsal) simply were what they were, while the actors presented characters. Thus, the actors were present in a symbolic way, as a *representation* of the characters. In contrast, at the premiere, the stage technicians, who also acted for us, acted as themselves – stage technicians – and not as characters. They kind of demonstrated for us what stage technicians tend to do when a theater rehearsal is underway. This gave them a status somewhere between presence and representation; let us call this the mode of *presentation*.

| | | | | | |
|---|---|---|---|---|---|
| Non-acting | | | | | Acting |
| | (mere) Present | Presence | Presentation | Representation | |

These modes show a possible subdivision of the continuum between non-playing and playing. Their categories are not sharp, but overlapping, like colours of a continuous spectrum.

Present: This mode of perception describes the actual, pure, ostensibly untainted state of affairs. Things are simply there or they are not. This can encompass subjects, persons, ambience, and processes as well as imaginings and hallucinations. In this mode, it does not strike us that this fleeting momentariness is conveyed by our perception. We perceive everything directly; our perception is simple, self-evident and transparent. We talk about 'recognizing' objects – we have a *that-perception*; we see a blue field, and it is a blue field for us. We see a glass of water and may even stretch out our hand to drink from it without thinking anything of it, perhaps without even remembering it afterwards. It is simply a glass of water; that is that, and we cannot say anything more about it.

Presence: If, however, we become aware of the fact that we have the *perception* of a blue field (of, say, the moment when it became for us a blue space, indicative of a specific blue-ness) or of the fact that we have the perception of a glass of water (perhaps because we get the impression that it feels a certain way to perceive this glass of water), then the glass of water or blue field acquire a presence for us. We notice *how* the glass looks, *how* it feels, *how* the water in it tastes and *how* it sounds when we put it back. This is a felt perception, a *how-perception* (a perception that somehow feels), a perceived perception, or, if you like, a perception squared. Many scholars thus pleonastically call this "aesthetic perception." I would rather like to call this mode of presence the aesthetic *sensing*[2]. This mode of aesthetic sensing is not at all limited to art. On the contrary, aesthetic sensing constantly accompanies us as a part of our perception, although it often flares up only for short moments of time before immediately disappearing again from our awareness.

Presentation: In the presentational mode, we understand things, persons, ambience and processes *as* something. They appear to us to be in a specific relation to us or to our surroundings – for example, as a tableau (a blue wall actually being a painting) or as a function (a door serving as the entryway); as a role (Mr. Hofmeyer being an actor, Mr. Neumayer a stage technician); in relation to something else (a glass of water being *my* glass), in illustrative reproduction (a photo being a photo *of* a glass of water) or in some other referential context (a glass of water being the third from the left and not having been there yet yesterday).

Representation: In the representational mode, objects are no longer just themselves but acquire an additional level as well.[3] They become an icon, representing something that does not itself necessarily have to be present. We lend them a meaning that we are able to understand or misunderstand, attribute to them a sense that we can access and develop or interpret them as the expression

2 I propose 'aesthetic sensing' as the appropriate correspondent term to 'ästhetisches Erleben' instead of the common phrase 'aesthetic experience', because the German 'Erleben' stresses more the here-and-now liveness in a basic sensuous perception in opposition to the more complicated 'Erfahrung' (which also translates as 'experience'), which should remain reserved for higher (namely artistic) modes of perception – see the explanations later in this article.

3 There are also, of course, non-aesthetic representations. These are distinguished from the aesthetic representations listed here by means of the fact that they are not present for us (which, according to the above-mentioned illustrations, is the same in meaning as the property of being aesthetic) – or, the non-aesthetic icons seem to us to be transparent in terms of their subjects. This also applies for non-aesthetic presentations.

of something or someone else. In this manner, the photo of a half-filled glass of water remind us of optimism, the work of the stage technicians exhibit for us the illusory nature of being, the blue of the blue wall becomes a commentary on Yves Klein's *International Klein Blue*, and the actors become for us Shakespeare characters (Erika Fischer-Lichte calls this their "semiotic corpus", emphasizing that both the presence of an actor and the representation of a character are processes of embodiment that permeate and overlap one another[4]).

| | *Present* | *Presence* | *Presentation* | *Representation* |
|---|---|---|---|---|
| *Things* | Here-and-Now | Effect | Show | Signify |
| | Concreteness | Embodiment | Relationality | Designation |
| *Persons* | Recognize | Experience | Perceive | Access |
| | Enter | Seem | Fulfill | Enact |
| | To do | To perform | To play | To act |
| *Pictures* | Figure | Picture | Image | Icon |
| *Texts* | Printed/Written | Seen | Read | (Mis-)Understood |
| *Processes* | Ongoing | Event | Gesture | Simulation |
| *Sounds* | Sound | Tone | Motive | Signal |

Similar descriptions can also be found within other genera, like the examples in the table above. All these categories are modes of perception, and do not describe object-like properties. As we have seen, they can occur occasionally with the very same contents.

4 Fischer-Lichte: *The Transformative Power of Performance.*

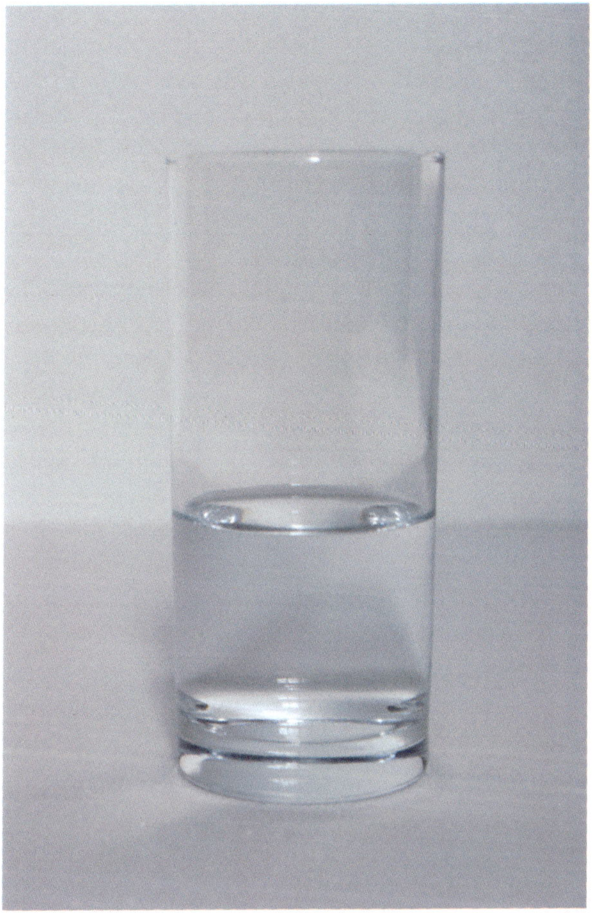

Fig. 1: Manuel Klein, A Glass, 2009.

## Interlude: Meta, or the Art of Perception

But when objects gain those statuses by our perception, why do we then often distinguish between categories of objects, as if their attributes were their inherent properties? An aesthetics as a theory of perception should be able to describe both the processes of aesthetic sensings in all their subjectivity and the physical properties of object-like matter in our communication on experiences, while expending the least possible amount of theoretical effort. Thus, an aesthetic theory should also be able to describe *how* individual aesthetic sensings can turn through our communication into the properties of objects that seem to be free of perception (while remaining relative), and how, in turn, these properties retroactively affect the experience of perception and thus our construction of reality. In particular, this means that an aesthetic theory should be dynamic and relativistic.

In the past century, the field of physics was faced with a comparably similar problem. Many of the properties supposedly belonging to physical particles were actually dependent on the observer. Physicians and philosophers sought for an explanation, attempting to establish how the stable properties of the macroscopic objects could possibly be based on the observer-dependent state of quantum objects they consist of. The theoretical solution was: Physical systems outside of laboratory conditions are not isolated enough from their surroundings to aggregate in coherent quantum superposition. With increasing volume of their surroundings (in terms of the degrees of freedom), these effects disappear in a process of *decoherence.* The macroscopic objects attain their observer-independent properties via the redundancy of information present in their surroundings. In other words, the 'weird' behavior of quantum objects can only take place if the surroundings 'know' relatively little about the observed system. Therefore, many of the supposed properties of objects must be interpreted as a product of the measurement process. While this means many of the classic properties are actually relative (dependent on the form of observation), it also allows for a gauge of the 'objectivity' of a state, namely, the *redundancy* with which the surrounding of an object register the object's state.

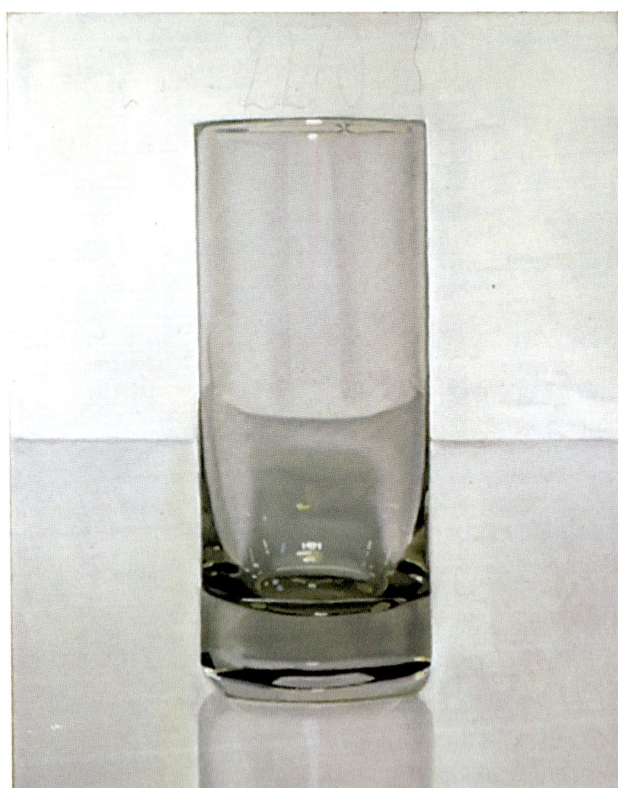

Fig. 2: Peter Dreher,
The Glass, 2004.

So where is the analogy to the aesthetic? An aesthetic sensing serving as the mode of perception is subjective and very difficult to access from the outside – often even for the person experiencing it. It cannot be directly observed. Yet often, a categorization is still made afterwards: One picture of a glass is just an illustration of a theoretical essay (like on page 125, fig. 1); the other is a piece of art, namely a photo of the 2270$^{th}$ painting in the project by Peter Dreher entitled "Das Glas" (page 126, fig. 2).[5] Arthur C. Danto, in his "Transfiguration of the Commonplace", describes the exhibition of a collection of nine square red panels unable to be distinguished from one another in terms of appearance and materials – some of which Danto treats as artwork, some of which he does not.[6] This might lead us to ask what would happen if the works were to be switched when they were returned to their original owners? It is worth noting that distinctions like this between red artwork and red nonsense are often made in connection with the greater surroundings, whether that be the art market, a public discourse or the cultural practices of a specific group. Yet all intersubjective categories of aesthetic experiences are grounded first and foremost in the subjective, individual aesthetic sensings of each individual. But the communication about these experiences is a process of interdependencies containing a mostly increasing amount of redundancy, a process in which many individual subjective experiences are involved; while these experiences, when observed in isolation, seem to be independent of objective categories – but all together forming stable systems of intersubjective cultural constructs.

Coming back to our spectrum of playing, we are able to interpret the dimension of the progression: the variable responsible for this process might be *redundancy.*

## Second Act: From Perception to Object

Since Nelson Goodman's formulation "When is art?"[7], at the latest, we have considered the question as to whether an object is art or not to be just as unanswerable as is the question of whether an electron is actually a particle or a wave;

5 http://www.peter-dreher.de/.

6 According to Danto, one of these panels is a painting described by Søren Kierkegaard of the Israelites crossing the Red Sea; two paintings entitled 'Red Square' (one of the Red Square in Moscow, one being just a geometrical red square), one comes from Giorgione, who unfortunately passed away after finishing the first coating of red for a planned painting 'Conversazione Sacra'; yet another is from Danto's dilettantish friend J., who entitled his work 'Untitled'; and one is simply "a thing with color on it." Danto: *Transfiguration of the Commonplace*, pp. 1ff.

7 Goodman: "When Is Art?"

for none of these properties are so much attributable to the objects as they are to be described as *processes* – an artistic method of perception in the one case, and a physical measurement in the other. *Art*, however, is not a property belonging to an object, but a perceptive process mode. For this reason, let us introduce another variant to the description of our continuum between present and representation: concepts that have more to do with the process of perception and emphasize its procedural nature, even if they happen to partially describe the same phenomenon. The advantage is that they are less predetermined by expressions that do not keep in mind the relativity of the aesthetic.

| **Present** | **Presence** | **Presentation** | **Representation** |
|---|---|---|---|
| Reception | Resonance | Frame | Refuge |

-> -> **Redundance** -> ->

*Reception*

In describing processes of perception, we must take note that there is a certain primacy of the first person perspective. In analyzing aesthetic processes, we have to consider at least three circumstances of perception: its general limitations, its constructivity and the filtering of perceptual processes.

Limitations: All perceptions are naturally limited by the functioning of senses. Our senses provide us with an access to the outside world, and this access is not always congruent with others. For example, the failure of one sense often leads to a change in the other senses (e.g. a sharpened sense of hearing in the darkness).

Constructivity: At first, even if all of the individual senses are in agreement with each other, the subsequent sensory stimuli processing can still differ. Tonal pieces of music, for example, sound different to people with absolute pitch than to people with relative pitch; people with absolute pitch would know by ear if a pianist were to play the Prelude in C major from Bach's "Well-Tempered Clavier" in, say, B major. Secondly, we construct interrelationships first and foremost in accordance with that to which we are accustomed, even if we know that our impression is not in agreement with 'reality'. This fact is supported by numerous examples of illusions – which are actually not so much illusions as they are very logical constructions reflecting the world in which we live. Take, for example, the many *Trompe l'œil* works, which are able to pass as three-dimensional illusions because we, in our perception of the construction of these objects, do not approach them with the assumption that they are two-dimensional pictures.[8] A left-footed amateur soccer player has a different sense for a free kick seen on

8 The illusionist street pictures by Julian Beever appear three-dimensional when viewed at a specific angle: http://users.skynet.be/J.Beever/.

television than does a right-footed one – or than someone who has never even attempted to make a free kick.[9] Third, quite often, our perception is also very creative; we are able to see things we know are not there, such as optical illusions that seem to be moving.[10] These also provide us with a good example of situations in which we suddenly become aware of our own perceptions without necessarily having intended to do so. We do not just see something but also note how this seeing *feels*, even without actively wanting to – we are simultaneously assaulted and surprised by this process of aesthetic sensing.

Filtering: It is our own awareness that defines the content of our perception. Probably the most-cited example exhibiting the power of our abilities to filter is the film of a basketball game by Simons and Chabris (1999);[11] typically, at least half of the people who view it do not even notice a person, uninvolved in the action on which the film focuses, strolling through it in a gorilla costume. This phenomenon is called *inattentional blindness*. Our own awareness defines the content of our perception (everything else becomes invisible to us, perhaps even despite our knowledge of its existence).

### *Resonance*

*Resonance* is a simple, yet helpful model for the analysis of perceptual processes: instead of 'senders' and 'receivers' we can speak of *agent* and *resonator;* the resonance functions with some degree of fuzziness, since the agent and the resonator do not have to have all properties in common for a successful resonance; and the *medium* of transmission enables the modeling of feedback and reflexivity. Resonance provides us with a precise model for perceptual processes, particularly as the agent needs have no intentions regarding the resonance: The resulting oscillation depends on the current conditions of both the agent and the resonator. Lastly, the agent itself can also be a resonator, which is often the case in artistic contexts. The resonance model is able to integrate many phenomena of perception, such as pareidolia (the ability to recognize shapes within amorphous structures), as well as the dependency of recognition on our experiences and expectancies – our resonance oscillations, so to speak.

9 Lozano, Hard and Tversky: "Putting motor resonance in perspective".

10 An example is the Rotating Snake by Akiyoshi Kitaoka: http://www.ritsumei.ac.jp/~akitaoka/rot snake.gif.

11 Simons and Chabris: "Gorillas in Our Midst"; the film can be seen at http://viscog.beckman.illinois.edu/flashmovie/15.php.

## *Redundancy*

We are able to make our way around in this world with ease because we learned the ability of categorizing early on in our lives. In order to be able to form categories, we require repetition, or more precisely, similar but not identical repetition: redundancy. We tend to order the world in compartments – we are taxophiles and taxomaniacs. In any case, categories do not help us to recognize *exactly* what we are dealing with, but they help us to exclude what cannot be meant. Elements of a category neither have to exhibit all features nor do they have to fulfill minimum requirements. Also which individual elements we consider as prototypical varies greatly.[12] We acquire our categories either depending on others or independently, but in any case they form the structure of our realities. One example of this constructivity of our perception is Diana Deutsch's recording entitled "So Strangely"[13]. In it, a segment of a sentence is continually repeated so often that it mutates into song by means of its sheer repetition. Here the escalation of redundancy creates a jump in our perceptive categories.

## *Feedback*

The way feedback takes place in the resonance model can be used for further modeling of aesthetic processes. Different types of feedback can be distinguished from each other in at least three dimensions: subjective-intersubjective, independent-interdependent and synchronous-diachronous. At first, the kinds of feedback we collectively, intersubjectively create when communicating with each other (verbally and nonverbally) regarding our perceptions are different from the kinds of feedback we individually and subjectively create without sharing it or entering into an exchange of ideas about it with others. In a second dimension, both of these respective kinds of feedback can be formed either independently of others, relying mostly on one's supposed 'own' experiences, or interdependently with others, in the sense that one's construction of reality is based on assumptions regarding the other's experiences.

If *I* have visited a large enough number of dress rehearsals in the theater, *I*, too, will no longer be startled by the hustle and bustle on stage shortly before the beginning of a rehearsal, but will just "know" that the stage technicians are readying the stage and the actors are warming up. We like to generalize within this independent, subjective and diachronous categorization from the very beginning.

In an interdependent and synchronous case of subjective feedback, we have the impression that others have a particular perception and would like to join in having it as well (amplification) – and if we do take on that perception, we are

12 Cf. Goldstein: *Sensation and Perception.*

13 Deutsch: *Phantom Words and other Curiosities.*

reaffirmed by the impression that everyone else actually has the very same perception we ourselves have. Alternately, we might decide to avoid this very consonance of perception (dampening).

The intersubjective exchange of ideas is also a form of feedback that influences current and future perception – and even past perception as well, since our memories of experiences change with every new activity. This kind of feedback, too, can take place either independently or interdependently. On the one hand, we tend to conform to the behavior of a group unified in agreement within itself, even if this runs contrary to our own intuition. On the other hand, one's own opinions based on aesthetic experiences often seem to be particularly "out of the question." Thus *you* and *I* could discuss at great length whether or not the preparations of the technicians and the actors were staged and perhaps never reach a conclusion, *I* with my subjective (independent) experience, based on many rehearsals, that the preparations always looked exactly the same, and *you* with your subjective (interdependent) conviction that everyone else had watched the preparations as if they had belonged to the whole.

## *Framing*

Objects, processes and persons do not appear isolated to us but are always found within surroundings; only in contrast to those surroundings are they accessible to us as objects, processes or persons. Even if we do not know exactly what (or who) we are dealing with, we often know to a large extent what we are *not* dealing with. We might not know exactly whether the liquid in a glass is water, but since we do know it has no color, it must not be orange juice. We might not know exactly awaits us within the framework of a Shakespeare performance, but we assume with a fairly large degree of certainty that no one will be continuing to build the stage props or working out their lines. If our conviction, however, proves incorrect, we feel slightly affronted and react defensively (perhaps refusing to drink colorless lemonade with orange flavoring or demanding our money back because of the unfinished staging).

Between the physical reality of an object (its irreducible corporeal presence, its resonant corpus) and its external boundaries (the convictions and opinions we hold about it) there is room, sometimes more, sometimes less, for various transformations and superimpositions (literally stated, room for play). That means these boundaries have an internal and external surface area, and between them is a dimension that is sometimes infinitesimal and sometimes voluminous. We interpret the things *to be* something when they present themselves to us *as* that something. Frameworks are often decisive factors in artistic work, and thus, they often provide a vital tool in the creation process.

There are many reasons to define the artistic (in contrast to the purely aesthetic) mode of perception on the level of the framing. In the artistic mode of perception, having an artistic experience means simultaneously finding yourself outside of a framework while still being inside that framework. This can be understood as a process that is analogue to the aesthetic sensing (the aesthetic sensing being that of sensing the perception) on the level of the framing. If the framework more or less continues 'all the way through us,' we are capable of feeling that. Erika Fischer-Lichte calls this a *liminal* state, a "betwixt and between."[14]

The artistic way of seeing the world encompasses an awareness that we find ourselves in a reality outside of that which we regard as the content of our perception. A sort of brink exists for us, an edge separating us from 'the other reality,' whether that be 'the assumed reality' or 'the invented reality.' This does not mean that a 'real' reality is less constructed than an 'invented' one, nor does it mean that we are 'more' in the 'real' reality than we are in the 'invented' one (on the contrary!); it solely means that we know ourselves to stand with one of our feet in one reality while operating within another reality.[15]

This distinguishes the artistic mode from other modes of framing, like the framework of a game. In a non-aesthetic game, we typically find ourselves *completely* within the framework of the game – as a soccer player, as a chess player or as a ballroom dancer. If a portion of our awareness, however, is still watching the framework from the outside, it is *precisely this* that forms the artistic part of our perspective; the point at which we see ourselves as being within a second framework is always the point at which we observe ourselves from the outside and thus from an artistic perspective. In an event parallel to the aesthetic sensing, we become aware of how it *feels* to enter the framework.

The artistic way of looking at things is a perceptual mode that accompanies us constantly and everywhere, just as aesthetic sensing does. Because of this, art (as a means of observing reality) cannot be separated from perception, since it is always present at the very least as a possibility – even outside of art-works and art-places. This is the main reason to speak of *artistic experience* instead of art in the sense of works or artifacts.

A further analogy proves interesting at this point. Cognitive scientists are currently discussing some of the networks found in the brain about which comparatively little is known, including a network encompassing what is called the *medial anterior prefrontal cortex* and its projections (a frontal region resting just behind the forehead). The functions brought into play by this part of the cortex include *introspection*, the 'parking' of *meta-intentions* and the simultaneous *representation* of multiple identities for the very same content (*decoupling*).[16] The question as to which common roots are behind all these functional effects remains unexplained. However, the finding that the very same network is responsible for each of these capabilities shows that they are closely interrelated. As it is

14 Fischer-Lichte: *The Transformative Power of Performance.*

15 Cf. Klein: "On Relativity".

16 Cf. Frith and Frith: "Development and Neurophysiology of Mentalizing"; Ramnani and Owen: "Anterior Prefrontal Cortex".

most certain that a large number of cognitive functions are needed for the artistic experience, defining a specific 'art network' within the brain may be a very ambitious project, but this example still at least provides evidence strongly affirming the idea that three means of experience and behavior are decisive to the artistic perspective: *reflection* on oneself or on one's individual perspective, purposefully framed observations of the world on a *meta-level*, and the multiplied presence of objects and/or persons that appear simultaneously in various embodiments *inside and outside* a framework. These three capabilities, according to the research, appear to be closely linked to one another not only in terms of the artistic experience but also functionally.

## *Refuges*

Mostly we have multiple frameworks available that interfere with one another. For this reason, we are often especially thankful for stable frameworks that define conventions. These stable frameworks grant us the feeling that we can 'understand' things. This is why we yearn for a hideaway, a safe haven, a place of refuge. Refuges are stable, highly redundant frameworks that have cultivated conventions of representation. In terms of art, concert halls, museums, theaters, movie theaters and books provide such safe havens. Or, also, discourses, social groups, rituals, and institutions. One important property of refuges is their *insularity*.[17] Conventions and representations are only valid within a protected sphere, and entry into it is often marked by material or virtual thresholds. Only in terms of such conventions are we able to make a distinction between form and content, inside and outside, regular and irregular behavior, norms and the abnormal, correct and incorrect understanding, and superior and poorer workability. All these evaluations are relative to the refuge from which we view things, persons and processes. And only within a refuge we are in the position to attribute such properties to objects. When changing between systems, the extensions, representations and logical values also change their contents alongside the changing perspective.

We always want to know what it is we are dealing with, to know the essence conclusively. Yet this kind of security cannot be guaranteed, because the meaning of things is relative to the framework within which we are confronted by them. This referential relativity is important. Refuges are not related hierarchically, and they have no comparative value from the outside. They are referential systems that are equal to each other in value and able to interfere with one other. We can enter and leave safe havens of refuges, and upon entry, we appropriate the refuge's frameworks, and we usually strip them off again when leaving the refuge. None of these standards are 'better' or 'worse' than each other; none are

17 Gumbrecht: *Production of Presence.*

'more appropriate' or 'more adequate' or are in any integral, objective way able to weighed up one against the other. Each refuge defines for itself a kind of system of coordinates, a gauge system in which things appear in different shapes. Sometimes this includes artistic models, sometimes not. The really interesting questions are: What is the reason behind each case of entering the artistic mode? What circumstances provoke particular modes of perception? How does content change in the process?

Artistic action likes refuges; on the one hand, wherever conventions are established, they allow themselves to be creatively used, served, avoided, expanded, and demolished. On the other hand, there is a consistent tendency for frameworks within refuges to become so stable that they no longer allow themselves to be moved or reshaped. Generally, such stiff frameworks allow only very little space between their internal and the external, a space in which we might tarry and play within an artistic mode. As a result, we only either enter or exit, and they no longer provoke us to enter the artistic mode. Once the redundancy becomes great enough to create stable representations, genuine artistic experience becomes less likely; because we tend to establish ourselves within the stable meanings. However, if every new event (including complex processes such as Shakespeare pieces) is just one more redundant confirmation of a meaning already known – that is to say, if we begin to know what the things are and stop asking about their possible frameworks and meanings because we already *understand* everything – that then marks the end of art.

## Finale: Towards an Artistic Theory of Relativity

We now have, on the one hand, the concept of *art* (which is a mode of our perception), and on the other, of course, that of specific *works* (the result of a chain of intentions on the part of the persons involved). But now we run up against the fact that there is no such thing as a category for specific creations that all have in common the property of being art. Thus, by avoiding the term and concept of 'artwork', it becomes possible for us to recognize the relativity of artistic observation as being a mode of our perception. A meaningful re-definition of the concept would be as follows: The intentionality of our artistic observation serves as the foundation for the 'work' that shapes the content of our perception into art.

Taken as a whole, the question as to whether a blue wall or a glass of water is art is dependent on our use of it and our perspective, just like the question as to whether a bicycle is a sports equipment. Riding a bicycle always has elements particularly inherent to sports, such as bodily exertion; but whether or not we see it as a sport depends on such things as the extent to which we undertake it for its own sake whenever we go on a bike ride and what we otherwise associate with the concept of the sport. Often enough, the sport mode is also mixed with other modes, such as when we ride our bicycle to work for the sake of the sport instead of driving the car. Also, in asking the question, "Sport or non-sport?", the distinction depends not so much on which bicycle is actually involved but the perspective from which we are describing it.

But what did we mean the whole time, then, when talking about 'artworks'? Well, against the backdrop of all our thoughts and considerations, we can now formulate an answer: 'Artworks', or, even better, 'art objects', are a category of perceptual experience brought forth by means of stable, redundant societal processes that we typically encounter in safe havens of refuges. According to this answer, an 'art object' is not literally an object but a constructed category of perceptual experiences – like an aesthetic equivalence class of perceptions.

Representatives of such classes might come in the form of scripts (e.g. musical scores), of imaginings (e.g. individual or collective memories), of crystallizations (enactments or objects) or of verbalizations (such as contemporary reports). The works of Shakespeare, for example, do not just consist of letters printed in books, but are living organisms with variform members that all make a contribution to its existence. The text of a drama only marks a region of what belongs to a class, more through setting certain limitations than in defining properties, because on the other hand, such a text clearly fulfills one of its purposes in an enactment. The most suitable model for the structure of one such meta-object is an arrangement of various embodiments all making reference to one another while forming a larger, open-ended whole.

## *Reprise*

We began by visiting a theater rehearsal, thus entering into the framework of the 'theater rehearsal' refuge. In doing so, there was no particular reason for us to aesthetically experience the activities of the stage technicians. Our observations of the preparations for the rehearsal did not constitute an art process; we had completely entered into the theater rehearsal framework, so we did not view ourselves and the stage from outside. There was, in our perception, no art taking place. This provides an example of how a stable representation may serve to repress the artistic mode, even in such a veritable temple of art as the theater.

It is therefore neither necessary nor possible to classify the doings of the stage technicians in the Shakespeare rehearsal into the categories of 'playing' or 'non-playing' – and also not necessary or possible to classify them as 'art' or 'non-art' – because the simple result of our analysis must be that it can be both at once, depending on the observer's perspective and framing.

Art – or better, the artistic – is a mode of our perception, a way of seeing and dealing with the world. Art is a process that we can support or avoid; art is the act of playing with frames – or a framed aesthetic experience, or an aesthetic experience of frameworks, or the perception of framed perceptions, whichever order best describes to the situation at hand. In any case, in the artistic mode, a framework and a doubled perception come into play, interacting with each other. No we have come to the point where we can notate the formula of the artistic relativity theory – so please stand with the drum roll: *Art equals framed perception of perception.*

$$\mathbf{A = f\,p^2}$$

## Coda: The value of aesthetic relativity

We should not only make a distinction between *art* and *work* but also between the terms *value* and *judgment*, because an object (whether physical or a perceptual category) can only have aesthetic value relative to an observer, a group of observers or a refuge. Qualitative evaluation, therefore, is always relative to this. A judgment, however, mostly claims objective or at least factual validity. I hold the combination of both to reach a "value judgment" to be categorically senseless and contradictory. Does this mean an objective (observer-independent and intersubjective) judgment of art processes is impossible? No. It only means that this objective judgment cannot be based on an *aesthetic* value, as it can only exist relative to the observer's perspective. An objective judgment regarding aesthetic experience, that is, art, is impossible if it is not related to an experiential perspective. The aesthetic sensing itself exhibits a value that we might, with good reason, be able to see as absolute.

After all, why is the artistic perspective mostly so fun? Perhaps because it is so vitally essential. In the artistic mode, we play with the framework of our perception because only in a situation we experience from within and without at the same time are we able to experience how our reality is constituted from perception. In the end, we use art not for art's own sake but because without it we would not have a sufficient concept of reality. Without an individual perspective and a chosen framework – which above all needs our own individual engagement – we would be unable to encounter the world. The artistic perspective is the human means of finding our bearings in such a world.

## References

Danto, Arthur: *Transfiguration of the Commonplace*, Cambridge MA (Harvard University Press) 1981.

Deutsch, Diana: *Phantom Words and other Curiosities*, La Jolla CA (Philomel Records) 1995.

Fischer-Lichte, Erika: *The Transformative Power of Performance*, New York (Routledge) 2008.

Frith, Uta and Christopher D. Frith.: "Development and Neurophysiology of Mentalizing", in: *Philosophical transactions of the Royal Society of London*, Series B Biological sciences (2003) pp. 459–473.

Goldstein, E. Bruce: *Sensation and Perception*, Belmont CA (Wadsworth) 2001.

Goodman, Nelson: "When Is Art?", in: *Ways of Worldmaking*, Cambridge MA (MIT Press) 1978.

Gumbrecht, Hans-Ulrich: *Production of Presence: What Meaning Cannot Convey*, Stanford (Stanford University Press) 2004.

Klein, Julian: "On Relativity", in: *Janus* 17 (2004), pp. 26–29.

Klein, Julian (ed.): *per.SPICE! – Wirklichkeit und Relativität des Ästhetischen*, Berlin (Theater der Zeit) 2009, pp. 104–134.

Lozano, Sandra, Bridgette Martin Hard and Barbara Tversky: "Putting motor resonance in perspective," in: *Cognition* 196 (2008), pp. 1195–1220.

Ramnani, Narender and Adrian M. Owen: "Anterior Prefrontal Cortex" in: *Nature Reviews Neuroscience* 5 (2004), pp. 184–194.

Simons, Daniel and Christopher Chabris: "Gorillas in Our Midst: Sustained Inattentional Blindness for Dynamic Events", in: *Perception 28*, pp. 1059–1074.

# Attention
# How the Brain Enables Perception

ALEXANDER THIELE

## Abstract

Attention is a rich psychological and neurobiological construct which influences almost all aspects of cognitive behavior. Without attention most events in our external world remain unnoticed. Attention enables enhanced processing of behaviorally relevant stimuli at the expense of irrelevant stimuli. At the neuronal level, attention up-modulates the firing rates of neurons representing attended objects or stimulus features, while down-regulating the firing rates of neurons that represent unattended objects or stimulus features. These changes in neuronal activity in sensory areas are mediated by feedback connections that arise in higher cortical areas, areas that are more directly engaged in the control of cognitive functions. These feedback connections may depend on the simultaneous presence of the neuromodulator acetylcholine, as recent work demonstrates that a finely tuned balance of acetylcholine is also a critical component of attentional enhancement. This paper reviews some of the recent findings, which illuminate how attention may be implemented in the brain.

## Introduction

Remember your way home from work yesterday? Were there kids playing in the street? Did a dog bark? How about remembering events from only 5 minutes ago. Was there a new flier on the wall? What was your colleague wearing? Most likely even the latter enquiries will draw a blank. This is because you may not have attended to those details. Without attention we are largely unaware of the sensory information that enters our brains. Consequentially most aspects of the external world are neither noticed nor remembered. While this may seem unfortunate, as we remain unaware of many events in our daily lives, it is a necessary consequence of our ability to focus on relevant events. Attention helps us tune out irrelevant information, enhance perceptual abilities and increase our readiness to respond appropriately. Some of the neuronal mechanisms behind this highly efficient selection process have been delineated over the last 25 years, and this article will focus on some of them.

Attended objects or locations are processed more efficiently, which is achieved by increased sensory representation of the attended objects at the neuronal level.[1] These results have originally led to the 'spotlight of attention' model. As the name indicates, it argues that attention works akin to a torchlight that illuminates relevant aspects in the environment, which would otherwise be invisible to our awareness. More recently, the 'biased competition model of attention' has been put forward to explain attentional selection mechanisms.[2] The 'biased competition model of attention' proposes that objects in the visual field continuously (and automatically) compete for processing resources. Attention then serves to allocate processing resources to the attended object at the expense of the unattended object in a push-pull manner. Consequently, attended objects or locations will be processed more efficiently, while unattended objects (or locations) in the immediate vicinity will be processed less efficiently. Attention that activates biased competition can thus be compared to a filter, which ensures that irrelevant information is tuned out.[3]

Single cell recordings in behaving monkeys have revealed neuronal correlates of 'biased competition of attention'. If, in the absence of attention, a preferred stimulus is presented inside a neuron's receptive field, the neuron will respond with a high firing rate. If, however, a non-preferred stimulus is presented inside a neuron's receptive field, the neuron will respond with a low firing rate. If both stimuli are presented simultaneously, the neurons will respond with a firing rate that is approximately the average of the firing rate elicited by the two individual stimuli (figure 1). If the animal is now required to attend to one of the two stimuli, then the neuron's firing rate is similar to a situation where the attended object is presented in isolation.[4] Thus, attentional effects can also be described as a shrinking of the neuron's receptive field around the attended location.[5] While these effects of attention on

1 Moran and Desimone: "Selective Attention Gates Visual Processing"; Reynolds/Chelazzi/Desimone: "Competitive Mechanisms Subserve Attention"; Motter: "Focal Attention Produces Spatially Selective Processing"; Spitzer/Desimone/Moran: "Increased Attention"; Treue and Maunsell: "Attentional Modulation of Visual Motion Processing"; Roberts et al.: "Attention Alters Spatial Integration"; Roelfsema/Lamme/Spekreijse: "Object-Based Attention".

2 Moran and Desimone: "Selective Attention Gates Visual Processing"; Reynolds/Chelazzi/Desimone: "Competitive Mechanisms Subserve Attention"; Kastner and Ungerleider: "The Neural Basis of Biased Competition".

3 Roberts et al.: "Attention Alters Spatial Integration"; Connor et al.: "Responses in Area V4"; Roberts and Thiele: "Attention and Contrast"; Lu/Lesmes/Dosher: "Spatial Attention".

4 Moran and Desimone: "Selective Attention Gates Visual Processing"; Reynolds/Chelazzi/Desimone: "Competitive Mechanisms Subserve Attention"; Spitzer/Desimone/Moran: "Increased Attention"; Chelazzi: "Serial Attention Mechanisms"; Chelazzi et al.: "A Neural Basis"; Luck et al.: "Neural Mechanisms".

5 Reynolds/Chelazzi/Desimone: "Competitive Mechanisms Subserve Attention"; Roberts et al.: "Attention Alters Spatial Integration"; Luck et al.: "Neural Mechanisms".

neuronal activity in sensory areas are well studied, they do not provide insight into the sources of attention, i.e. they do not tell us 1) which parts of the brain control where to attend to and 2) how neuronal effects of attention are enabled.

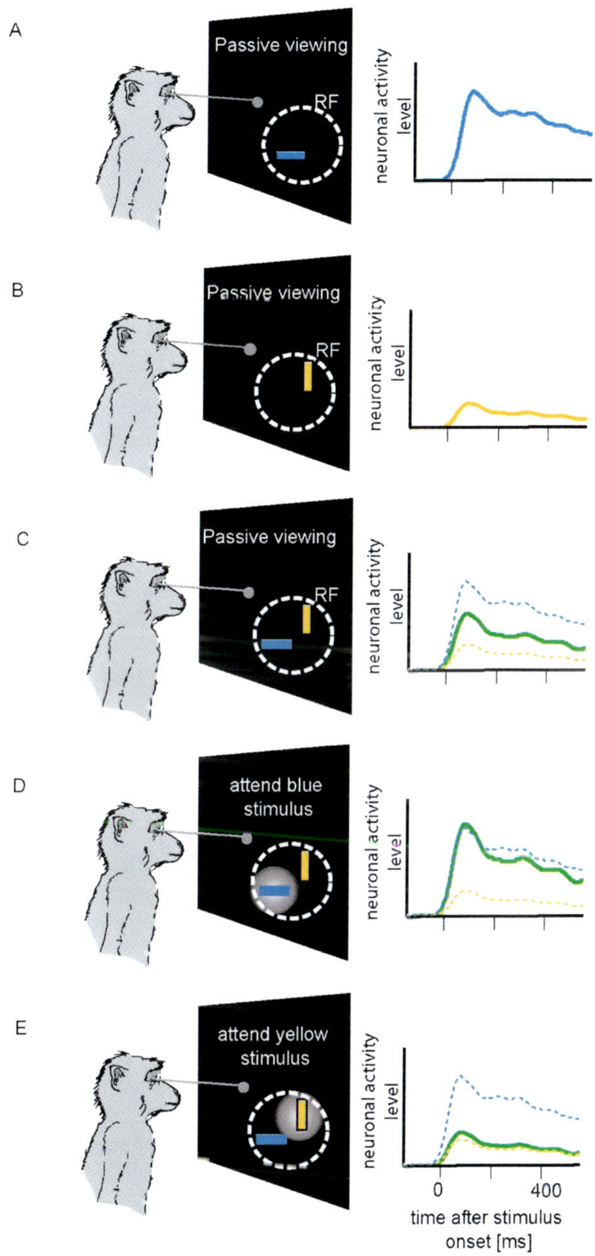


Fig. 1:A) Spatial attention and its effect on stimulus 'filtering' in single-cell recording of V4 neurons from the brain of a behaving monkey. In the absence of directed attention, the monkey passively looks at the fixation spot (grey circle) presented on a monitor. If, under these conditions a preferred stimulus (c.g. a blue bar) is presented inside the neuron's receptive field (represented by the dashed circle, corresponding to a spatial position that the neuron is responsive to), a large response by the neuron will be elicited (blue line in the graph on the right). B) If a non preferred stimulus is presented inside the neuron's receptive field a small response will be elicited. C) If both stimuli are presented simultaneously, a response intermediate to the two individual responses will be elicited. Note that the combined response is not a sum of the individual responses. D) If the animal is now required to covertly attend to the blue stimulus (whereby it still has to fixate the central grey spot on the screen, i.e. monitor the blue stimulus without moving its eyes away from the fixation spot, the response of the neuron will be very similar to the condition when only the blue stimulus was presented. E) If attention is covertly directed to the yellow stimulus, the neuron's response is very similar to the condition when only the yellow stimulus was presented. Thus, attention effectively removes the influence of the unattended stimulus; it is almost as if it were not present. The grey shaded area represents the focus of attention.

## Sources of Attention

To understand how attention is implemented in the brain it is important to distinguish the control signals responsible for the generation and maintenance of attention (which originate in so called higher 'source' areas) from their effect on sensory processing and perception (which occur in sensory areas as described above). Attentional control signals are mediated and maintained within circumscribed networks, which are largely localized in the frontal and parietal cortex (figure 2). Sources of attention in humans can be localized by means of functional magnetic resonance imaging, a technique that measures changes in blood flow to those parts of the brain that are active during specific cognitive tasks. These changes (increases) in blood flow are an indirect marker for increased neuronal activity. Voluntary attention activates the human dorsal fronto-parietal network, and parts of the extrastriate cortex.[6] These non-invasive measurements in humans are backed by single cell electrophysiology measurements in macaques, which have provided evidence that areas of the parietal cortex[7] and the frontal/prefrontal cortex[8] are crucial for attentional control.

6 Shulman et al.: "Two Attentional Processes"; Kincade et al.: "An Event-Related Functional Magnetic Resonance Imaging Study"; Corbetta and Shulman: "Control of Goal-Directed and Stimulus-Driven Attention".

7 Steinmetz and Constantinidis: "Neurophysiological Evidence"; Duncan/Humphreys/Ward: "Competitive Brain Activity"; Kusunoki/Gottlieb Goldberg: "The Lateral Intraparietal Area"; Cook and Maunsell: "Attentional Modulation of Behavioral Performance"; Li et al.: "Inactivation of Macaque Lateral Intraparietal Area"; Bisley and Goldberg: "Neuronal Activity in the Lateral Intraparietal Area"; Constantinidis and Steinmetz: "Posterior Parietal Cortex".

8 Lecas: "Prefrontal Neurones"; Bon and Lucchetti: "Attention-Related Neurons"; Boussaoud and Wise: "Primate Frontal Cortex"; Thompson and Schall: "The Detection of Visual Signals"; Everling et al.: "Filtering of Neural Signals"; Everling et al.: "Selective Representation of Task-Relevant Objects"; Moore and Fallah: "Microstimulation of the Frontal Eye Field"; Moore and Armstrong: "Selective Gating of Visual Signals"; Armstrong and Moore: "Effects of FEF Microstimulation"; Armstrong/Fitzgerald/Moore: "Changes in Visual Receptive Fields"; Armstrong and Moore: "Rapid Enhancement of Visual Cortical Response".

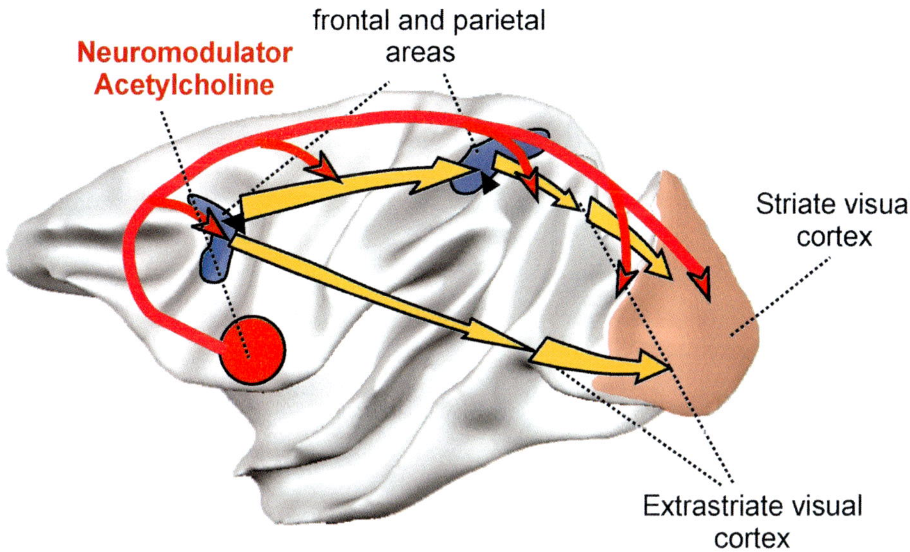


Fig. 2: Mechanisms that may contribute to attention. Voluntary attention is controlled by 'higher' cortical areas in the frontal and parietal cortex. These areas can influence sensory processing (e.g. in striate and extrastriate cortical areas) by means of their 'feedback' connections, i.e. they can influence which parts or features of the visual world are more effectively processed. Additionally, it has been proposed that the brain chemical acetylcholine contributes to our ability to attend. Acetylcholine is generated by neurons in the basal forebrain (symbolized by the red dot) which can exert its influence in almost all cortical areas. Note that this is a cartoon; thus anatomical locations are not correct locations in a 3-D brain.

The parietal and frontal areas that control attentional selection are assumed to influence sensory processing and perception via feedback projections to the sensory areas (figure 2), and direct evidence for this idea is mounting.[9]

9 Moore and Armstrong: "Selective Gating of Visual Signals"; Armstrong and Moore: "Effects of FEF Microstimulation"; Armstrong/Fitzgerald/Moore: "Changes in Visual Receptive Fields"; Armstrong and Moore: "Rapid Enhancement of Visual Cortical Response"; Gregoriou et al.: "High-frequency, Long-Range Coupling".

## The Role of Neuromodulators

In addition to feedback, it has often been argued that the neuromodulator acetylcholine (ACh) contributes to attention (figure 2). Attentional states are associated with activation of the cholinergic system originating in the basal forebrain.[10] Disruption of the cholinergic system in humans can lead to selective spatial attention deficits.[11] Moreover, application of cholinergic antagonists (substances which block the action of acetylcholine) into the parietal cortex affects attentional orienting in macaque monkeys[12] and systemic application of cholinergic antagonists affects attentional orienting in humans.[13]

Despite a wealth of data in support of a role of acetylcholine in attentional modulation, it is unclear how ACh contributes to neuronal processing in sensory areas during selective attention. What are the cellular mechanisms by which ACh enables different aspects of attentional processing? Does ACh affect firing rates in a manner similar to attention? Predictions in relation to these questions can be based on *in vitro* brain slice studies, data from anaesthetized animals, as well as on some recent data from our lab in task-performing macaques. The slice studies have demonstrated that ACh applied to the sensory cortical areas increases the efficacy of the input that comes from the sensory organs (e.g. retina, skin, ear; this type of input is often termed 'feed-forward') and reduces intracortical processing.[14] It could thereby contribute to changes in firing rates and spatial filtering, as receptive fields should in principle shrink when lateral intracortical interactions are down regulated and firing rates should increase when the feed-forward drive is increased (figure 3).

From these results, it is tempting to speculate that ACh increases the representation of stimuli at the current attentional focus, and protects it against interference from competing stimuli, thus resulting in reduced distractibility. Thereby task relevant information would be processed more effectively, which comes at the expense of irrelevant information. Recent data from our lab in the anesthetized and awake primates are supportive of this idea.

10 Marrocco/Witte/Davidson: "Arousal Systems"; Witte/Davidson/Marrocco: "Effects of Altering Brain Cholinergic Activity"; Robbins: "Arousal Systems and Attentional Processes"; Voytko: "Cognitive Functions of the Basal Forebrain"; Voytko et al.: "Basal Forebrain Lesions"; Dalley et al.: "Distinct Changes in Cortical Acetylcholine"; Sarter/Bruno/Turchi: "Basal Forebrain Afferent Projections"; Sarter/Givens/Bruno: "The Cognitive Neuroscience of Sustained Attention"; Gill/Sarter/Givens: "Sustained Visual Attention".

11 Parasuraman/Greenwood/Alexander: "Alzheimer Disease".

12 Davidson and Marrocco: "Local Infusion of Scopolamine".

13 Bentley et al.: "Cholinergic Enhancement"; Thiel/Zilles/Fink: "Nicotine Modulates Reorienting of Visuospatial Attention".

14 Gil/Connors/Amitai: "Differential Regulation of Neocortical Synapses"; Kimura: "Cholinergic Modulation of Cortical Function".

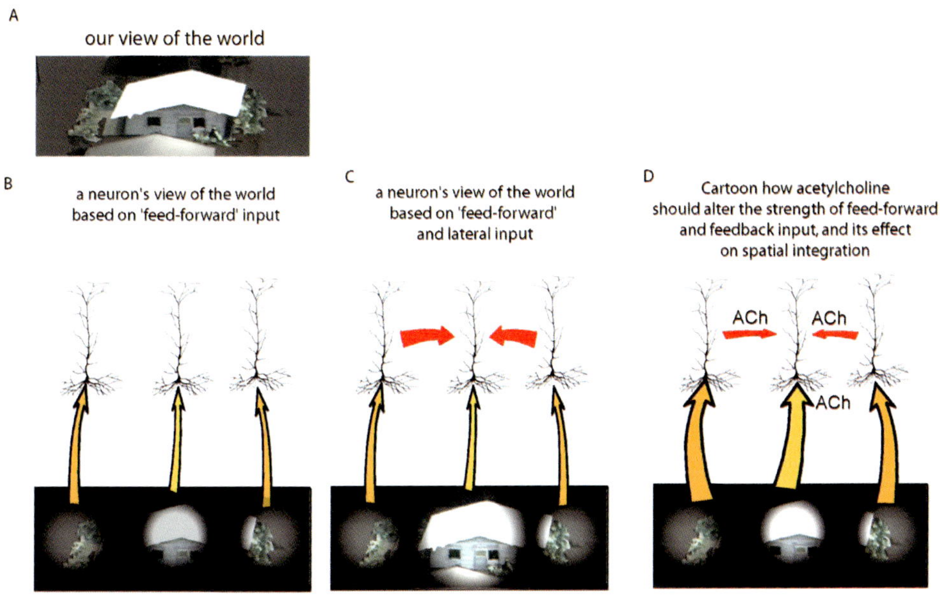


Fig. 3: Cartoon delineating how neuronal integration is affected by input from the senses, by intracortical integration, and by the neuromodulator acetylcholine. A) We see pictures holistically (a cutting from a panting by Dirk Skreber). B) Neurons in visual cortex see only parts of the picture, referred to as the classical receptive field. The information from those parts is provided through feed-forward projections from relay stages, which have direct input from the sensory organs (here, the retina). C) In addition to this feed-forward input, neurons within the cortex are heavily interconnected, enabling them to receive additional information. These connections enable a neuron to see the 'bigger picture'. D) The neuromodulator acetylcholine affects the relative strength of feed-forward and intracortical connections, thereby making the cortex more reliant on information that comes from the senses, and likely decreasing the spatial integration of neurons.

## The Role of Acetylcholine in Spatial Integration

Based on the *in vitro* studies mentioned above, we argued that ACh might alter the flow of feed-forward and lateral/feed-back information in the cortex. In the primary visual cortex, feed-forward inputs from the thalamus are largely responsible for the response properties of the neuron's classical receptive field [CRF],[15] while influences from areas immediately surrounding the receptive field (called the non classical receptive field [nCRF]) are mostly mediated by lateral and feed-back connections.[16] Thus, ACh applied *in vivo* should reduce the impact of sti-

15 Dragoi/Sharma/Sur: "Adaptation-Induced Plasticity".

16 Angelucci/Levitt/Lund: "Anatomical Origins"; Cavanaugh/Bair/Movshon: "Nature and Interaction of Signals"; Das and Gilbert: "Topography of Contextual Modulations".

muli presented in the nCRF while increasing the effect of stimuli placed within the CRF. Figuratively speaking, it should cause a shrinkage of the receptive field, as surround influences are reduced. This proposal was investigated in V1 of anesthetized marmoset monkeys[17] by measuring the neuronal spatial summation properties, i.e. how much the response to a stimulus presented inside the neuron's CRF was affected by stimuli simultaneously presented in the nCRF. A simple way to investigate this is to measure how well a neuron responds to stimuli of different lengths. It is well known that neurons usually give the largest response to stimuli that are larger (longer) than the diameter of their CRF, as nCRF influences from just outside the CRF can boost neuronal responses further. Thus, the preferred length is a useful parameter to investigate how well neurons integrate influences from the CRF and the nCRF. We predicted that the preferred length should be reduced when ACh was externally applied compared to when it was not applied. In line with this prediction we found that application of ACh resulted in a significant reduction of a neuron's preferred length and this was mediated by reduced spatial summation (figure 4).

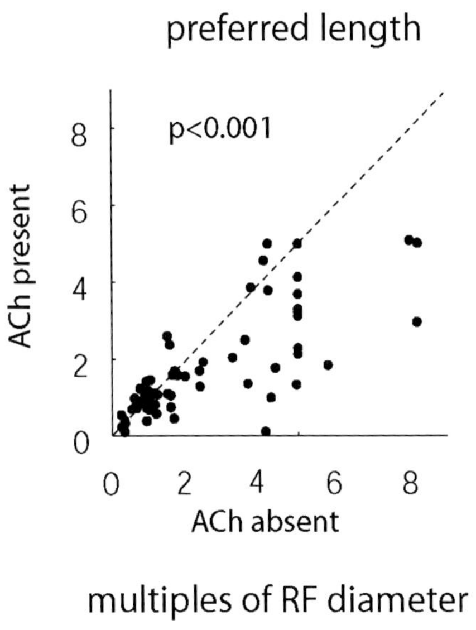


Fig. 4: Preferred length (a proxy of spatial integration) of V1 neurons for the condition when acetylcholine was applied (y-axis) and when it was not applied (x-axis). In the presence of acetylcholine applied, neurons preferred shorter bars, and effect which was mediated by reduced spatial integration. This effect is apparent by the systematic offset of the data points to the right of the diagonal.

17 Roberts et al.: "Acetylcholine Dynamically Controls Spatial Integration".

## Attention and Spatial Integration

If acetylcholine contributes directly to attentional modulation, then attention should result in reduced preferred length and reduced spatial summation at the perceptual and at the neuronal level. Testing spatial integration in the presence and absence of attention in humans confirmed that attention reduces spatial summation at the perceptual level.[18] To investigate whether neuronal spatial summation is affected in a similar way by attention, we trained macaque monkeys to attend to one of two possible locations (one location was always covered by the receptive field of the neuron under study). Monkeys had to detect a small stimulus that was superimposed on bar stimuli of varying lengths, thus allowing us to measure spatial integration with and without attention. In line with our prediction we found that attention could cause reduced spatial summation[19] in a manner very much similar to the application of acetylcholine.

## Cholinergic Receptors Involved in Attentional Modulation in V1

The results described above mirrored the results of acetylcholine application in V1 from the anesthetized primate,[20] suggesting that acetylcholine is critically involved in the neuronal mechanisms of attention. To test this proposal more directly, we recorded neurons while monkeys performed the attention-demanding task, and simultaneously applied acetylcholine.[21] Acetylcholine acts on two different receptors in the brain, and we wanted to determine which of the two might be involved in the process of attention. Therefore, we also applied selective receptor blocking agents. The receptors investigated were the muscarinic and the nicotinic receptor which can be blocked by the antagonists' scopolamine and mecamylamine, respectively.

When we applied low doses of acetylcholine, we found increased attentional modulation of V1 neurons (fig. 5). We also found a systematic effect of ACh application on the animal's performance. These were most prominent when the animals attended to a location that was not represented by neurons influenced by our ACh application. The animal's performance was reduced under those conditions. It was as if the animals had difficulties disengaging their attention from the location represented by the neurons that were influenced by our ACh application (figure 6).

18 Roberts and Thiele: "Attention and Contrast".
19 Roberts et al.: "Attention Alters Spatial Integration".
20 Roberts et al.: "Acetylcholine Dynamically Controls Spatial Integration".
21 Herrero et al.: "Acetylcholine".

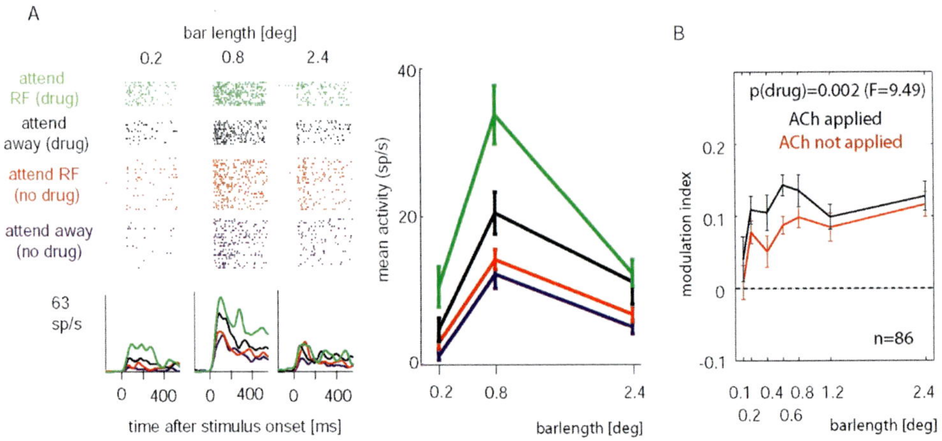


Fig. 5: Influence of acetylcholine on attentional modulation in V1. A) Example of a single cell where the application of acetylcholine resulted in enhanced attentional modulation. In the absence of acetylcholine application, attentional modulation was small but significant ($p<0.05$). Left plot shows single trial neuronal activity for the 4 conditions and the corresponding peri-stimulus time histograms. Right plot shows mean activity obtained from the time period of 200-500 ms after stimulus onset. B) Attentional modulation was quantified by the modulation index, a normalized measure that basically shows the difference of the mean activity levels in the presence and absence of attention. The larger the modulation index, the stronger the influence of attention. The figure shows the mean attentional modulation index for our population of V1 cells when acetylcholine was applied. Attentional modulation was significantly increased in the presence of externally applied ACh.

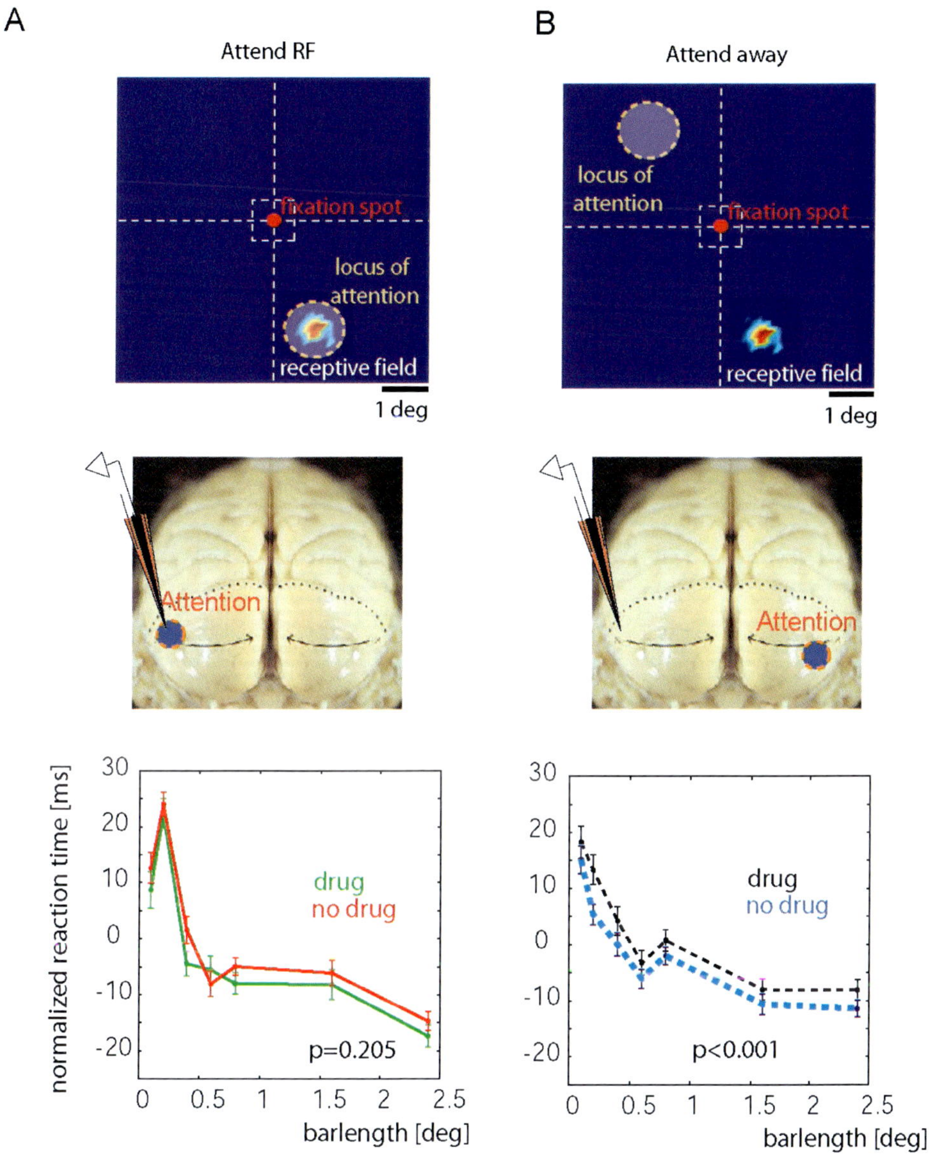


Fig. 6: Effect of acetylcholine application on reaction times. A) Condition when the animal attended to the part of the visual field that was represented by the neurons we recorded from. In this condition the animal had to 'listen' to the neurons that were influenced by the drug, provided it was applied. This is indicated by the middle panel, where the attentional focus is at the location of our recording electrode and our pipette. Under these conditions, application of acetylcholine slightly reduced the animals reaction time (i.e. the animal was faster), but the effect was not significant. B) Condition when the animal attended to the part of the visual field that was not represented by the neurons we recorded from. In this condition the animal had to 'listen' to neurons that were not influenced by the drug. This is indicated by the middle panel, where the attentional focus is at a location represented by neurons in the hemisphere opposite to our pipette location. Under these

conditions, application of acetylcholine resulted in increased reaction times, while acetylcholine was actually applied to neurons the animal should '**not** listen to'. It was almost as if the animal had difficulty disengaging its attention from the location that was represented by the neurons influenced by acetylcholine.

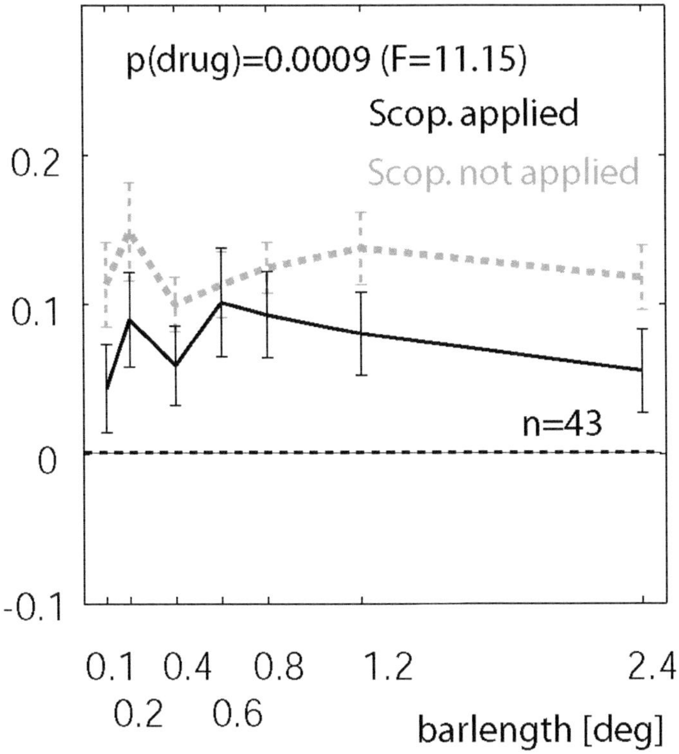


Fig. 7: Mean attentional modulation index for our population of V1 cells when muscarinic receptors were not blocked by scopolamine and when they were blocked by scopolamine. Attentional modulation was significantly reduced when muscarinic receptors were blocked.

When we applied the selective muscarinic receptor antagonist scopolamine, attentional modulation was significantly reduced in V1 neurons (figure 7). Interestingly, the nicotinic antagonist mecamylamine had no systematic effect on attentional modulation, while it reduced the overall neuronal gain. Thus, these data demonstrate that acetylcholine contributes to attentional modulation of sensory information in primary visual cortex through muscarinic receptors. Whether nicotinic receptors contribute to attentional modulation in higher areas remains to be determined. We believe it likely to be the case as there is a well known contribution of nicotinic receptors to attention at the perceptual level.

# Outlook

Studies over the last 30 years have provided insight into how attention affects neuronal processing in the brain and recent data also provide insight into the mechanisms by which it does so. Attention-induced firing rate changes in V1 depend on cholinergic activation of muscarinic receptors. In this paper I have neglected one mechanism by which attention influences neuronal processing. This mechanism relates to neuronal synchronization. It has been shown that attention increases the ability of neurons to fire synchronously, whereby their influence on their targets may be enhanced.[22] This process could be compared to an audience that claps in synchrony, thereby increasing the volume of the clapping, affecting the performer and maybe coaxing him/her for an 'encore'. Within this review I have focussed on how acetylcholine affects attention-induced firing rate changes, but future work on the mechanisms of attention might focus on delineating whether acetylcholine contributes to changes in cortical synchrony during states of attention in addition to its contribution to firing rate changes.[23] Moreover, it will be important to determine what additional mechanisms are at work to influence neuronal synchrony. It will also be important to investigate how acetylcholine contributes to attentional modulation in other cortical areas, and identity the interaction between acetylcholine input and feedback connections from higher cortical areas. It is almost certain that other well known neuromodulators (such as dopamine, noradrenaline, serotonin) also play a role in attentional modulation, but this may be dependent on the cortical area that is investigated. Thus, to obtain a full and mechanistic understanding of attention, all these aspects need to be studied and delineated.

The questions outlined in this review, although challenging, can now be addressed directly in task-performing monkeys. Such experiments will provide specific insights into the mechanisms of attention and other cognitive functions such as working memory, decision making etc. The approaches are ideally informed by detailed model predictions, but effectively these are empirical questions, which have to be tested experimentally. Ultimately it will be necessary to study how different neurotransmitters contribute to cognitive function in many (if not all) cortical and sub-cortical areas. And in each of these areas the specific roles of different receptors will have to be delineated. Finally, we need to understand how the different transmitter systems contribute to rate and/or synchrony coding schemes in order to understand cognition at the mechanistic level. While there is much more to be learned, we now at least understand some of the brain mechanisms that govern cognitive functions.

22 Fries et al.: "Modulation of Oscillatory Neuronal Synchronization"; Womelsdorf et al.: "Gamma-Band Synchronization".

23 Herrero et al.: "Acetylcholine".

## References

Angelucci, A., J. B. Levitt, and J. S. Lund: "Anatomical Origins of the Classical Receptive Field and Modulatory Surround Field of Single Neurons in Macaque Visual Cortical Area V1", in: *Prog Brain Res* 136 (2002), pp. 373–388.

Armstrong, K. M. and T. Moore: "Rapid Enhancement of Visual Cortical Response Discriminability by Microstimulation of the Frontal Eye Field", in: *Proc Natl Acad Sci U S A* 104 (2007) 22, pp. 499–504.

Armstrong, K. M. and T. Moore: "Effects of FEF Microstimulation on Competing Visual Representations in Macaque Area V4", in: Proceedings of the *SFN* 2004 (San Diego).

Armstrong, K. M., J. K. Fitzgerald, and T. Moore: "Changes in Visual Receptive Fields with Microstimulation of Frontal Cortex", in: *Neuron* 50 (2006) 5, pp. 791–798.

Bentley, P., et al.: "Cholinergic Enhancement Modulates Neural Correlates of Selective Attention and Emotional Processing", in: *Neuroimage* 20 (2003) 1, pp. 58–70.

Bisley, J. W. and M. E. Goldberg: "Neuronal Activity in the Lateral Intraparietal Area and Spatial Attention", in: *Science* 299 (2003) 5603, pp. 81–86.

Bon, L. and C. Lucchetti: "Attention-Related Neurons in the Supplementary Eye Field of the Macaque Monkey", in: *Exp.Brain Res.* 113 (1997), pp. 180–185.

Boussaoud, d. and S. P. Wise: "Primate Frontal Cortex: Neuronal Activity Following Attentional Versus Intentional Cues", in: *Experimental Brain Research* 95 (1993), pp. 15–27.

Cavanaugh, J.R., W. Bair, and J.A. Movshon: "Nature and Interaction of Signals from the Receptive Field Center and Surround in Macaque V1 Neurons", in; *J Neurophysiol* 88 (2002) 5, pp. 2530–2546.

Chelazzi, L., et al.: "A Neural Basis for Visual Search in Inferior Temporal Cortex", in: *Nature* 363 (1993), pp. 345–347.

Chelazzi, L.: "Serial Attention Mechanisms in Visual Search: A Critical Look at the Evidence", in: *Psychol Res* 62 (1999) 2–3, pp. 195–219.

Connor, C. E., et al.: "Responses in Area V4 Depend on the Spatial Relationship Between Stimulus and Attention", in: *Journal of Neurophysiology* 75 (1996), pp. 1306–1308.

Constantinidis, C. and M. A. Steinmetz: "Posterior Parietal Cortex Automatically Encodes the Location of Salient Stimuli", in: *J Neurosci* 25 (2005) 1, pp. 233–238.

Cook, E. P. and J. H. Maunsell: "Attentional Modulation of Behavioral Performance and Neuronal Responses in Middle Temporal and Ventral Intraparietal Areas of Macaque Monkey", in: *J Neurosci* 22 (2002) 5, pp. 1994–2004.

Corbetta, M. and G. L. Shulman: "Control of Goal-Directed and Stimulus-Driven Attention in the Brain", in: *Nat Rev Neurosci* 3 (2002) 3, pp. 201–215.
Dalley, J. W., et al.: "Distinct Changes in Cortical Acetylcholine and Noradrenaline Efflux During Contingent and Noncontingent Performance of a Visual Attentional Task", in: *J Neurosci* 21 (2001) 13, pp. 4908–4914.
Das, A. and C. D. Gilbert: "Topography of Contextual Modulations Mediated by Short-Range Interactions in Primary Visual Cortex", in: *Nature* 399 (1999) 6737, pp. 655–61.
Davidson, M. C. and R. T. Marrocco: "Local Infusion of Scopolamine Into Intraparietal Cortex Slows Covert Orienting in Rhesus Monkeys", in: *J Neurophysiol* 83 (2000) 3, pp. 1536–1549.
Dosher, B. A., et al.: "The Spatial Window of the Perceptual Template and Endogenous Attention", in: *Vision Res* 44 (2004) 12, pp. 1257–1271.
Dragoi, V., J. Sharma, and M. Sur: "Adaptation-Induced Plasticity of Orientation Tuning in Adult Visual Cortex", in: *Neuron* 28 (2000) 1, pp. 287–298.
Duncan, J., G. Humphreys, and R. Ward: "Competitive Brain Activity in Visual Attention", in: *Curr Opin Neurobiol* 7 (1997) 2, pp. 255–261.
Everling, S., et al.: "Filtering of Neural Signals by Focused Attention in the Monkey Prefrontal Cortex", in: *Nat Neurosci* 5 (2002) 7, pp. 671–676.
Everling, S., et al.: "Selective Representation of Task-Relevant Objects and Locations in the Monkey Prefrontal Cortex", in: *Eur J Neurosci* 23 (2006) 8, pp. 2197–2214.
Fries, P., et al.: "Modulation of Oscillatory Neuronal Synchronization by Selective Visual Attention", in: *Science* 29 (2001) 5508, pp. 1560–1563.
Gil, Z., B. W. Connors, and Y. Amitai: "Differential Regulation of Neocortical Synapses by Neuromodulators and Activity", in: *Neuron* 19 (1997) 3, pp. 679–686.
Gill, T. M., M. Sarter, and B. Givens: "Sustained Visual Attention Performance-Associated Prefrontal Neuronal Activity: Evidence for Cholinergic Modulation", in: *J Neurosci* 20 (2000) 12, pp. 4745–4757.
Gregoriou, G. G., et al.: "High-Frequency, Long-Range Coupling Between Prefrontal and Visual Cortex During Attention", in: *Science* 324 (2009) 5931, pp. 1207–1210.
Herrero, J. L., et al.: "Acetylcholine Contributes through Muscarinic Receptors to Attentional Modulation in V1", in: *Nature* 454 (2008) 7208, pp. 1110–1114.
Kastner, S. and L.G. Ungerleider: "The Neural Basis of Biased Competition in Human Visual Cortex", in: *Neuropsychologia* 39 (2001) 12, pp. 1263–76.
Kimura, F.: "Cholinergic Modulation of Cortical Function: A Hypothetical Role in Shifting the Dynamics in Cortical Network", in: *Neurosci Res* 38 (2000) 1, pp. 19–26.
Kincade, J. M., et al.: "An Event-Related Functional Magnetic Resonance Imaging Study of Voluntary and Stimulus-Driven Orienting of Attention", in: *J Neurosci* 25 (2005) 18, pp. 4593–4604.

Kusunoki, M., J. Gottlieb, and M. E. Goldberg: "The Lateral Intraparietal Area as a Salience Map: The Representation of Abrupt Onset, Stimulus Motion, and Task Relevance", in: *Vision Res* 40 (2000) 10–12, pp. 1459–1468.

Lecas, J. C.: "Prefrontal Neurones Sensitive to Increased Visual Attention in the Monkey", in: *Neuroreport* 7 (1995), pp. 305–309.

Li, C. S., et al.: "Inactivation of Macaque Lateral Intraparietal Area Delays Initiation of the Second Saccade Predominantly from Contralesional Eye Positions in a Double-Saccade Task. Effect of Reversible Inactivation of Macaque Lateral Intraparietal Area on Visual and Memory Saccades. Deficits of Visual Attention and Saccadic Eye Movements After Lesions of Parietooccipital Cortex in Monkeys", in: *Exp Brain Res* 137 (2001) 1, pp. 45–57.

Lu, Z. L., L. A. Lesmes, and B.A. Dosher: "Spatial Attention Excludes External Noise at the Target Location", *J Vis* 2 (2002) 4, pp. 312–323.

Luck, S. J., et al.: "Neural Mechanisms of Spatial Selective Attention in Areas V1, V2, and V4 of Macaque Visual Cortex", in: *J Neurophysiol* 77 (1997) 1, pp. 24–42.

Marrocco, R. T., E. A. Witte, and M. C. Davidson: "Arousal Systems", in: *Current Opinion in Neurobiology* 4 (1994), pp. 166–170.

Moore, T. and K. M. Armstrong: "Selective Gating of Visual Signals by Microstimulation of Frontal Cortex", in: *Nature* 421 (2003) 6921, pp. 370–373.

Moore, T. and M. Fallah: "Microstimulation of the Frontal Eye Field and Its Effects on Covert Spatial Attention", in: *J Neurophysiol* 91 (2004) 1, pp. 152–162 (Epub 2003 Sep 17).

Moran, J. and R. Desimone: "Selective Attention Gates Visual Processing in the Extrastriate Cortex", *Science* 229 (1985) 4715, pp. 782–784.

Motter, B.C.: "Focal Attention Produces Spatially Selective Processing in Visual Cortical Areas V1, V2, and V4 in the Presence of Competing Stimuli", in: *Journal of Neurophysiology* 70 (1993), pp. 909–919.

Parasuraman, R., P. M. Greenwood, and G.E. Alexander: "Alzheimer Disease Constricts the Dynamic Range of Spatial Attention in Visual Search", in: *Neuropsychologia* 38 (2000) 8, pp. 1126–1135.

Reynolds, J. H., L. Chelazzi, and R. Desimone: "Competitive Mechanisms Subserve Attention in Macaque Areas V2 and V4", in: *J Neurosci* 19 (1999) 5, pp. 1736–1753.

Robbins, T. W.: "Arousal Systems and Attentional Processes", in: *Biol Psychol* 45 (1997) 1–3, pp. 57–71.

Roberts, M., et al.: "Attention Alters Spatial Integration in Macaque V1 in an Eccentricity-Dependent Manner", in: *Nat Neurosci* 10 (2007) 11, pp. 1483–1491.

Roberts, M. J. and A. Thiele: "Attention and Contrast Differently Affect Contextual Integration in an Orientation Discrimination Task", in: *Exp Brain Res* 187 (2008) 4, pp. 535–549.

Roberts, M. J., et al.: "Acetylcholine Dynamically Controls Spatial Integration in Marmoset Primary Visual Cortex", in: *J Neurophysiol* 93 (2005) 4, pp. 2062–2072.

Roelfsema, P. R., V. A. Lamme, and H. Spekreijse: "Object-Based Attention in the Primary Visual Cortex of the Macaque Monkey", in: *Nature* 395 (1998) 6700, pp. 376–381.

Sarter, M., B. Givens, and J. P. Bruno: "The Cognitive Neuroscience of Sustained Attention: Where Top-Down Meets Bottom-Up", in: *Brain Res Brain Res Rev* 35 (2001) 2, pp. 146–160.

Sarter, M., J. P. Bruno, and J. Turchi: "Basal Forebrain Afferent Projections Modulating Cortical Acetylcholine, Attention, and Implications for Neuropsychiatric Disorders", in: *Ann N Y Acad Sci* 877 (1999), pp. 368–82.

Shulman, G. L., et al.: "Two Attentional Processes in the Parietal Lobe", in: *Cereb Cortex* 12 (2002) 11, pp. 1124–1131.

Spitzer, H., R. Desimone, and J. Moran: "Increased Attention Enhances Both Behavioral and Neuronal Performance", in: *Science* 240 (1988), pp. 338–40.

Steinmetz, M. A. and C. Constantinidis: "Neurophysiological Evidence for a Role of Posterior Parietal Cortex in Redirecting Visual Attention", in: *Cereb.Cortex* 5 (1995), pp. 448–456.

Thiel, C. M., K. Zilles, and G. R. Fink: "Nicotine Modulates Reorienting of Visuospatial Attention and Neural Activity in Human Parietal Cortex", in: *Neuropsychopharmacology* 30 (2005) 4, pp. 810–820.

Thompson, K. G. and J. D. Schall: "The Detection of Visual Signals by Macaque Frontal Eye Field During Masking", in: *Nat Neurosci* 2 (1999) 3, pp. 283–288.

Treue, S. and J. H. R. Maunsell: "Attentional Modulation of Visual Motion Processing in Cortical Areas MT and MST", in: *Nature* 382 (1996), pp. 539–541.

Voytko, M. L.: "Cognitive Functions of the Basal Forebrain Cholinergic System in Monkeys: Memory or Attention", in: *Behav. Brain Res.* 75 (1996), pp. 13–25.

Voytko, M. L., et al.: "Basal Forebrain Lesions in Monkeys Disrupt Attention But Not Learning and Memory", in: *J Neurosci* 14 (1994) 1, pp. 167–186.

Witte, E. A., M. C. Davidson, and R. T. Marrocco: "Effects of Altering Brain Cholinergic Activity on Covert Orienting of Attention: Comparison of Monkey and Human Performance", in: *Psychopharmacology (Berl)* 132 (1997) 4, pp. 324–334.

Womelsdorf, T., et al.: "Gamma-Band Synchronization in Visual Cortex Predicts Speed of Change Detection", in: *Nature* 439 (2006) 7077, pp. 733–736.

# *Different Minds*

# Emil Post against Turing Machines
# Models of a Plural Mind[1]

PIERRE CASSOU-NOGUÈS

## Abstract

This paper concentrates on Emil Post's critical analysis of Turing machines and on the alternative models of the mind that he attempts to define. Without going into Post's technical results, I rely on the logician's unpublished notebooks to show that, though he has anticipated Turing's thesis, Post criticizes, after 1938, Turing machines on the ground that the mind as represented in Turing's analysis is essentially linear. States of mind succeed one another. They come one after the other. On the other hand, Post aims at describing the mind as essentially plural, with different lines of thoughts developing in parallel or different "workers", various homunculi so to speak, acting together. I discuss two informal models, which may be found in Post's notebooks, for this plurality of the mind.

## Emil Post against Turing Machines: Models of a Plural Mind

My paper concerns the critical analysis that E. L. Post offers of Turing machines and the alternative models of the mind that he attempts to define. As is well known, the concept of a machine that the logician Allan Turing introduced in 1937 represented the main model of the cognitive mind at least until the 1990s. The identification of the mind with a Turing machine does not necessarily imply the reduction of the mind – mental phenomena, as they appear in the first person – to a mechanism such as that of the brain. A Turing machine is, so to speak, an abstract mechanism, defined by certain properties and which may apply to mental phenomena as well as to the mechanism of computer. Turing machines may

1 Acknowledgments: Post's notebooks are quoted with permission of the Library of the American Philosophical Society, which I was able to visit thanks to a fellowship from this institution in August 2006 and May 2007. I wish to thank all the staff for their kind help during my stay. The entries in Post's notebooks are dated in the American fashion: month/day/year. I have converted them in the system: day/month/year.

be considered as a model describing the mind as it is given in the first person. In fact, it is impossible to distinguish the cognitive mind from a Turing machine by indicating a precise task which the mind could accomplish, but not a Turing machine. We do not know how to define a precise task that the human mind could accomplish but that a Turing machine could not. It is, of course, possible to criticize Turing machines from a philosophical point of view, as regards the adequacy of this model to the actual operations of the human mind, but we cannot literally prove that the human mind is not equivalent to a Turing machine. Second, up to the 1990s and the introduction of dynamical systems, which are continuous, all the models elaborated in cognitive science, including connectionist models, can be translated in terms of Turing machines. They can be implemented or mimicked, so to speak, on Turing machines. Thus, at least before the use of dynamical systems, Turing machines remained an essential reference in the program of cognitive science.

Now Emil Post, in his logical research in the 1940s and early 1950s, tried to refute Turing's thesis and give alternative models of the mind. I will discuss two of these models. The first model distinguishes two instances in the mind: one is conscious and can be identified to a Turing machine, while the other one usually remains unconscious, or as Post sometimes phrases it, subconscious, and works on an entirely different basis. The emphasis – I believe – should not be put on the opposition between conscious and unconscious, but on the duality between two instances, two characters so to speak, like Jekyll and Hyde, who do not communicate with each other. The second model also stresses the plurality of the mind. Imagine that I start working on a certain proof and arrive at an alternative, either A or B. In Post's model, I would split into two workers which work in parallel, one on A and the other one on B. And each would again be able to split or – as Post phrases it – "reproduce by fission", and so on. Eventually, the cognitive mind appears to be a kind of factory with different workers sometimes organized hierarchically, sometimes without interactions.

Post did not publish this research. I will rely on the notebooks on which Post worked daily. These notebooks, which remain unpublished, are kept at the Library of the American Philosophical Society in Philadelphia. Besides, these models – as I have just outlined them – are not fully formalized, and rather constitute images that underlie Post's logical research.

Nevertheless, they have, to me, a twofold interest. First, they point to various weaknesses in Turing machines conceived as models of the mind. In particular, the mechanism of a Turing machine is linear in the sense that its operations may be ordered. The operations follow one another. The Turing machine takes one step after the other. What Post intends to stress is that, on the contrary, several things may happen at once in the mind. I may be thinking of dinner while writing this paper. If I were a Turing machine, these operations would have to take place one after the other, as if writing this paper made think of dinner, and this idea of dinner brought me back to my paper. Obviously, this is not how it works: I entertain the prospect of a nice dinner at the same time that I write my paper, in two parallel trains of thoughts. However, the description that Post gives of this plurality, or the model that Post gives for this plurality, remains bizarre: I do not spontaneously think of myself as a kind of factory: with one part of me virtually cooking dinner while another one writes a paper, and several other parts doing still other things which I may not be conscious of. As Post himself sometimes acknowledges, his models seem to be related to his own personality and severe psychic problems. A tentative interpretation of Post's research would be that, while dealing with logic, Post is in fact speaking of his own problems, speaks of his anguish of falling into madness or investigates in a phantasmatic mode the mechanism of his falling into madness: his breakdowns, as he calls them.

The question, therefore, is not that of the adequacy of Post's models to the actual operations of our thinking. The point is rather that Post's models bring to light aspects of thinking that the Turing machine covers up or occults. One would be tempted to conclude that one of the reasons for our adhesion to Turing machines as a model of the mind is precisely that this model occults and renders impossible these aspects of thinking. The mind as a Turing machine goes through definite states, which follow each other linearly. Such a model of the mind completely eliminates the danger of an uncontrollable plurality, which fascinated Post. In the light of Post's alternative models, the Turing machine seems to be inadequate but reassuring. The question would be whether this reassurance does not play a role in our identification with Turing machines.

## 1. Who is Post?

Emil L. Post was born in 1897 in Poland. The family immigrated to the United State in 1904. Unlike logicians who emigrated from Central Europe to the USA in the 1930s, such as Gödel or von Neumann, Post went to school and to university in USA.

His dissertation of 1920 introduces truth tables at about the same time as Wittgenstein's *Tractatus*. After this, Post embarks on an ambitious program, trying to define generally what he calls "finite processes": procedures of thought following unequivocal and deterministic rules, rules that prescribe unequivocally at each step the operation to be accomplished. Now this question that Post raises in the early 1920s is exactly the question of "computability", which Church, Gödel and, finally, Turing answer in the 1930s. A "finite process" in Post's sense is what we would call a computation, and the notion is a defined by Turing machines. A procedure following unequivocal and deterministic rules is a procedure that may be implemented on a machine of certain characteristics: a Turing machine. There is good reason to think that in the early 1920s Post anticipated some aspects Turing's thesis. However, before he publishes anything, Post has a first breakdown – to use his own expression – in 1921, and a second one in 1924, which basically removes him from the field of logic until 1936.

When he comes back, Turing has not yet stepped in, but Post discovers that Gödel and Church have to a great extent answered the problems that bothered him in the 1920s. He still draws on the material of his earlier notebooks to formulate an alternative definition of the notion of computation. Post's formulation involves a worker in front of a chain – as in chain work in a factory – and obeying orders from a boss. It is very similar, and equivalent, to Turing's formulation, which uses a machine programmed for certain actions instead of a worker obeying a boss. Post sends his text to Church at about the same time as Turing. But it is Turing's formulation, which is clearer, which will be used as the standard formulation.

After 1938, and for reasons which I cannot go into here,[2] Post attempts to refute these definitions of computability which he has himself contributed towards establishing. He attempts to show that there are definite thought procedures – computations, so to speak – that cannot be implemented or mimicked on a Turing machine. It is in this perspective that he develops the two models of the mind to which I have alluded. What Post aims at is what he calls a formulation 2 – by opposition to the standard definition, or formulation 1, of computable procedures – which is more extensive. He does not succeed in finding a procedure following definite rules which cannot be implemented on a Turing machine. He does publish various important papers – in particular, he gives a solution to the problem of Thue and an influential paper on degrees of insolvability. However, his attempt at defining alternative model of the mind is from a logical point of view. It nevertheless fills an important part of Post's notebooks.

Indeed, Post wrote a kind of logical-philosophical diary from 1938 up to his death in 1934. They were not meant for publication, and Post's style is sometimes ungrammatical. When there is no ambiguity as to the meaning, I will not attempt to correct Post's writing. The logician wrote each day for 2 hours, and never more, because extensive work seemed to precipitate his breakdowns. These diaries express very vividly Post's struggle against his breakdowns – I will give several examples. They are sometimes interrupted for several months when "it" happened.

Post died in 1954 after a heart failure following an electroshock treatment.

2 See Cassou-Noguès: *Les démons de Gödel*, chapter IV.

## 2. An analysis of what goes on in the mind

> I see my work as a complete and scientific psychical system – the first (Mechanics is such a physical system[3]

This first quotation shows clearly that Post's aim is to analyze what goes on in the mind during a computation. It is extracted from a paper that Post wrote in 1941 and which was only published in 1965 by his student M. Davis. Post quoted his diaries from the 1920s, which are now lost.

The second quotation shows that Post does hope to find a definition of "finite processes" more extensive than the standard (here called formulation 1) and which would include procedures not computable by Turing machines (or which require a "growing" machine and therefore not a Turing machine in the strict sense). However, this goal is secondary, and Post rather stresses the adequacy of the formulation that he is working on with the actual mental processes.

> Doubt if formulation 2 corresponds to a growing Turing machine, i.e. could get a fixed machine in the ordinary sense – I think – doing the same: a universal machine, yes, but simpler and not as universal machine but only as machine. *Really corresponds to our mind, but limited to specific reactions, as only machine*. Project really a must for me, success of some sort assured [...] A must because *I don't like machine idea.* [...] What I want is where human (sub!) is the machine [...] *Point of formulation II is not more power but to take care of formulation I's deficiency, i.e. a simple formulation to be the standard.*[4]

## 3. The unconscious: a first model of a plural mind

As H. Putnam showed,[5] Turing machines are in a sense conscious of their internal states. A Turing machine may be in a finite number of internal states. Say, it has three possible internal states: it may be 'happy, 'sad' or 'angry'. The machine can be programmed to print the state in which it currently is, so that there is no possibility of mistake. Each time the machine is 'happy', it prints: "I am happy". H. Putnam compares this ability with introspection. The machine might not be able to enunciate the rules that it follows. In this sense, it does not 'know' what determines its change of mind, what determines its being 'happy' or suddenly becoming 'sad', but it can always indicate its internal state. Taking Turing machines as a model of the mind, one could say that the mind, seen as a Turing machine, is conscious of its states but unconscious of the rules it follows.

3 Post: "Absolutely Unsolvable Problems", p. 440.
4 Notebook *Theory of Finite Processes*, vol. XI, p. 150, 29/07/48. My emphasis.
5 In particular, Putnam: "Minds and Machine".

Now Post seems to attempt to analyze this role of the unconscious in the thinking process. This analysis is related to Post's view on symbols and meaning. Post's idea is that, when considering a symbol, the mind may consciously grasp part of the meaning, or grasp no meaning at all, while it unconsciously grasps a deeper or more extensive meaning associated with the symbol. It is an old idea of Post that can be found as early as in the 1920s notebooks:

> [Meaning] as subconscious perception of things associated with symbol [...] The symbol is like an island which rises above the sea of the unconscious and is itself connected with the vaster regions below. [...] The unconscious is the seat of birth of new ideas.[6]

> Back in 1921–2 had idea of symbolization as symbol in conscious field connected to its meaning in the subconscious.[7]

From this perspective, it seems that, while consciously observing a certain symbol, the mind may unconsciously grasp its full meaning and then act according to this full meaning without knowing why. More precisely, Post imagines the following model. The mind may be in two different possible states. For clarity, I will call them 'happy' and 'unhappy': in state 1 (say when it is 'happy'), the mind only considers the symbols and computes on them according to certain rules, mechanically; in state 2 (say when it is 'unhappy'), the mind considers the meaning of the symbols and may then read a new rule for the computation, a new order from the boss so to speak: a message that is addressed to the unconscious and that the conscious, the mind in state 1, does not understand. Thus the mind goes back to state I and takes up the computation with this new rule. So the rules of the computation have changed, but the mind in its normal state (state 1, state 'happy') does not know anything about this change of rules which took place when it was in a different state.

> A sequence [of symbols] [can] be viewed with the mind in two possible states i.e. state 1 viewing it as it is, state 2 viewing it at as what it means. [...] Now the mind can also have two states, 1 passive, so that it looks at a complex if under state 1 gathers the impression, if under state 2 gathers meaning [and] if that meaning is an order follows that order [...]. Perhaps as it were orders itself at a later time to do things in state 1.[8]

> When c [a symbol] is observed, we consider M [the mind] to be in one of two states of receptivity
> receptivity of form let us say
> receptivity of meaning

6 Post: "Absolutely Unsolvable Problems", pp. 438–439.
7 Post: Notebook *Creative Logic*, vol. VII, p. 23 3/2/43.
8 Post: Notebook *Creative Logic*, vol. III, p. 7, 21/2/39.

> States 1 or 2 of M cause c to effect M correspondingly. Effect is the consciousness of the form of c on one case, the meaning of c in the other. [...] Only in state 2 will M be activated i.e. become a cause of action.[9]

The question would be to find out what determines these changes of states. What makes the mind go into state 2? Some particular symbol, for example, might make the mind 'click' into state 2 – as if a particular thing had the property to make the mind suddenly 'unhappy' – or it might 'charge' the mind, which then discharges itself when it falls back into state 1.[10]

This model is interesting in its ambiguity. It has a logical motivation. This distinction between state 1 and state 2 is intended to give an account of how the rules of a computation might be changed during the computation, so as to obtain a process which on the whole would not follow a definite set of rules or a set of rules that could be computed by a Turing machine. But one could also look at this distinction as a – probably unconscious and oversimplified – model for the mechanism of Post's own breakdown: something suddenly brings him into a different state, with an otherwise unconscious meaning appearing, and without himself knowing why the rule of his behaviour changes.

## 4. "The split personality picture"

As early as in the previous model, Post distinguishes two instances in the mind (the mind in state 1 *versus* the mind in state 2, or the conscious mind that considers the symbol *versus* the unconscious mind that considers its meaning) which act separately. Putting emphasis on the distinction between the two instances, rather than on the opposition between the conscious mind and the underlying unconscious, one could already see in this model a split of personality, such as that which takes place between Jekyll and Hyde. The mind is divided in two modules, which alternately takes hold of one's behaviour.

In any case, the idea of a division of the mind is at the centre of Post's attempts to go beyond Turing. As already noted, a Turing machine works linearly: it accomplishes one operation after the other. Now Post's idea is that our mind operates in parallel: there can be several processes going on at the same time. If I encounter an alternative, either A or B, I may follow up the consequences of A and of B in parallel. It is as if I split up in two halves, so that one half of me deduces the consequences of A and another half deduces the consequence of B.

9 Post: Notebook *Creative Logic*, vol. II, p. 71–72, 19/10/38 (wrongly dated 1932 by Post).

10 For the "clicks", see Post: Notebook *Creative Logic*, vol. XVI, p. 9, 12/11/1947. For the "charges/discharges", see Post: Notebook *Creative Logic*, vol. II, p. 71–72, 19/10/38 (wrongly dated 1932 by Post).

Post offers vivid descriptions of this plural mind. In the quotation below, the mind becomes a universe with different centres of activity. Generally speaking, Post opposes the "monogenic" process of the Turing machine to the "polygenic processes", which go on in our mind, and hopes to discover a polygenic process which could not be translated into a monogenic process computable by a Turing machine.

> In polygenic processes activity goes on at many points. Suppose assume one time + a sort of pump throughout universe and each time pump is pushed a next step takes place at each active focus. Not too unnatural to say each time pump is pushed a wave of activity passes along till one by one those steps are done.[11]

In the next extract, Post tries various images to illustrate his idea of parallel processes, the idea that there is a multiplicity of trains of thoughts in the mind, a multiplicity of workers operating at the same time. The first image is theological. The second turns the mind into a kind of factory where different workers coexist. Elsewhere, Post mentions the "boss" and his "subordinates". Post also acknowledges that this split personality picture is related to his own psychiatric problems.

> An unholy thought: if allow multiplicity of workers have a miniature of a philosophy of God working his will by at one time being himself and simultaneously also being each and every one of his creatures [...] Hope this isn't a hint I should drop present analysis for a while. [...] Have to imagine for my polygenic purposes that I can be in many places at once. For, in the polygenic process, it will be at many points that something may happen which requires when it happens a certain something to be done. [...] Try split personality picture: not for me but for my worker. [...] Let me say (and I hope that this won't split my personality) [...]: At the ringing of the bell, half of me keeps going, the other half goes back to [its the previous task] where left off. [...] When that first half gets to another point where bell is ringing it splits again. [...When the initial task is finished] what is left of me dies as it were with the *finis*. But my dichotomous division descendants as it were keep on. [...] A worker suffering reproduction by fission [...].[12]

Post sees this ability to split in two instances as forming the very foundation of our mathematics. In particular, it accounts for our idea of an infinite set. How can natural numbers be considered as a set? Well, I can count 1, 2, 3 and I split in two: one half of me continues to count endlessly and the other half leisurely imagines the result of the indefinite work of my first half.

> At bottom, the basic human ability of for example doing things for a while in a certain way, seeing this can be continued and sort of splitting off from real self, a sort of robot self which is imagined to keep on doing so for ever. Discussed this elsewhere.[13]

11 Post: Notebook *Calculus of finite processes*, vol I, p. 47, 25/8/44.
12 Ibid. p. 112 ff., 11/12/44.
13 Post: Notebook *Creative Logic*, vol. XV, p. 180, 4/11/47

> [The] worker becomes self conscious. Thus can imagine himself split in two à la movies. The real self stays a free agent, the other obeys the rule. [The real self] can thus imagine time going forward and himself holding back and so a concept of result of following a rule. [...] [The real self] can picture time to be speed up and à la bouncing ball imagine what the process engaged in by his other self would be even if unending [...]: infinite object. [...] [I] really have in mind bouncing ball completing infinite number of bounces in finite time[14]

This "split personality picture" also enables Post to come back to his idea of analysing the way in which the rules of a computation can be changed during the computation. The mind is divided in several workers, each taking care of a certain type of operation. A first one will work on numbers. He will accomplish certain operations on numbers. But a second one will work to determine the operations that the first one is ordered to accomplish. He will so to speak supervise the first worker and deal not with numbers but with operations on numbers.

> Prescription for a mathematical adventure. Here is involved the mind whose adventure is described and the mind which does the describing. Various next steps. First separate the time of one and the time of the other. Describing mind can picture as it were biography of described mind for all of later time. A la bouncing ball.[15]

Now, one could imagine a third worker who again would work to define the operations that the second worker will carry on. Eventually, Post describes his worker as a kind of tortoise with a shell on which another worker may calculate: "Picture the thing as a kind of tortoise, robot or organism [...] with a sort of metal frame [...] like a tortoise shell."[16] The result is that a second worker, working on the shell of a first worker, determines the actions of the first worker. This second worker may himself have a third worker operating on his back, and so on.

We have here a rather bizarre representation of what goes on in our mind. If the idea of studying the way in which one might modify the rules of a computation during a computation may have logical motivation, one must acknowledge that this picture of the tortoises working on each other's back is a surprising model of our mind.

## 5. Conclusion

The question is not whether Post's descriptions are adequate to the reality of mental processes. Post's models are bizarre and, as he acknowledges himself, related to his psychiatric problems. Nevertheless, they do point to some weak-

14 Post: Notebook *Creative Logic*, vol. II, p. 185–186, 2/11/38.
15 Post: Notebook *Creative Logic*, vol. III, p. 7, 20/2/39.
16 Post: Notebook *Theory of finite processes*, vol. XI, p. 177, 4/8/48.

nesses in Turing machines conceived as models of the mind. Though I can hardly picture my mind as a mental factory hosting a whole team of workers, it is true that I may think at several things at once or follow various trains of thought simultaneously. Or, again, though it does seem slightly exaggerated to distinguish two separate modules in the mind, a conscious personality, so to speak, and an unconscious one which would grasp a meaning to which the conscious personality has no access whatsoever, but which will eventually determine our behaviour, at the same time it is hardly possible to deny that our behaviour may depend on an unconscious understanding of certain events, an understanding which under normal circumstances we cannot formulate.

The point is that the Turing machine, with its operation linearly ordered, with this succession of internal states governed by fixed rules, does not account for this multiplicity of the mind, which so fascinated Post and which he seemed to fear so much. One could even say that it occults this possible multiplicity and, in this way, offers a reassuring model of the mind.

In the words of Dr. Jekyll,

> [...] man is not truly one, but truly two. I say two, because the state of my own knowledge does not pass beyond that point. Others will follow, others will outstrip me on the same line; and I hazard the guess that man will be ultimately known for a mere polity of multifarious, incongruous and independent denizens.[17]

It is also what Post believed and attempted to use against Turing machines.

## References

Cassou-Noguès, Pierre: *Les démons de Gödel. Logique et folie*, Paris (Seuil) 2007.

Cassou-Noguès, Pierre: "Gödel et la thèse de Turing", *Revue d'histoire des mathématiques*, 14/1 (2009), pp. 77–111.

Davis, Martin (ed.): *The Undecidable*, Hewlett (Raven Press) 1965.

De Moll, Liesbeth: "Closing the Circle: An Analysis of Emil Post's Early Work", *Bulletin of Symbolic Logic*, 12/2 (2006), pp. 267–289.

Grattan-Guiness, Ivor: "The Manuscripts of Emil L. Post", *History and Philosophy of Logic*, 11 (1990), pp. 77–83.

Post, Emil: *Solvability, Provability, Definability: The Collected Works of Emil L. Post*, ed. by M. Davis, Berlin (Birkhäuser) 1994.

Post, Emil: *Absolutely Unsolvable Problems and Relatively Undecidable Propositions: An Account of an Anticipation,* in: ibid.

17 Stevenson: *Dr Jekyll and Mr Hyde*, p. 307.

Post, Emil: *Theory of Finite Processes*, unpublished notebook. Library of the American Philosophical Society.

Post, Emil: *Creative Logic*, unpublished notebook. Library of the American Philosophical Society.

Post, Emil: *Calculus of Finite Processes*, unpublished notebook. Library of the American Philosophical Society.

Putnam, Hilary: "Minds and Machine" (1960), in: Hilary Putnam, *Mind, Language and Reality*, Cambridge (Cambridge Univ. Press) 1975, pp. 362–386.

Turing, Allan: "On computable numbers, with an application to the *Entscheidungsproblem*" (1937), reprinted in Martin Davis (ed.): *The Undecidable*, Hewlett (Raven Press) 1965, pp. 115–153.

Stevenson, Robert L.: *Strange Case of Dr. Jekyll and Mr. Hyde* (1886), in: *The Complete Stories of R. L. Stevenson*, New York (Modern Library) 2002.

# *Cognitio animi experimentalis* Intoxication, Hallucination, Imagination, and Modernity

GERHARD SCHARBERT

Claude Lévi-Strauss exemplified in *Science et conscience de la société*[1] how the myths die as a transformation of mythological contents in analogy to the camera obscura. After passing by a narrow strait of communication in form of minimal assertion they get back their former capacity on the other side, but the picture stands finally overhead, like rays of light, which are forced to pass a small hole to arrive in a dark room and are crossing thereby. Regarding the relationship between life sciences and the birth of an esthetical modernity since 1800, there seems to be a similarity. The emergence of experimental neurophysiology in nineteenth century France did not accidentally encounter with eminent changes in the way of thinking about consciousness, not at least in the field of literature.

The term modernity originates in that historical moment. Both appear in the reversed telescope of colonial desires which had overwhelmed Paris in suite of Napoleon the First. But both appear also strangely isolated in discourses of literary criticism or history of sciences.

For that reason I will start from a special constellation where the encounter of experimental psychiatry and poetics produces modernity. I understand this as a contribution to a certain kind of archaeology of cultural techniques which connects both aspects of modernity that are seemingly far away from each other.

Modernity as a specific term coined by Charles Baudelaire and the experimental groundings of Medicine, Psychiatry, and Neurology in Nineteenth century are linked together not in a hazardous way. I suppose that a historical exact constellation of literature and experimental psychophysiology represents the *Urszene* of esthetic Modernity, so the medical *Experimentalkultur* of the first half of the Nineteenth century is via physiology and neurology directly related to the phenomenon in which poetry could say "Me is another"[2] and case reports later may be read as poetry.[3]

After Albrecht von Haller, but in spite of him, neurophysiology was understood as a superior paradigm of a dynamic medicine. This aspect sometimes dominates the other fields of medical research. William Cullen, author of the word neurosis reinterpreted the Hallerian categories of sensibility and irritability,

1 Lévi-Strauss: *Science et conscience de la société*, Vol. 1, pp. 131–141.
2 Rimbaud: *Œuvres Complètes*, p. 249.
3 Freud: *Gesammelte Werke,* Vol 1, p. 227.

which were formerly only used to describe quantitative functional properties in small structures of the ligature of the nervous and muscular apparatus, as qualitative states,[4] followed by Pierre Cabanis.[5] For a soul projected on a net of nerves and brain, sensibility and irritability become sources of disorder. The word *Seelenstörungen* (soul-disorders), a term of the nineteenth-century medicine, describes in this matter not a deficit of mind but a superfluity in its bases. By the appearance of the nervous and neurotics it would be possible to associate the most important anthropological sign of man and his soul, the ability to produce language, with a medical semiotic of symptoms.

Condillac mentioned the remarkable habitude of human beings to link any imaginations with arbitrary signs, "l'habitude de lier quelques idées à des signes arbitraires."[6] From the shouts of nature, "cris naturels"[7] of necessity arose first the order of language, then thought. So the lingual expression is determined by an order and every expression of imagination has to be measured by that standard. Pierre Cabanis, the *médecin-philosophe,* who has built up the medical administration of revolutionary France until he was dismissed from his public functions by Napoleon protected Philippe Pinel and this made such opinions constitutive for nosological and therapeutical models of French medicine around 1800.

I suggest that the linguistic model of sign later follows these lines of pathology.

I only mention Ferdinand de Saussure's remarks on this subject in his *cours de linguistique générale*.[8] But nevertheless I consider such a disgression of medical semiotics to other fields as a media effect.

In the Nineteenth century the immanent redundancies of the "reine Verstandesbegriffe"[9], mentioned by Leibniz a long time ago, became obvious in their own medium. Writing books as a testament of a more real nature of man based on religion, now suggests the limits of artificial memory as an overflow of endless possibilities for the recently alphabetized subjects. But these limits foreshadow some others: The medico-biological treatment of the bases of mind and the organic premises of philosophical anthropology offers a new way to perceive "the thought petrified in the printed brain of society,"[10] as the French paleoanthropologist André Leroi-Gourhan said.

The leadership of french Neurology in that era is illustrated by a sentence of Robert Castel: The Golden Age of Psychiatry, *L'Âge d'or de l'aliénisme*.[11]

4 Cullen: *Synopsis nosologiae methodicae.*
5 Cabanis: *Œuvres Philosophiques*, Vol. 2.
6 Condillac: *Essai sur l'origine des connaissances humaines*, p. 114.
7 Ibid., p. 114.
8 De Saussure: *Cours de Linguistique Générale.*
9 Leibniz, G.W.: "αποκατάστασις (πάντων)", pp. 27–34.
10 Leroi-Gourhan: *Hand und Wort*, p. 329.
11 Castel: *L'ordre psychiatrique.*

According with Philippe Pinel and Dominique Esquirol a psychiatry that argues physiologically but is not working in the same way, becomes a solid part of European medicine especially in its claim to elucidate moral and mental behaviour on a basis of new biological knowledge about man without any metaphysical ballast.

Realities which were formerly imagined by the époque through poetry or an exotic journey, "now encounter manifest to the researcher's perceptions" to mention a sentence of the German physician and poet Gottfried Benn.[12]

Nietzsche has denunciated this "[...] scientific lust of man on his own behalf as *lust for the extraordinary*"[13] and consequently this desire looks after such extraordinary cases, for example in sign-systems.

Philippe Pinel and Dominique Esquirol were sure that the hypertrophies of cognition and imagination belong to the general prognostic instruments of neuropathology. This had been the opinion of some of such famous forerunners like William Cullen and also the Scottish Psychiatrist and Neurologist Sir Alexander Crichton. He had taught first, that every single faculty of the mind like attention, memory, judgement, imagination could become ill separately.[14] Pinel's pupil, Victor Broussais, wrote in 1828 in his main work *De l'irritation et de la folie* a long chapter about the validity of signs, *valeur des signes*, where he was denying this validity of signs in respect of any self-description of psychical phenomena. His judgement is disastrous for this subject. Terms like *moi, intelligence, imagination, conscience* should be considered as the helpless trial to explain various physiological states of the nervous system. Nevertheless, the book takes a well known imperative mood: "Lisez!" (Read!)[15]

Not so much later Charles Baudelaire subsumes in the opening poem of *Les Fleurs du Mal* with the title *Au lecteur*, to the reader, logically not only the production but also the reception of poetry as forms of not-normality.[16] An esthetic theory that declares exactly these states of cognition as its subject, which Broussais was in doubt about the validity of lingual signs to describe them, is able to inscribe a new beauty into the stony deserts of the mega cities and the oscillations of consciousness more bizarre than all the dreams of spiritualists. The naked real and the operations on it.

In this view, the famous address to the reader of *Les Fleurs du Mal* "hypocrite lecteur", etymological ὑποκρίτης *lector*, is a metonymic, a displacement.

This is rather concrete because of the existence of a real background, known only as a spooky footnote, which encounters the random phenomena of the new sciences with a very old practice of sign-production.

12 Benn: "Beitrag zur Geschichte der Psychiatrie", p. 417.
13 Nietzsche: *Nachgelassene Fragmente*, Vol. 11, p. 38.
14 Crichton: *An Inquiry into the nature and origin of mental derangement.*
15 Broussais: *De l'Irritation et de la Folie*, Vol 1, pp. 489sqq.
16 Baudelaire: *Œuvres Complètes*, Vol. 1, pp. 5sq.

While the French colonial armies in Algiers are preparing themselves to "re-civilize" the orient, the neurologist Jacques-Joseph Moreau de Tours brings back another gift to Paris, which he had learned about on one of the journeys with patients of his teacher Esquirol. This substance promises to excite the deregulations of other sides of cognition and imagination in an experimental manner. Now it seems possible to classify, to describe and to recapitulate them. This substance was Hashish.

Moreau became acquainted with it through Louis Aubert-Roche, who had formerly lead a military hospital in Egypt. Aubert described the psycholytic potential in context of his book about the treatment of typhus, published in Paris in 1840.[17] This disease was more dangerous for French colonial armies than the precise fire of the royal Navy and the less precise of the Osmanian troops or of the Arabians. Thus there was an urgent need for research. Aubert-Roche classified typhus as a nervous disease according to his famous predecessors. As I have mentioned before, Hashish would become the chosen *pharmakon*, because it works powerfully on the nervous system.

This could be observed in many natives of northern Africa, where consumption of hashish was nearly endemic.

Moreau de Tours was testing the new substance first in series of self experiences, but soon he thought about an experimental and therapeutically use. His research started from a previous reflection about the physiological phenomena of sleep and dreams traditional in France, which he wanted to systematize.

Moreau is radicalizing these theories by a supposed unity of dream and madness both caused in a kind of twilight state, *état crepusculaire*, which also can be the cause of all forms of madness.[18]

The crème of contemporary French intellectuals representing literature and the fine arts was subject to Moreau's experiments with Hashish at the *Île St-Louis* in the so called *Hôtel Pimodan*, an old city palace. Based on the data from these meetings Moreau de Tours was defining the *aliénation mentale* as a state, where the incommensurable worlds of inner and outer perception unite.[19]

Broussais' diagnosis that the self would be disposable was a mise-en-scène by Moreau; with a little help from his friends and the *cannabis sativa sive indica*, as well as the discernment that self-perception is an inner physiological sense, called "sens intime" by Moreau.[20]

This seems to be a little uncanny not only for the Neurologists. The shock and the trauma of a monstrous mega city modernity, bringing any traditional self to burst asunder via techniques of traffic, metropolitan topography and working began to condense in a literary esthetic, which was later identified with these ruptures in a strange way. But the poets, deeply impressed by Moreau's experi-

17 Aubert-Roche: *De la Peste ou typhus d'Orient.*

18 See: Moreau de Tours: *Du Hachisch et de l'aliénation mentale.*

19 Ibid., p. 173.

20 Ibid., p. 31.

ments, Charles Baudelaire and Gérard de Nerval, were reflecting their own medium not without reason on the height of the contemporary sciences. Nerval invents a preliminary form of typewriter that enables him to write down directly literature in its given shape as discreet signs and to multiply it. He also reflects about theory and practice of Daguerreotypes.[21]

The double unhappy love story he speaks about in *Sylvie*,[22] one of the most beautiful of his stories called *Daughters of Flame*, reflects the concussions of consciousness, the undulations of dreaming Baudelaire spoke about later, on the height of Moreau's experiments. The melancholia of the former beloved girl's shy courting shows the poet's desire to come back to the places of youth and childhood in another way as a simply sentimental journey. The Rousseauian theatre which is played by the people of the highly artificial landscape in the text represents the literally pendant of this desire and of its vibrations.

"Tour à tour bleue et rose comme l'astre trompeur d'Aldébaran, c'était Adrienne ou Sylvie, – c'étaient les deux moitiés d'un seul amour. L'une était l'idéal sublime, l'autre la douce réalité."[23] (After the row blue and pink like the delusive star Aldebaran, was Adrienne or Sylvie, – these were two halves of one single love. The one was the related ideal, the other the sweet reality).

The split is exemplified by Nerval as an inevitable consequence following the trial to come back to the past. Any love that should fulfil the desires of the past and initiate the escape from it at the same time, must become an *astre trompeur*, a disaster.

It is possible to read *Sylvie* as a subtle resuming commentary to French romanticism which was so highly engaged in Rousseau's illusions about nature. The text fixed what was inscribed through this split into modernity: Physiological vacillations, troubles of cognition, uncertainty about mind and soul in the light of developing biology of brain and nervous systems. Under the shadow of this *désastre*, literature began to be marginalized. The work of Nerval is a testimonial and does not mention these developments, but sometimes is bearing their names: *Daughters of flame*, *Sylvie*, *Aurélia*.

Charles Baudelaire called his monograph about hashish *Poème* and so he signalizes formally very clear, especially in France that he wants to reflect the cannabis experiments of Moreau de Tours, published in 1845, in a theoretical and poetical manner.[24] In spite of the current doctrine of rime and verse, represented again and again for instance by Théodore de Banville, Baudelaire oriented his following latest poems in prose towards a principle of modular and segmental

21 These topics will be described in a further publication by the author, which will be published in 2010 by Wilhelm Fink Verlag München: *Dichterwahn. Über die Pathologisierung von Modernität.*

22 Nerval: *Œuvres Complètes*, Vol. III.

23 Ibid., p. 567.

24 Baudelaire: *Œuvres Complètes*, Vol. 1, pp. 401–441.

structure, following both the possible derangement of the self and the advanced iron building structures of the two greatest libraries in Paris.

In dedication to Arsène Houssaye he wrote:

> [...] I send you a small work, from which one without doing her wrong could not say that she has neither head nor tail, on the contrary, everything in her is exchangeable head and tail at the same time, alternately and mutually.
> Consider, please which admirable comforts this connection offers us to all, you, me and the reader.
> We can make a cut where we want, I in my daydreaming, you in the manuscript, the reader in his reading; because I don't stuck on his shrewed will not to the endless thread of a superfluous intrigue.
> Take away a vertebra, and both limbs of this [...] thing fit together easily again.
> Disassemble it in different parts, and you will see that everything can exist for itself.[25]

This is the poetic reaction that aims directly and consequently at a *cognitio animi experimentalis* just the way Moreau de Tours had put it *en scene* earlier on.

Contrary to Moreau, Baudelaire himself is very aware of the fact, that the *Other Sides of Cognition* provoked by intoxication will not prosper in the laboratory of the Hotel Pimodan alone:

> Who of us during his ambitious hours would have not dreamt of the miracle of a poetic prose that is musically without rhythm and rhyme, pliable and resistant enough to adapting itself to the lyrical movements of the soul, the undulations of the daydreaming, and the vibrations of the consciousness?
> It is the bustle of the gigantic towns before all things, it is the criss-crossing of her countless meetings what bears this obsessive ideal.[26]

Baudelaire himself has realised this programme in the writing to which the dedication for Houssaye formed the introduction; however, the contemporaries have not approved by the majority the consequence of this new poetry.

Thus the doyen at that time of the Parnasse Théodore de Banville ascertained still in 1872, the same year Nietzsche's *Geburt der Tragödie aus dem Geiste der Musik (birth of the tragedy from the mind of the music)* appeared, in his *Petit Traité de Poésie Française* apodictically, the overcome Poesy, "les rhythmes connus", the known rhythms, are just "tous les rhythmes qui existent", the only rhythms which there are.

And even in view of Baudelaire's prose poems he stuck to his narrow concept of poetry.

On the rhetorical question: "Peut-il y avoir poèmes en prose?" can there be poems in prose? he gave himself the rash answer: "Non, il peut pas y en avoir,

25 Ibid., p. 275.
26 Ibid., p. 275sq.

malgré […] les admirable *Poèmes en prose* de Charles Baudelaire", no, there cannot be any, in spite of the admirable *Prose Poems* of Charles Baudelaire.[27]

Thus a modern poetry developed *malgré* de Banville. The novelty of Baudelaire's prose poems, reached not only a Parisian public, but spread to the extreme periphery of France. In a pupil's room of the province, corresponded contents from Baudelaire's prose poem, *Le Confitéor de l'artiste,* in which he had tried to describe the dissoluton of the self and this time more radical: *Je, est un autre!* Me is another

Already Gérard de Nerval had written years earlier, under an engraved portrait Eugène Gervais had made of him: *Je suis l'autre*, I am the other. At least to the first contemporaries of modernity it seemed to make sense, that also poetically, nothing could remain as it was.

But it appeared that – as Hugo Friedrich marked very appropriately – "not yet everything was done for the genesis of speech of the modern soul."[28]

In the same letter from which also the famous *I am the other* was written, Rimbaud described how a poet creates such new poetry. After what he had already said about the form of true poetry, which consists of sound and rhythm, the experimental character of this plan is very clearly recognizable in the context of the contemporary sciences, in particular of an experimental psychiatry à la Moreau de Tours.

> The first aspiration of the person, who wants to become a writer, is an unlimited knowledge of himself; he searches his soul, investigates it, researches it, and gets to know it. As soon as he knows her he must cultivate it. This looks easy: In every brain a natural development [...] completes itself – However, it is a matter of making the soul monstrous: [...] imagine somebody who implants warts in his face and cultivates them.
> The poet becomes a seer by a long, immense and rational Entregelung [dérèglement] of all senses. All forms of the love, the suffering, the insanity; he searches for his own ways; he exhausts all poisons in himself to preserve only their quintessence.
> He must make his inventions noticeably, handy, audible [...] finding language [...] weaklings could start to think about the first letter of the alphabet and lose themselves abruptly in madness! –
> [...] future will be materialist as you see; – Always fulfilled from number and harmony, such poems will be made to remain. – Basically this would be almost once again a sort of the Greek poetry. [...] The poetry will not rhythmicize any more the action; elle sera en avant. She will be ahead.
> [...] Baudelaire is the first seer, king of the writers, a true God.[29]

One must stylize oneself as a monster, in order to take note of the trends of the life sciences of the late nineteenth century and the vicinity of its encyclopaedic efforts; which has long ago integrated poetry as a statement of varying states of nervous brain matter into its catalogue of symptoms.

27 De Banville: *Petit traité de poésie française*, pp. 11; 14.
28 Friedrich: *Die Struktur der modernen Lyrik*, p. 94.
29 Rimbaud: *Œuvres Complètes*, pp. 251ff.

Arthur Rimbaud, shortly after his promising works influenced by the *Fleurs du Mal*, began with a dynamic criticism of the contemporary lyric which he discussed from the heights of his own critical and philological-poetic abilities.

After the new poems, in a simple folk tone unheard of in France, he presented a cycle of prose pieces that were deeply influenced by Baudelaire's *Poème du Hachisch.*

*A season in hell* is a composition of eleven texts in which a clear separation of prose from poetry is not possible. The intensity of the poems provoked a large variety of interpretations, which all appeal to what is said in the text because Rimbaud has produced an amazing simultaneousness of biographic, psychological-psychiatric, historical, religious, and erotic discourses.

They are hermetic, however, not incomprehensibly. If one considers the context of the experiment Rimbaud himself had called for in the seer's letters, it discloses alongside this simultaneousness which we find again in the psychiatric diagnoses of the intoxicated experience of Moreau de Tours and in the theories on hallucinations of his contemporary colleagues, clues of a radical subject criticism, religious criticism and literary criticism which should form the preparation for the even more basic experiment of the later *Illuminations*.

In the tone of a long ago grown pale recollection the *Saison* begins in a dialogue with Satan who presents the telling or writing self with a narcotic overdose, already Baudelaire's Satan, to whom these sheets of this *carnet de damné*, diary of a damned, are given.[30]

In this cryptic tribute to the Baudelaire of the *Petits Poèmes en prose* Rimbaud leads to his characterization of the hashish as "un parfait instrument satanique", a perfectly satanic instrument what also puts the coming pages of the *Saison* under this spell and already rejects every version for the sole purposes of biographically-religious *confessio*: The writer will neither describe nor teach. On the contrary, due to the drug related inducement, even the structure of the *Saison* contradicts every kind of *cogito*; it is possible to read them as an alternative draught to *Descartes Discours de la Méthode* who turns his intentions around, in such a way that truth and beauty arise causally from a controlled Derailment of all "senses".

Arthur Rimbaud at least writes his "*Illuminécheunes*"[31] on single sheets of paper without backside or order. One of these pieces, MATINÉE D'IVRESSE, shows the connections not only with Hashish itself but also with Baudelaire's hashish poem clearly enough.

Indeed, the preliminary callings "*Ô mon Bien! Ô mon Beau!*" are quoting Baudelaire's sentences from part four of the *Poème du Hachisch*: "– toutes ces

30 Ibid., p. 93.

31 This is how Paul Verlaine describes the English pronunciation of "Illuminations" in a letter to Sivry (27.Oct. 1878).

choses ont été créées pour moi, pour moi, pour moi!" (All these things were created for me only! For me, for me!)[32]

The following verses mention a tune, the children's laughing all beginning and ending with – the well known initial effect of the drug – and the harmony too is thought regarding the end: "Ce poison va rester dans toutes nos veines même quand, la fanfare tournant, nous serons rendus à l'ancienne inharmonie."[33]

The poison will remain in the organism of the intoxicated when the sound of a new harmony is long over and the drunken is fallen back into the missed harmony of sobriety. This is an observation which is absolutely correct. The active substance could be indicated in blood still weeks later through its metabolites when any shadow of intoxication has vanished long ago: "Cela commençait par toute la rustrerie, voici que cela finit par des anges de flamme et de glace."[34]

What begins as nonsense like the biographical episode described by Ernest Delahaye, when Rimbaud first takes hashish and had called it "un paradis artificiel exactement raté"[35], an artificial paradise that failed precisely, ends as a vision of angels made of flames and ice. This seems to be a good description of the irritations of protopathical sensibility. And in the end there is sensible and theoretical evidence resulting from the base of intoxication.

> Nous t'affirmons, méthode ! Nous n'oublions pas que tu as glorifié hier chacun de nos âges. Nous avons foi au poison.[36]
>
> (We state, method! We do not forget that you have glorified yesterday each of our age. We have confidence in poison.)

Is this a confirmation of the *methode d'analyse*, the analysis method, which Moreau de Tours had learned from his academic teacher Esquirol like he had learned it from Pinel, but has modernized it with psychopharmacological additions?

Maybe Rimbaud reflects in this poem the thoughts of Moreau about the unity of drug delirium and madness in respect of experimental methods:

> Ô maintenant nous si digne de ces tortures! rassemblons fervemment cette promesse surhumaine faite à notre corps et à notre âme créés : cette promesse, cette démence ! L'élégance, la science, la violence![37]
>
> (Oh, now we, so worthy of these tortures! let us collect this superhuman promise which is made in our created body and soul: this promise, this insanity! The elegance, the science, the violence!)

32 Rimbaud, Arthur: *Œuvres Complètes*, p. 130.
33 Ibid., p. 131.
34 Ibid.
35 Delahaye: *Souvenirs familiers à propos de Rimbaud*, p. 162.
36 Rimbaud: *Œuvres Complètes*, p. 131.
37 Ibid.

Discourse and practice of experimental simulation of psychical phenomena indicates an exact question about the medium of description and places it on the agenda of modern poetry. This is why I have sketched how in the medium of writing phenomena of introspection and medical impression of brain and nervous systems leads to a theory of modernity which takes these impressions seriously.

The dissociation of perception and cognition finds its way into the work of Nerval Baudelaire and Rimbaud as a technical writing of processes related to the physiology of cognition and psychopharmacology.

Stéphane Mallarmé demonstrated later how poetry could be considered as a medial resonance of nervous oscillations in an optical field.

He did this in accordance with the contemporary experimental physiology not only of the brain but also of the apparatus of perception.

Mallarmé started in *crise de vers* with the concussion caused by his own crisis of writing when he was young and transformed it into a negative diagnosis of the contemporary poetry using elements of the doubts about it, which are related with mathematics and music. He knows very exactly "that music to the verse finds the way back to form poetry since Wagner,"[38] like he said in the same oration, but he answers in a way not only rhetorically, what would confirm the deficit of poetry against the soundscapes of post-Wagnerian orchestra. The key words are *transposition* and *structure*.[39] Also Mallarmé knows according to his century, that less or more all books are simply the fusion of certain sets of countable repetitions,[40] literature in a narrow sense is nothing as a reduced form of theory of combination.

But in this gap or interregnum something is marching in that accepts the vanishing of the poet, who is a pretext for reflexes of nervous irreducible movements.

At least the melody of every speech is transformed into an overwhelming non-hazard of the printed page, where "a middle extension of words is constellated under the computing regard and so silence."[41]

The poet's death by a nervous crisis and the end of poetry in the crisis of verse both are leading to a resurrection of word art as a radical practice consequently reduced to printed paper. Leo Bersani wrote that the strategic use of musical metaphor leads step by step away from the rhythmical and prosodic qualities of speaking to an exclusion of any sound in poetry.[42] Mallarmé confronts the evidence of hearing with the *virtualité*[43] of reading.

38 Mallarmé: *Œuvres Complètes*, p. 365.

39 Ibid., p. 366.

40 Ibid., p. 367: […] *que, plus ou moins, tous les livres, contiennent la fusion de quelques redites comptées*[...].

41 Ibid., p. 364: […] *une moyenne étendue de mots, sous la compréhension du regard, se range en traits définitifs, avec quoi le silence.*

42 Bersani: *The Death of Stéphane Mallarmé*, p. 44.

43 Mallarmé: *Œuvres Complètes*, p. 368.

These thoughts should not be misunderstood as esoteric. But exactly in the field of experimental anatomy of brain and nerves they deeply correlate in the second half of the nineteenth century with fundamental inventions.

Like Arthur Rimbaud in one of the *lettres du voyant*, like Mallarmé himself in *crise de vers*, Paul Flechsig wrote in 1896:

> In the construction of our mind, in the big persisting characteristics of his arrangement the architecture of our brain is reflected clearly and precisely.[44]

The proof of this thesis was brought about with the first anatomical and embryological demonstration of an ontogenetic grounded ordering principle of the *Leitungsbahnen* Flechsig did himself.

The time-shifted myelinisation of nervous fibers allow during the ontogenesis the absolute complete unveiling of the sensory lines of their entry into the central organ, up to their final sites in the brain bark.[45]

Because of this exploration it is possible to differentiate distinct cortical areas in their functions and there appear great cortical areas which are not innerved for sensorial tasks only, called association centres by Flechsig.

From the formerly known sensorial areas there are tracing a great number of association fibers in these areas which are spread over the whole cortex.

From the association centres are running again bundles of nerves which are connecting nearer or farer cortical areas. The function of the association centres Flechsig describes as "deren Tätigkeit [...] die Erregungszustände verschiedenartiger Sinnessphären zu assoziieren."[46] (To associate their activity with the states of excitement of various sensory spheres.)

Such finer structures of the brain are denying a generalised theory of psycho-pathology based only on one single neurophysiologic state, such as Cesare Lombroso or Max Nordau who have used something of it to classify Mallarmé.[47]

44 Flechsig, Paul: *Die Localisation der geistigen Vorgänge*, p. 3: "Im Aufbau unseres Geistes, in den großen beharrenden Zügen seiner Gliederung spiegelt sich klar und deutlich die Architektur unseres Gehirns wider."

45 Ibid., p. 13: "[...] die völlig lückenlose Darlegung der Sinnesleitungen von ihrem Eintritt in das Zentralorgan bis zu ihren Endstätten in der Hirnrinde." This method of Flechsig Sigmund Freud uses as an embryological and anatomical straight line for his own findings in the anatomy of the brain he published in 1885 and 1886: "Zur Kenntnis der Olivenzwischenschicht" [Neurologisches Centralblatt 4, Bd. 12 (1885), pp. 268–270] and in collaboration with Darkschewitsch: "Über die Beziehung des Strichkörpers zum Hinterstrang und Hinterstrangskern nebst Bemerkungen über zwei Felder der Oblongata" [Neurologisches Centralblatt 5, Bd. 6 (1886), pp. 121–129].

46 Ibid., p. 60.

47 Cesare Lombroso, who provided Max Nordaus *Dégénérescence*, in which among other things Mallarmé's small conchae are judged as being a sign for his "degeneracy" – "Entartung" – and others with key words, holds forth about Rimbaud and Mallarmé in longer passages of his work [Lombroso, Cesare Ezechio Marco: *L'homme de génie, traduit sur la VIe édition italienne par Fr. Colonna D'Istria et précédé d'une préface de M. Ch. Richet* Paris 1889, pp.

In spite of this the contemporary experimental Psychology observes more and more in daily life, some kind of physiological, non-pathological nervous restlessness, a special kind of backside or underground of cognition.

Since for example Benno Erdmann and Raymond Dodge in 1898 had totally atomized the reading process by a technical mechanism,[48] what could be more consequent than to translate the terms of psyche to these of the apparatus?[49]

This was also a remark of Mallarmé. In which he describes restlessness, vibrations, shimmer and discontinuity not merely in his own beginnings in literature but was able according to his time, to give a reference to experimental physiology of the optical perception. The emergence of the theory of neurons is another part of this history.

There were many serious reasons to consider modern literature as a nervous action of its own right and structure, the domain of poetry changes from writing hand to computing letters. The discrete Charm of typography, *the pure notation*![50]

Seen from this angle, modern poetry has really been another side of cognition, leading out from the field of psychiatry and experimental psychology of its time and accounting for a different concept of language – a concept taken up later on by linguistics and psychoanalysis.

## References

Aubert-Roche, Louis Rémy: *De la Peste ou typhus d'Orient, documens et observations recueillis pendant les années 1834 à 1838, en Égypte, en Arabie, sur la mer rouge, en Abyssinie, à Smyrne et à Constantinople. Suivis d'un essai sur le hachisch et son emploi dans le traitement de la Peste [...]* (Paris 1840).

Baudelaire, Charles: *Œuvres Complètes*, ed. by *Claude Pichois* Paris (Gallimard [Bibliothèque de la Pléiade]) 2004.

340–348]; in the case of other publications, the title speaks for itself: *La poésie décadente devant la science psychiatrique* (Émile Laurent, Paris 1897), *L'aliénation poétique. Rimbaud, Mallarmé, Proust* (Jean Fretet, Paris 1946). The list could be much longer, because the "[...] Stiftung eines Zusammenhangs zwischen Genie und Wahnsinn ist französischen Ursprungs" (the foundation of the relation between genius and mental illness is of French origins (Leibbrand and Wettley: *Der Wahnsinn*, p. 671)).

48 Erdmann and Dodge: *Psychologische Untersuchungen.*

49 The important consequences in the field of media history and theory were described by Friedrich Kittler.

50 Mallarmé: *Œuvres Complètes*, p. 368: *la notion pure.*

Benn, Gottfried: "Beitrag zur Geschichte der Psychiatrie", in: *Autobiographische und vermischte Schriften*, ed. by Dieter Wellershoff, Stuttgart (Klett-Cotta) $^{3}$1978.

Bersani, Leo: *The Death of Stéphane Mallarmé*, Cambridge (Cambridge University Press) 1982.

Broussais, Victor: *De l'Irritation et de la Folie, ouvrage dans lequel les rapports du physique et du moral sont établis sur les bases de la médecine physiologique* (Paris 1828).

Cabanis, Pierre-Jean-Georges: *Œuvres Philosophiques*, ed. by Claude Lehec and Jean Cazeneuve, Vol. 2, Paris (Presses Universitaires de France [Corpus Général des Philosophes Français, Auteurs Modernes, Vol. XLIV,1]) 1956.

Castel, Robert: *L'ordre psychiatrique. L'Âge d'or de l'aliénisme*, Paris (Minuit) 1976.

Condillac, Etienne B. de: *Essai sur l'origine des connaissances humaines, éd. établie par Raymond Lenoir*, Paris (Armand Colin) 1924.

Crichton, Alexander: *An Inquiry into the nature and origin of mental derangement. Comprehending a concise system of the physiology and pathology of the human mind. And a history of the passions and their effects* (London 1798).

Cullen, William: *Synopsis nosologiae methodicae [...]* (Leiden 1772).

De Banville, Théodore: *Petit traité de poésie française* (Paris 1872).

De Saussure, Ferdinand: *Cours de Linguistique Générale*, Lausanne-Paris (Payot) 1916.

Delahaye, Ernest: *Souvenirs familiers à propos de Rimbaud, Verlaine, Germaine Nouveau*, Paris (Albert Messein) 1925.

Erdmann, Benno and Raymond Dodge: *Psychologische Untersuchungen über das Lesen auf experimenteller Grundlage* (Halle 1898).

Flechsig, Paul: *Die Localisation der geistigen Vorgänge insbesondere der Sinnesempfindungen des Menschen* (Leipzig 1896).

Fretet, Charles: *L'aliénation poétique. Rimbaud, Mallarmé, Proust*, Paris (J. B. Janin) 1946.

Freud, Sigmund: *Gesammelte Werke chronologisch geordnet*, ed. by Anna Freud et al., Vol. 1, Frankfurt am Main (S. Fischer) 1999.

Friedrich, Hugo: *Die Struktur der modernen Lyrik. Von der Mitte des neunzehnten bis zur Mitte des zwanzigsten Jahrhunderts,* Hamburg (Rowohlt) $^{9}$1979.

Laurent, Émile: *La poésie décadente devant la science psychiatrique* (Paris 1897).

Leibbrand, Werner and Annemarie Wettley: *Der Wahnsinn. Geschichte der abendländischen Psychopathologie*, Freiburg im Breisgau (Karl Alber) 1961.

Leibniz, G.W.: "αποκατάστασις (πάντων)", in: Max Ettlinger: *Leibniz als Geschichtsphilosoph. Mit Beigabe eines bisher unveröffentlichten Leibnizfrag-*

*mentes über «Die Wiederherstellung aller Dinge»*, München (Rösel und Pustet) 1921.

Leroi-Gourhan, André: *Hand und Wort. Die Evolution von Technik, Sprache und Kunst*, Frankfurt am Main (Suhrkamp) [3]1984.

Lévi-Strauss, Claude: *Science et conscience de la société. Mélanges en l'honneur de Raymond Aron*, Paris (Calman Lévy) 1971.

Lombroso, Cesare Ezechio Marco: *L'homme de génie, traduit sur la VIe édition italienne par Fr. Colonna D'Istria et précédé d'une préface de M. Ch. Richet* (Paris 1889).

Mallarmé, Stéphane: *Œuvres Complètes*, Paris (Gallimard [Bibliothèque de la Pléiade]) 1996.

Moreau de Tours, Jacques-Joseph : *Du Hachisch et de l'aliénation mentale. Études psychologiques* Paris 1845.

Nerval, Gérard de : *Œuvres Complètes en trois volumes. Édition publiée sous la direction de Jean Guillaume et de Claude Pichois et al.* Paris (Gallimard [Bibliothèque de la Pléiade]) 1989–1993.

Nietzsche, Friedrich: *Nachgelassene Fragmente 1884–1885* (= *Kritische Studienausgabe*, Vol 11), ed. by Giorgio Colli and Mazzino Montinari, Munich / Berlin / New York [2]1988.

Rimbaud, Arthur: *Œuvres Complètes*, Paris (Gallimard: [Bibliothèque de la Pléiade]) 2005.

# The Physiology of Thought
# Neuroplasticity in Lancelot Law Whyte's Model of "Unitary Thought" and Richard Hamilton's 1951 *Growth and F*orm Exhibition

ISABELLE MOFFAT

> Aesthetics is no longer an isolated science of beauty; science can no longer neglect aesthetic factors. Aspects of Form discusses this rapprochement from several specialized points of view, and the editor, Mr. L.L. Whyte, brings the whole discussion within the focus of that unitary principle which is emerging as the explanation of all phenomena within the range of human perception and understanding.[1]
>
> Herbert Read, Preface to *Aspects of Form*, edited by Lancelot Law Whyte, accompanying Growth and Form.

Like many institutions in London and around the country, the Institute of Contemporary Arts [ICA], with which members of the Independent Group were already involved, actively participated in the 1951 Festival of Britain. The ICA organized two exhibitions that loosely corresponded to the Festival's themes of national stock-taking, good-natured technological optimism, and vernacular scientism. One of them was a historical survey entitled *Ten Decades – A Review of British Taste 1851–1951*, duly recalling the earlier *Great Exhibition* which, with the immense image-making success it had provided England in the previous century, originally inspired the Festival, before circumstances forced a national rather than international celebration of a new Britain.

The ICA's first exhibition to open during the Festival summer, though, was the rather less conventional one-room installation largely conceived and executed by Richard Hamilton, *Growth and Form*. Like his later show, *Man, Machine and Motion*, *Growth and Form* was an attempt to make the modern spectator aware of the changes human life, and with it human perception, had undergone. "Growth and Form," as Hamilton later said, "dealt with the natural world," whereas *Man, Machine and Motion* was "a survey of appliances invented by men to overcome the limits imposed on them by the physical attributes provided by nature."[2] In other words, *Growth and Form* explored the impact of science on our

1 Read: *Aspects of Form*, p. vi.
2 Hamilton: *Collected Words: 1952–1982*, p. 18.

perception of nature, and *Man, Machine and Motion* the impact of technology on our perception of the moving world.

In his first proposal written for Herbert Read in 1949, Hamilton discussed the importance D'Arcy Thompson's book had for him and how he wanted to translate the book's key principles visually. Hamilton's lively interest in form and in the laws of its creation and his confidence in finding answers in Thompson's theses come across at once:

> The initial stimulus for the proposed exhibition was provided by Thompson's book *On Growth and Form*. The visual interest of this field, where biology, chemistry, physics and mathematics overlap was considered an excellent subject for presentation in purely visual terms. The laws of growth and form pertaining to the processes of nature are quite contrary to the processes of artistic creation. However complex the form (accepting Thompson's hypothesis) it is the result of very precise physical laws; the complexities of art, on the other hand, are the products of involved psychological processes.[3]

What is at stake here for Hamilton is the difference between art and organic form and the processes of their creation. "The complexities of art," as he says, "are the products of involved psychological processes;" organic form, however, is free of psychology and intentionality. Hamilton draws a distinction between the naturalness and inherent laws of necessity underlying organic creation, represented in Growth and Form by photographic depictions taken from the world of science, and the deliberately created work of art. Moreover, the images themselves, produced by scientists with scientific apparatuses, are considered entirely in visual terms. Cleansed by science, Hamilton suggests, these forms are free of any connotative meanings and guarantee a kind of directness that he sought also to translate into his art.

Accompanying Hamilton's exhibition was *Aspects of Form*, a book edited by Lancelot Law Whyte. The book included texts by a broad range of thinkers on topics ranging from mathematics, organic chemistry, the early study of brain waves to physics and plant life.[4] The contributors to *Aspects* who were not strictly speaking scientists were in the minority: Konrad Lorenz, Rudolf Arnheim and Ernst Gombrich.

Analyzing how these distinct positions could gather around this show – at this historical moment and its intellectual climate – is the goal of the larger project from which this text is taken. Each position has a longer history, dating

3 Hamilton: *Growth and Form Exhibition, First Draft Schedule*, reprinted in Jacob: *Die Entwicklung der Pop Art in England*, p. 166. (Jacob dates it 1949; the pages have no date, but the cover page preceding the text in the file reads "20 December 1950.")

4 A survey of the list of contributors reads like a collection of the eminent scientists of the time, among them, J. Needham, C.H. Waddington, C.C.L. Gregory, F.C. Gregory, A. Dalcq, H.B. Cott, W. Grey Walter, S.P.F. Humphreys-Owens; several of them were also on the organizing committee of *Growth and Form*, in addition to Jacob Bronowski, J.R.M. Brumwell, A. Comfort and, of course, Lancelot Law Whyte.

back to idcas about science and perception, from the influence of logical positivist ideas on the Bauhaus, especially Moholy-Nagy, and the later popularization of those ideas in England through A.J. Ayer; from German Romanticism, Neo-Kantian philosophy and Gestalt psychology to Gombrich's adaptation of certain ideas of Karl Popper's – and they continue their divergent trajectories after this brief intersection. What is important in the context of this project is to examine what made *Growth and Form* so legible for many different points of view, and in this regard Whyte represents an important position in postwar England, not because of the permanence of his influence, but because of the hybridity of his position and its brief but ardent popularity at this moment in time.

Herbert Read's circa 350-word preface to *Aspects of Form* that precedes this essay conveys his hope for the ability of a universalizing aesthetics to account for the role of form in naturc and in the form-giving activities of man. Densely packed with some of the assumptions found in Read's work on poetry, his introductions to the history of art, and his wartime political tracts, the preface, together with his foreword to the small brochure for *Growth and Form,* may offer the most confident formulation of his interest in scientific thought.

What is particularly striking however is the importance Read gives to Whyte's work. Even the casual style with which this short text claims profoundly new ground cannot quite dampen the hyperbole of Read's final statement in this preface: "Mr. L.L. Whyte brings the whole discussion within the focus of that unitary principle which is emerging as the explanation of all phenomena within the range of human perception and understanding."[5] Read's certainty in the "intellectual promise" of the unitary principle is startling. Not least because, as compelling as it seemed to Read then, Whyte's ideas entirely disappeared from intellectual debate as the vogue for holistic models for making sense of the world temporarily abated.

Who, then, was this man and what gave Read the confidence to make these claims?

In a decade in which "everyone" and "everyman" wanted to be a scientist, wanted to reform their discipline into a scientific endeavor, Whyte was – if only for a few moments – a perfect hybrid.[6] He had the legitimizing credentials of a

5 Read: preface to *Aspects of Form*, p. vi.

6 By training, Whyte was a scientist, but he had abandoned Physics for a career in the jet engine industry. In the late twenties he began writing about the interdependence of the natural sciences, philosophy and psychology, but it was not until 1944, with his *The Next Development in Man*, that he fully articulated his notion of unitary thought. Between 1944 and 1954 he published six books, all expanding on this idea. The following decade he spent teaching at Harvard and, later, at Stanford. At first his appointments were in physics and biophysics, but later on his disciplinary affiliations were less straightforward, as, for instance, at Stanford where he was a Fellow at the Center for Advanced Studies in the Behavioral Sciences; in the 1960s his published works seem to hover in the interstices between religious mysticism and scientific inquiry. When, in 1972, he died, he had traveled to the periphery of academia but was still writing popular essays and giving lecture tours in the Unites States. His death was

scientist and of an ostensibly scientific method, and what further distinguishes Whyte in the context of *Growth and Form* and the *Aspects of Form* book is the eclecticism of his point of view which sought to relate matter (a subject he had first studied as a young man at University with Russell), the psyche (he was greatly influenced by Freudian and Jungian psychoanalytic theories and in 1960 he published a book on the *Unconscious Before Freud*), and form. The combination could not have been more appropriate for these two projects.

In the late forties and early fifties Whyte was at his heyday.[7] His programmatic books, *The Next Development in Man* and *Everyman Looks Forward*, published in England in 1944 and 1946, respectively, abound with hopeful enthusiasm for a new future of man. His ringing declarations, laced with apocalyptic fears, foresee a communal future, but one without the burdens of communist politics; accordingly he writes, "the historical trend which is now forming the unitary world is the expression neither of idealism nor of animal self-interest, but of the formative vitality of the community and its members."[8] The utopian tenet of Whyte's thought collapses under the pressures of practical application, yet this helplessness should not obscure his momentary influence.

In a contemporary review of *The Next Development in Man* in *The Philosophical Review*, Harold A. Larrabee called the book a combination of a "philosophical tract and [an] exercise in prophecy."[9] Larrabee was not entirely convinced by Whyte's book and remonstrated its author for failing to back up his plea for "unitary man" with practical solutions for bringing about this change. "Now it is one thing to join in the general clamor for the integration of the sciences and the humanities," Larrabee complained,

> but it is another to show how it may be brought about in practice….it seems at times as if Mr. Whyte were relying much too heavily on the magic of "the uttered word, 'unitary,'" rather than upon the scientific evidence of which he speaks so highly.[10]

Larrabee concludes his review of Whyte's book by noting about the author: "as a prophet, he is stimulating but vague; as a critic of ideas, or philosopher, he leaves much to be desired."[11] Indeed, the book's conflation of physiological processes, psychology, scientific-sounding analyses, and mysticism is so eccentric and arbitrary at times, that one can understand the exasperation of reviewers.

mourned predominantly in specialized publications such as *Isis* and *The British Journal for the History of Science*.

7 Several of his books were published in short succession during this period: *The Next Development in Man*, *Everyman Looks Forward, The Unitary Principle in Physics and Biology*, *Aspects of Form*, and *Accent on Form*.

8 Whyte: *The Next Development in Man*, p. 244.

9 Larrabee: "Review of *The Next Development in Man*", pp. 386f.

10 Ibid., p. 387.

11 Ibid., p. 387.

At the same time, Whyte's eclecticism served a purpose in the immediate postwar decade and this daringness to cross interdisciplinary borders, combined with his passionate style, gained him some influence and also won him passionate admirers. Just as the impact of A.J. Ayer's *Language, Truth, and Logic* has often been attributed to the style of the book – the deeply-felt conviction it exuded and the youthful enthusiasm it managed to inspire – Whyte's writings must be seen in light of a similar emotional charge; as in the case of Ayer's book, the conviction of Whyte's prose initially determined its success, not its theoretical rigor or lack thereof. Whyte was an expansive and original thinker, who drew together aspects from different disciplines and linked ideas that other thinkers could or would not combine. As one commentator wrote: "Scientists tend to complain that Whyte's ideas are difficult to grasp, often closer to metaphysics than to science, and supported by too little experimental evidence. Others, however, even when they do not accept his arguments, are stimulated by the 'brilliance and daring' of his thought, his willingness to grapple with really fundamental questions."[12] Or, as Arthur Koestler wrote in the introduction to Whyte's book on the unconscious,

> from physics he turned to biology and published a series of unorthodox but scholarly and well-documented books which turned him into a minor cult-figure among scientists discontented with the prevailing reductionist *Zeitgeist*. In spite of his heretical views, he was elected Chairman of the Philosophy of Science group of the British Society for the History of Science and held office from 1953 to 1955; [...]. He possessed great charm, equalled only by his insatiable intellectual appetite.[13]

Koestler ends his brief introduction to the 1978 reprint of *The Unconscious Before Freud* with a quote from Whyte's obituary which appeared in *The British Journal for the Philosophy of Science*. It was the perfect epitaph, Koestler notes, and indeed it corresponds closely with the image I have been trying to paint:

> Although it is too soon to say which of Lancelot Whyte's many ideas will bear fruit, the catholicity of his interests and the unorthodoxy of his views, coupled with his infectious enthusiasm, acted as an intellectual stimulus. He was a fascinating talker and had an unrivalled gift for bringing together people with similar interests who, but for him, would probably never have met. Many of us owe him a great debt for encouraging us to look at old problems in a new way.[14]

This discussion of Whyte's "unitary thought" does not want to decide the success or failure of its philosophical argument nor pass judgment on the merits of its scientific credibility. My objective is not to judge the veracity of Whyte's model, but rather to give a sense of his theory, his terminology, and of the urgency and

12 No author: "Whyte, Lancelot Law", p. 1545.

13 Koestler: Introduction to Whyte: *The Unconscious Before Freud*, no page number.

14 From an obituary notice by Professor Whitrow, quoted in Koestler: Introduction to Whyte: *The Unconscious Before Freud*, no page number.

conviction he managed to communicate with his texts. It is not always easy to summarize his trains of thought succinctly, because they are not succinct. Any attempt to rephrase his theories in one's own words acts a little bit like a disenchantment – the spell is broken and the magic dissipates. When his critic spoke of "the magic of the uttered word, 'unitary'" the analogy was apt; Whyte's language enacts his theory's analogy between the workings of the smallest organisms with human development, constantly invoking the metaphorical significance of the formal characteristics of cellular symmetry, harmony and order, making his texts a rich mixture of Romantic notions of unity, organicist holism and the philosophy of science.

Whyte's *The Next Development in Man* is all that his critics allege: it is messy, idealistic and eclectic. In it, Whyte constructs an intellectual history in which he opposes analytic thought with a new form which he calls unitary thought. His model postulates that "unitary thought" has become necessary because only an understanding of man's unity with nature and all its processes will save man from extinction. "Analytic thought" has been too static and too atomist to allow this new kind of thought to develop. He writes:

> The analytical method studies permanence and conservation, the unitary method development.... The analytical method has to its credit the cumulative achievements of more than two thousand years of thought and experiment, yet it cannot account for the development of form. It was developed first because, as we shall see, it corresponded to the structure of thought during one stage of the development of mind.[15]

For Whyte that stage of intellectual evolution has come to an end and it is time for a fundamental shift in human intellectual development: "Humanist man was an explorer; he tore aside the veil of religion and rejoiced in the expansion of his powers. Unitary man is an organizer; he sets out to order his finite world."[16] Previous (analytic) models of thought with their binary oppositions, Whyte holds, have warped the human psyche and poisoned our minds, both metaphorically, and as he will later on explain in terms of the physiological strain they exerted, literally.

Science, in this model, is an all-cleansing, all-forgiving power and it is the ordering power of science that will solve humanities *dilemma.* But his notion of science is a specific one: while traditional religion cannot satisfy the needs of unitary man, it now will be based on science, just as science will no longer be at a remove from life because it will become one with feeling and action. "The human need for unity first created subjective religion, then objective analytical science; now it corrects the partiality of these attitudes by substituting one complete doctrine."[17]

15 Ibid.
16 Whyte: *The Next Development in Man*, p. 263.
17 Ibid., p. 218.

According to Whyte, the single aim of science is "the search for unity in diversity and for continuity in change."[18] The ability of science to act as a kind of filter, eliminating the clutter of human subjectivity and guaranteeing a kind of innocence of intent have made scientific method the harbinger of Whyte's unitary thought. He writes: "Science is the elimination of the arbitrary ....the scientific attitude recognises the diversity in detail and yet seeks to find a single ordering principle." [19] Whyte's emphasis is on the systematization of knowledge, as it was for Neurath or Moholy-Nagy. But in Whyte's text science is given even an even greater power to unify and pacify. The "innocence" of scientific knowledge Whyte asserted earlier is an active, a therapeutic one. In his model science is reconfigured as holistic process in which discovery and knowledge have become one: "Static thought divided scientific prediction into two part: the identification of a system, and the discovery of its laws. But unitary thought, by postulating one universal law, combines these into one: the identification of the particular form whose development characterizes the system."[20] Whyte's hopes go much further though when he writes in a later chapter: "subjective attitudes have to be tested against [unitary conviction] and the facts of analytical science re-interpreted through it so that the duality of subjective and objective knowledge may disappear. From this restoration of the unity of thought there comes a new vigor: knowledge from science becomes inseparable from knowledge for action, and thought no longer delays but kindles action."[21] Whyte alludes to the connection between thought and physiology; in such a model the right thinking and knowing will in itself be curative: "Unitary thought is a guide to correct thought because it organises knowledge in conformity with the laws of nature."[22] Whyte believes he can change the way humanity thinks and, with it, humanity itself.

## The Physiology of Thought

When Whyte subsequently writes "The chief task of unitary thought in the organic world is the study of the failure of proper organic development and its interpretation as the consequence of some other overriding process of development,"[23] he means much more than a molecular process, namely, the human psyche or a social system. Apart from this methodological analogy between a molecular process

18 Whyte: *The Next Development in Man*, pp. 17f.
19 Ibid.
20 Ibid., p. 240.
21 Ibid., p. 218. Whyte's notion of unity is also reminiscent of Husserl's notion of regaining the "primordial oneness of all consciousness." See Jay: *Downcast Eyes*, p. 268.
22 Whyte: *The Next Development in Man*, p. 30.
23 Ibid., p. 41.

and a social organization, Whyte strives for a greater unity yet: one of matter and mind.

> We are now in a position to approach the main dualism of European and western thought: the antithesis of matter and mind. In unitary thought these are regarded as names to aspects of process and the relation of the two has to be found through a unitary interpretation, not of these abstracted nouns, but of the adjectives *material* and *mental*. These terms, as used in unitary thought, do not imply any general dualism, because they are defined in relation to one universal form of process.[24]

We find Whyte distinguishing between a right and a wrong way to think. In this case he is referring to its "pattern," a term one might consider to include concepts, ideas, and ideologies. "If the general scheme of the pattern is wrong" he says, "we see confusion" where we should recognize the unity of nature. His plan is to ensure that the correct scheme will determine our perceptions. This correction is, of course, unitary thought:

> The unitary method of thought has this natural magic [to bring out the true form of nature]; it throws immediate light on certain aspects of the general arrangement of nature. It leads at once to simple universal principles, as relevant to man as to the rest of nature.[25]

But the human mind has already been affected by its thought processes, in particular, by the dualistic structure at the basis of Western humanist and analytical thought which, according to Whyte, originated in physiology: "The cardinal duality expresses itself in a dual development of the central nervous system which, in intellectual man, has broken out as a damaging dualism." Whyte develops an ingenious split, based on the separate functions of "retentive nerve masses of the brain" and "conducting fibres of the sensori-motor system." Whereas the former preserve form in time, the latter transport it in space. Whyte's physiological approach to time and space leads him to make far-reaching speculations about the evolution of man's brain. He notes:

> As the nervous system developed in the higher mammals, the nerves conducted more quickly and the brain became more retentive, the organism being thus better linked both to environment and to its own past. This specialisation of function was controlled by the formative tendencies of the dominant organising processes (in the brain and elsewhere) so that two types of structure co-operated, the interaction of past records and present stimuli producing new responses.[26]
>
> But the divergent tendency of the specialised structures constituted an organic weakness, which sooner or later was bound to make trouble, as it did finally in intellectual man. Each structure tended to dominate the system. The higher brain, with its organised record of the

24 Whyte: *The Next Development in Man*, pp. 41f.
25 Ibid., p. 44.
26 Ibid., pp. 46f.

> past, tended to organise behaviour by facilitating the deliberate repetition of processes which had successfully organised behaviour in the past. But the afferent nerves, perpetually drawing the attention of the individual to present stimuli, tended to produce swift responses and to challenge the control of the deliberating head. A proper differentiation of the nervous system thus was converted into the conflict of cortex and hypothalamus, of reason and instinct, of slow deliberate responses based on continuity with the rationally organised experience of the past and immediate instinctive responses to present situations. Yet in man instinct plays a reduced role. If certain special conditions had not prejudiced the integrity of the organising processes, this duality in the nervous system might never have become the dualism which lies so deep in the experience of European man.[27]

With this physiology of the intellectual development of Western man, Whyte has established a connection between molecular and organic development. By implication Whyte is suggesting that the "proper" thought can still influence the physiology of the human brain.

## Aspects of Form

C'est la dissymétrie qui crée le phénomène. (Curie)

From the frontispiece of
*The Unitary Principle in Physics and Biology*

The discussion of *Next Development* shows the important role which form plays in Whyte's model as record of the process of development. His focus on form seeks to identify a single unitary principle. This he claims to have found in the decrease of asymmetry. Whyte's introduction to *Aspects of Form* constructs his unitary train of thought from inorganic to organic matter, to astronomy, biology, plant life and biochemistry, to embryology, animal form, and finally to the first of the three Gestaltist essays, Lorenz' "The Role of Gestalt Perception in Animal and Human Behaviour"; Arnheim's "Gestalt Psychology and Artistic Form" follows after an interlude on activity patterns in the human brain; the final essay is Gombrich's "Meditations." The sequence is intriguing: in a progression from the inorganic, to the organic, to plant and animal life, and finally human brain function and creative impulse, it enacts Whyte's theory of the unitary principle – the relatedness of the molecule to human behavior, through pattern, process, form, and shape.

"Exact science," Whyte notes, "seems to know much, and yet it has so far only got to grips with the simplest forms such as crystals and bubbles. Complex forms still baffle it. All the powers of science do not let us see into the growing point of a plant, or the dominant centers of an embryo, or the grey matter of the

27 Whyte: *The Next Development in Man*, pp. 46f.

brain, and understand exactly what is going on there when new forms develop. Our eyes look out on a complex world, but the brain unconsciously selects what interests us and makes it seem simple."[28] This an intriguing model, partially based on the instinct theory of the Gestalt psychologists; some forms, it suggests, are more "significant" than others, and are better recognized and understood, even though this process appears to bypass conscious thought.

There is no "scientific philosophy of form" Whyte holds and *Aspects* is an attempt to remedy this lack. The essays, Whyte explains, only deal with spatial form, not musical, abstract mathematical, or linguistic thought, psychology, or society, yet he gives no specific reason for the exclusion of, for example, music. He writes, "Common to the ideas of form, configuration, pattern, and structure, is the notion of an ordered complexity, a multiplicity which is governed by some unifying principle. Our theme is thus the *realisation of unity of spatial form in the complex processes of physics, biology, psychology, and art.* But "form" includes development and transformation."[29] Again, Whyte poses the problem in terms of long-standing binaries that now need to be overcome: the sets that have been posed as opposites in the debate are, firstly, "atomism – material analysis – quantitative precision" and, secondly, "form – unity – symmetry." This goes hand-in-hand with his proposals, voiced earlier in *The Next Development in Man*, and *Everyman Looks Forward*, that the time has come to erase the split between mind and matter, between object and subject. "There are signs that this antithesis must now be overcome, that if science is to advance it must discover how the ordering of parts gives form to the whole, in organisms for example."[30] The notion of a unifying principle is invoked here, but the allusion to some kind of all-encompassing system of belief is hard to suppress.

Only that Whyte doesn't seem to favor such an ideological solution. His is a mystical wholeness that is both of man and not of man. He is appealing to an inner logic that he takes in part from his discussions of form: the all-encompassing principle, as he said in *The Next Development in Man*, is the "decrease of asymmetry." That is a rather broad brush, but also one that obscures the potential for rigidity and authoritarianism that such a normative model, striving for a harmony considered "healthy" for the system, can entail. This authoritarian potential is shrouded in utopian credos when he writes that "the unitary tradition will not only satisfy the need for authority, but assuage the demand for mystery by revealing to a generation hungry for magic the scientific miracle of an unsuspected unity in nature."[31] Yet, this symmetrical healthfulness is contrasted with the "organic weakness" of the dualism of the human mind. As we have seen in *The Next Development of Man*, Whyte makes an even stronger case for the destructiveness of dualistic thinking. In that book it is considered both result of a

28 Whyte: Introduction to *Aspects of Form*, p. 1.
29 Ibid., p. 2. [his emphasis]
30 Ibid., p. 3.
31 Whyte: *The Next Development in Man*, p. 265.

physiological dualism and an evolutionary change resulting from a psychological dualism. The terminology is already somewhat alarming, but when the ordering principle becomes one of harmony, symmetry, order, and the decrease of asymmetry, as it does in his *Aspects* text, the memory of national-socialist terminology of racial health and degeneration comes to mind. It is, however, also consistent with the politics of consensus; it is an odd dream that is curiously appropriate for the cold-war climate in postwar Britain: a non-communist commune, a pacifist authoritarianism, and a benevolent and consensual conformism.

After introducing several of the more strictly scientific and specialized papers – from a physicist's view of the atom, an astronomer's discovery of conic sections in the heavens, the contrast between healthy and pathological biological forms, the interplay of external and internal forces in growth, to the role of *highly specialized molecular units* in the creation of organic form – Whyte's introduction comes to the article that had so inspired Read in his *True Voice*. About this essay, Albert Dalcq's "Form and Modern Embryology," he writes that the author "takes up the story of the *development of animal form and function* from the original fertilised egg," submitting "that the processes of embryological development in man seem to anticipate and prepare the subsequent development of the human mind,"[32] literally. It is a notion reminiscent of Whyte's earlier statement which suggested that knowing about the form of a protein would tell him more about the processes fueled by this chemical component to organic life and allow him to understand better, for example, the process of writing a sentence. It is a step on the route toward equating the thinking matter with thought, of accounting for thought and its shape by examining the physiology of thought.

The book gives the impression of being itself an attempt of Lancelot Law Whyte's to construct his unitary thought by bringing together these disparate realms of knowledge. His short summary of the texts reinforces this view as he constructs a narrative progression, culminating with Gombrich's essay on the roots of aesthetic form, the last in the collection. In Whyte's retelling, the article on brain patterns follows and he expects great discoveries from this "entirely new realm of knowledge" where "for the first time the processes of the brain and the activities of the mind, to use two descriptions of one thing [!], are subject to exact investigation and some degree of direct experimental control."[33] If, as Whyte suggests here, brain and mind are considered coterminous then thought, and with it consciousness, and the natural sciences are thought to be unified under a common principle.

In the introduction to *Aspects of Form* Whyte makes the link between the laws of form in nature and man's evolution and the laws of form in aesthetics explicit. "From these brain activity patterns [discussed in W. Grey Walter's essay] it is a small step to the rôle of the visually-perceived configuration in deter-

32 Whyte: Introduction to *Aspects of Form*, p. 5 [his emphasis]. This essay also plays a prominent role in Whyte's later book, *Accent on Form*.

33 Whyte: Introduction to *Aspects of Form*, p. 6.

mining aesthetic qualities. Arnheim shows how the *aesthetic significance* of a particular form depends not only on its actual shape and structure, but also on the formative processes of perception, the personal needs and tensions of the perceiver, and on his social and historical context."[34] The discussion of aesthetics in Gestaltist terms represents the evolution from nature to culture in this narrative Whyte has constructed. From the instinctual and behaviorist importance of form of which Lorenz speaks, to the "aesthetic significance" of Arnheim, ultimately, to Gombrich's amalgamation of biological and psychological needs in an emotionally-charged image. Hence Whyte writes: "Finally, to close our survey, Gombrich takes us for a ride on his hobby horse towards the conclusion that the root characteristic of aesthetic creation is not representation, image-forming, or abstraction, but simply the *making of a functional substitute*, an object which can serve in place an original (or desired) experience in respect of some function or need of the individual. Here again the significance of a form is seen to depend on the total organic situation within which it appears."[35] To some extent Whyte's narration of the consecutive texts follows, of course, the convention of the introduction to any book that includes several essays from different authors; still, Whyte gives them a coherence that they achieve only in his own, unitary method of thought.

In order to discuss the significance of Whyte's ideas for Read, *the Growth and Form* exhibition, and the Independent Group, let us highlight a few key points from the earlier more detailed discussion of Lancelot Law Whyte's unitary thought, as he presented them in *The Next Development in Man* and *Everyman Looks Forward*. Whyte's identification of the destructiveness of analytic thought and of any binary model of human consciousness prepares the way for his unitarism. Since the classification of behavior into good and evil, the separation of mind and body, of thought and action has had a degenerative effect on human ethics, thought, and on the human brain itself, this binary construction of human life and consciousness must be overcome. Once unitary thought has healed these rifts, the previous, dualistic model of man, thought, and world will be obsolete. According to this model all previously-held dualisms – such as those inherent in Christian doctrine and Western philosophy – will be meaningless. Binaries such as man/nature, mind/matter, thought/action, subject/object, will be distinctions erased by "unitary man."

According to Whyte, the catalyst for the momentous change from a dualistic world view to one of unitary thought is the ordering power of science. It will augment the power of the unifying principle underlying all and everything: one expression of this principle, so Whyte, is the "decrease of asymmetry." Importantly, the unitary principle is equally at work on a molecular as on a social level. In Read's words, they are "on an identical plane of enquiry."[36] This anthropo-

34 Whyte: Introduction to *Aspects of Form*, p. 6.
35 Whyte: Introduction to *Aspects of Form*, p. 6.
36 Read: *Aspects of Form*, p. vi.

morphic notion of cells (and vice versa, if you will) is an important assumption in this model and, again, according to Whyte, it is science that has begun to expose these connections and has made this step toward unitary thought possible.

For Read, as has been pointed out earlier, Whyte's model offered a scientific explanation of a Romantic notion of man and nature in (spiritual) unison. Moreover, it gave credence to his claims that thought has a physiologically constitutive function for the brain. The formative role Read claimed for art and creativity in the history of human civilization, finds its scientific equivalent in the claims of Whyte that thought not only has the ability to shape consciousness but has a physiological equivalent in brain patterns.

Hamilton's arrangement in *Growth and Form* of photographs, drawings, models and films of "atomic particle traces, crystal structures, chromosomes and cell divisions, marine larvae, skeletal structures, plant forms, and more presented on a free-standing frame system as well as on walls, ceiling and floor."[37] might be seen as part of a visual re-education. He thought of his exhibitions as "didactic," even if retrospectively he began calling them "installations," and he continued to stress his effort for an education of the viewer by "*forcing*" them to see. Judging from installation shots, it appears that the spectator must have had some sense of descending into cell structures themselves – a distinctly surreal impression of being reduced to the size of blood cells and wandering among multiplying minute organisms and cell clusters. One contemporary reviewer noted the darkness of the exhibition space, in which "shapes and forms move on screens on the ceilings or on the floor. Projected on the ceiling was the drama of crystal formation; on another screen, sea urchin's eggs divided themselves."[38] The sense of dislocation and spatial confusion that radiates from this reviewer's description is repeated in the visual and spatial tricks that will dominate Hamilton's later contribution to This is Tomorrow.

Lancelot Law Whyte's epistemological model insisted on the parallelism of molecular, human, and social processes. The integration of images from biology, chemistry and astronomy, then, is justified by the unitary principle inherent in and organizing all. The role as arbiter of unitary truth, so to speak, that Whyte has chosen for science, is carried through to *Growth and Form*, where the scientific credentials of the images constitute a conceptual umbrella under which the diversity is subsumed (i.e. the difference between X-ray and molecular model, between static image and filmed process). Moreover, the scientific ancestry of the imagery is understood to guarantee their objectivity and a complete absence of any political connotations – just as Whyte's model of unity professes the absence of any political ideology.

His notion of a physiology of thought, namely of a neuroplasticity corresponding to patterns of thought that could entail either productive, almost thera-

37 Whitham: *The Independent Group*, p. 45.
38 Ibid., p. 46.

peutic, effects on the one hand and "destructive" ones on the other, was one of the sources that allowed Hamilton to think of perception as malleable, both on an individual level and on a social level.

## References

Hamilton: "Growth and Form Exhibition, First Draft Schedule", in: *ICA Papers, Tate Gallery Archive TGA 955.1.12.26* [1949], reprinted in Jacob: *Die Entwicklung der Pop Art in England – von ihren Anfängen bis 1957: das Fine-Populart Art Continuum*, Frankfurt am Main/New York (Peter Lang) 1986, p. 166.

Hamilton, Richard: *Collected Words: 1952–1982*, London and New York (Thames and Hudson) 1982.

Jay, Martin: *Downcast Eyes, The Denigration of Vision in Twentieth-Century French Thought,* Berkeley (University of California Press) 1994.

Koestler, Arthur: "Introduction", in: Lancelot Law Whyte: *The Unconscious Before Freud*, London and New York (Julian Friedmann Publishers and St. Martin's Press) 1978.

Larrabee, Harold: "Review of *The Next Development in Man* by Lancelot Law Whyte", in: *The Philosophical Review*, Volume 58 (1949) Issue 4/July, pp. 386f.

Whitham, Graham: *The Independent Group at the Institute of Contemporary Arts: its Origins, Development, and Influences 1951–1961*, Ph.D. diss. University of Kent at Canterbury, 1986.

Whyte, Lancelot Law: *The Next Development in Man*, London (The Cresset Press) 1944.

Whyte, Lancelot Law: *Everyman Looks Forward* (1946), New York (Holt) 1948.

Whyte, Lancelot Law: *The Unitary Principle in Physics and Biology* (1949), New York (Holt) 1949.

Whyte, Lancelot Law (ed.): *Aspects of Form*, with preface by Herbert Read, London (Lund Humphries) 1951.

Whyte, Lancelot Law, *Accent on Form* (1954), Santa Barbara CA (Greenwood Press) 1973.

Lancelot Law Whyte: *The Unconscious Before Freud*, London and New York (Julian Friedmann Publishers and St. Martin's Press) 1978.

No author: "Whyte, Lancelot Law", in: Wakemann, John (ed.): *World Authors 1950–1970,* New York (H.W. Wilson Company) 1975.

# Reflexes in Brain Research
# Images, Practices and Diagrams[1]

YVONNE WÜBBEN

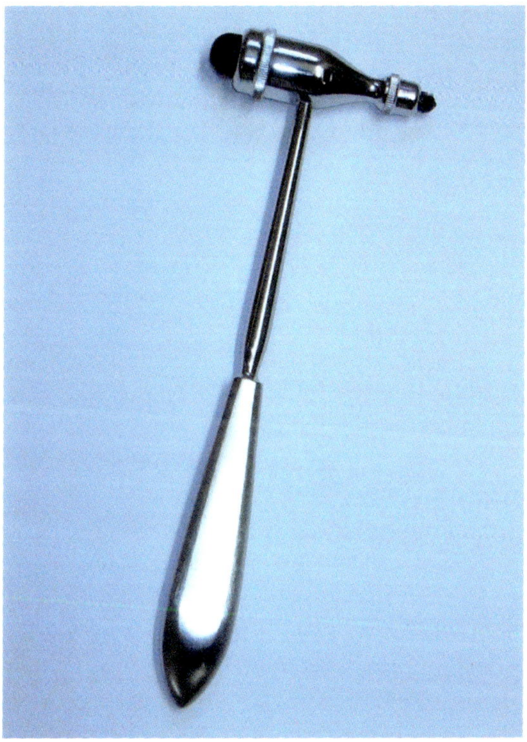

Fig. 1: A reflex hammer 'Modell Trömner'.

Like the stethoscope and other mobile diagnostic instruments, the reflex hammer can be considered an emblem of professionalization.[2] It symbolizes a diagnostic practice – testing reflexes – that has belonged to the basic inventory of determining neurological status since 1870 and has been included in clinical forms.[3] Testing reflexes is standard practice today. But of importance is not just the medical practice, but rather the fact that every test not only triggers a reflex, but also updates knowledge about reflexes. So, in terms of the history of knowledge, one could provocatively ask: which came first, the practices and images, or the knowledge about reflexes?

Knowledge about reflexes has evolved through history, and, as I would like to show in this essay, has developed above all along images and practices. In addition, and this is how my talk connects to the general theme of the conference, it is

1 This paper is a translated and extended English version of Yvonne Wübben: "Transhumane Physiologie. Bilder und Praktiken des Reflexes (Thomas Willis, Robert Whytt, Marshall Hall)", in: Christoph Lüthy (ed.): *Early Science and Medicine*, Vol 25. Leiden 2010, pp. 105–121.

2 Troemner: "Ein neuer Reflexhammer", and "Ueber Sehnen- resp. Muskelreflexe".

3 Gowers: *The Diagnosis of Disease of the Spinal Cord.*

not only knowledge about reflexes which was conveyed via images and practices, but at the same time knowledge about the brain. The fact that research on reflexes and research on the brain were very closely interwoven is demonstrated by the mechanical orientation of brain research in 19$^{th}$ century and revealed not least by programmatic titles such as Ivan Mikhaylovich Sechenov's work "Reflexes of the Brain," first published in Russian in 1863.[4]

I would like to demonstrate that the coupling of brain research and research on reflexes emerged co-evolutionary. Since the early modern period, the brain has no longer been merely an object of structural and descriptive anatomy and therefore just a place to be mapped. It has also been an object of physiology, that is, its functions were observed in relation to anatomical structures. Research on reflexes, more specifically: the practices and images of reflexes, were of central importance to the question of such functional cerebral relationships. In 1833, Marshall Hall defined the reflex as follows in his work "On the Reflex Function":

> This [new] property is characterized by being excited in its action, and reflex in its course: in every instance in which it is exerted, an impression made upon the extremities of certain nerves is conveyed to the medulla oblongata or the medulla spinalis, and is reflected along other nerves.[5]

This textbook definition is still valid today. In what follows, I would like to use this definition as a starting point to explain how practices and images have contributed to the forming of a concept of reflexes, and how Marshall Hall's concept became important in 19th-century brain research. My proposition is that the transfer between research on reflexes and brain research is based on traditions of scientific images of the early modern period as well as on the practices of research on reflexes.

Images and practices are important not only because they illustrate knowledge and serve to generate evidence.[6] They have contributed to the forming of knowledge because, as media or actions, they bear their own, non-discursive knowledge.[7] Without the experimental practices and without the images of the early modern period, I would like to argue, the reflex would not have developed into a concept, and the reflex model of the brain would not have become part of clinical research.

However, these aspects have hardly been taken into account in studies of the history of the concept of the reflex, for example those by Franklin Fearing of 1930 and George Canguilhem of 1955. These authors tended to look at the se-

4 Ivan Secenov: *Refleksy Golovnogo Mozga* (*Reflexes of the Brain*); Wübben and Vöhringer: *Phantome im Labor*.

5 Hall: "On the Reflex Function", p. 652.

6 Machamer: "17th Century Demonstrations".

7 Latour: "Drawing Things Together", p. 260.

mantic content, that is, the propositional knowledge, in research on functions relating to structures. Images and practices in their functions, as media of knowledge, were often neglected. Now, it cannot be argued that this applied to brain research to the same extent. There, the epistemic function of images has been emphasized many times. But this usually applied to the way anatomy depicted the brain, and less to the images and physiological practices of reflexes.

I ask you to join me in taking three steps: first to Thomas Willis, whose tractate on muscle movements formulates a central component of the concept of reflexes and who also includes the brain in his considerations, differentiating between the center and the periphery, as was the norm later on, too. I believe Willis's component of the concept of the reflex can be understood only if we also take account of the images of the day, images of the brain and pyrotechnics. Then, I will proceed to Robert Whytt's stimulus-response experiments. In his tractate on involuntary muscle movement, Whytt mentions practices which permit the concept of the reflex to be applied to functional brain research as well, as they lend the reflex response a new temporal dimension. And my final step is to Marshall Hall, whom I already quoted, and a physiological model of the brain which is based on the concept of the reflex and which takes up in a certain sense pictorial components of meaning of the early modern period, without, however, portraying the corresponding visualizations.

## I

I would like to begin my deliberations with the Oxford physician Thomas Willis, who introduced the term "motus reflexus" in his work "De motu musculari" (1680), and whom the reflex historian Georg Canguilhem named as the founder of the reflex in 1955.[8] Willis writes:

> motus utriusque generis est reflexus, qui silicet a sensione praevia tanquam causa evidenti aut occasione immediatius dependens, illico retorquetur.[9]

Willis called a movement "reflected" if it is preceded by a sensation and is "cast back" (retorquere) to the location of the sensation. Unlike Marshall Hall, he did not use the term in a functional way relating to structures, that is, he did not set it in relation to concrete anatomical conditions. On the contrary, Willis introduced

8 Canguilhem: *Die Herausbildung des Reflexbegriffes*.

9 Thomas Willis: *De motu musculari* [1644], quoted in: Canguilhem, *Die Herausbildung des Reflexbegriffes*, p. 86: "of these two movements we call the one reflected which follows a preceding sensation and which depends on this sensation as its cause or occasion."

an abstract classification of movements, much like Galen and Aristotle.[10] Reflex movements were characterized by being preceded by a cause (causa) or an occasion (occasio), and they consisted of two events that were basically distinct.[11] Willis used scratching in response to an itch as an example of such a reflex movement.[12] The stimulation is the sensation, and the scratching is the movement that follows. The passage quoted above has been interpreted as a precursor of the reflex concept, and the "casting back" has been understood as the switching over of the impulse in the spinal cord as described by Marshall Hall.[13] However, Willis's text lacks evidence that would justify such an interpretation at this point. For this reason, let us take another look at the text I just quoted. One of Willis's central examples of reflexes is the response of the heartbeat to warmth. It is true that Willis explained this movement physiologically. But he understood the contraction of the heart muscle as a kind of explosion,[14] thus making a connection between a phenomenon, the heartbeat, and an underlying physiological process. This connection, however, has no central consequences for the term "reflected" and thus for knowledge of reflexes understood in the specifically modern sense, as it applies to every process in the same way. For this reason, we must ask what the expression "cast back" means for reflexes in concrete terms.

Willis's figurative comparisons as well as the context of the time shed light on this question. When Willis compared muscle contraction with an explosion, he drew on the pyrotechnics of his day, as did Francis Glisson before him. It is likely that Willis was familiar with numerous images of pyrotechnics. I think that the relevance of pyrotechnics for Willis's physiology of movement and also the relevance of the component of the reflex – the "casting back" – can be understood only if we include contemporary images and their diagrammatic aspects. They show the spreading of the explosion as a relationship between center and periphery. Figure 2 shows a visualization of fireworks:

10 Aristoteles: *De motu animalium,* 703b2-21.

11 Willis: *Five Treatises*, p. 34.

12 Ibid.: "As to the original beginning of Motion, we shall take notice, that that which proceeds from the Brain, with a knowing and auspicious appetite, may be called Spontaneous or Voluntary; but that which is wont to be excited from the Cerebel where the Law of Nature presides, such as are Respiration, the Pulse, with many others, may be called merely Natural, or Involuntary; either of these is either direct, which is stirred up to it self, or primarily from this or that beginning, as often as the appetite requires this or that thing [...] or the motion of either kind is reflected, to wit, which depending on a previous sense more immediately, as an evident cause or occasion, is presently retorted, so a gentle titillation of the Skin causes a rubbing of it, and the more intense heats of the Praecordia stir up the Pulse and Respiration."

13 Canguilhem: *Die Herausbildung des Reflexbegriffes*, 86.

14 Willis: *Of Musculary Motion*, 45f.

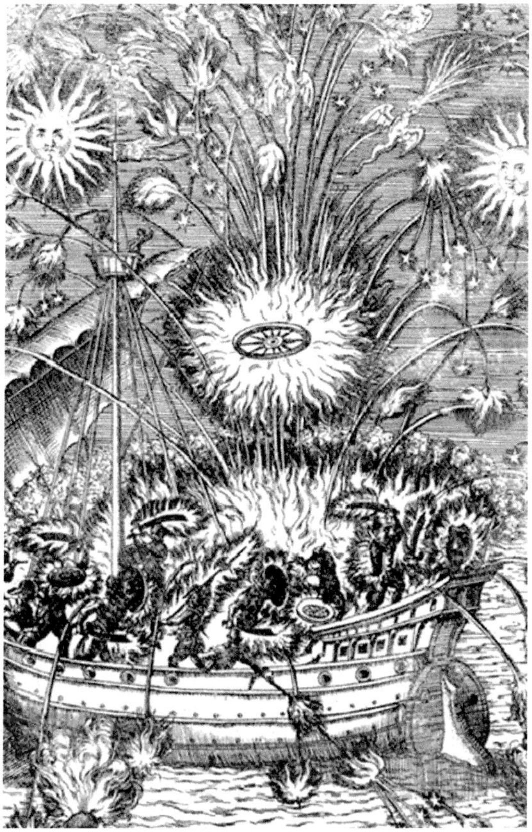

Fig. 2: Anonymus, Pyrotechnica, 17th century.

The explosion depicted here was taken from nautical science. On the one hand, explosions and muscle contractions – as Willis himself underlined – share the characteristic of instantaneity. At the same time, the movement of light depicted here can be interpreted as a casting back that points back to its origin, thereby visualizing the point of origin of the movement and its extensions. The transmission of light is depicted by a line here, a line which is cast back – just as a reflex is. This image could therefore be an important source to explain the otherwise unclear part of the meaning of being cast back which cannot be deduced using physiological terms. Precisely this aspect of the reflex is thus transported exclusively via images, via their spatial configuration or architecture. In addition, it shows how the center – of the movement – and the periphery enter into a relationship with one another.

Exactly this topological relationship of center and periphery can also be substantiated in other fields that now depict the brain. Willis compared the brain stem and the cerebellum with a fountain in his work "Anatome Cerebri".

> When some time past I diligently and seriously meditated on the office of the Cerebel [...] it occured, to wit, that the Cerebel is a peculiar Fountain of the animal Spirits designed for

> some works, and wholly distinct from the Brain. Within the Brain, Imagination, Memory, Discourse, and other more superior Acts of the animal Function are performed; besides, the animal Spirits flow also from the nervous stock, by which all the spontaneous motions, to wit, of which there are knowing and will, are performed. But the office of the Cerebel seems to be for the animal Spirits to supply some Nerves, by which involuntary actions (such as the beating of the Heart, easie Respiration, the Concoction of the Aliment, the protrusion of the Chyle, and many others) which are made after a constant manner unknown to us, or whether we will or not are performed.[15]

This comparison is founded upon a visual analogy that is initially constructed via topographical orders. This figure (3), from one of August Ramelli's "Schatzkammer mechanischer Künste", depicts a fountain. René Descartes also refers to it in his "Traité de l'homme".[16] Seven pipes, representing snakes, spring from the gazing ball at the top of the picture. The next image (fig. 4) is a portrayal of the brain from Willis's "Cerebri anatome". The cranial nerves coming out of the brain stem resemble the pipes of the fountain. And it is the distinctly discernible topographical similarities that organize the comparison of the cerebellum with a fountain, so that the fountain as the source of the image plays a decisive role for knowledge about the cerebellum. Only in a second step, these similarities are than transformed into functional observations. According to Willis, the brain is comparable to a pump in physiological terms as well, to a pump that guides the animal spirits through the nerve pathways, just as the fountain guides water through the pipes. I believe that these functional analogies and considerations are founded on the topographical ones. After all, the comparison is actually not supported empirically or by experiments. It is for the most part figurative. Nonetheless, it attained a position central to 18th-century experimental physiology, and it, too, transported the concept of the brain as a center that transmits impulses, substances or signals to the periphery.

15 Willis: *The Anatomy of the Brain and Nerves*, Vol. 1, p. 111.

16 Canguilhem: *Die Herausbildung des Reflexbegriffs*, p. 81.

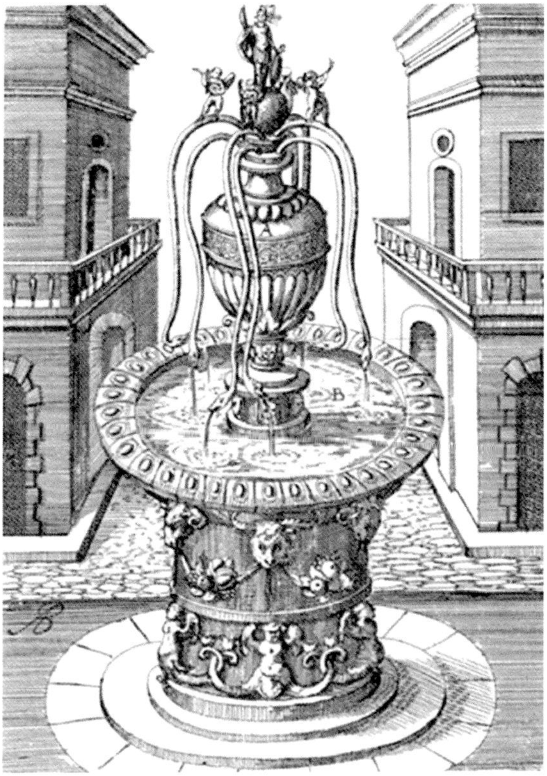

Fig. 3: Agostino Ramelli, Fountain, 1620.

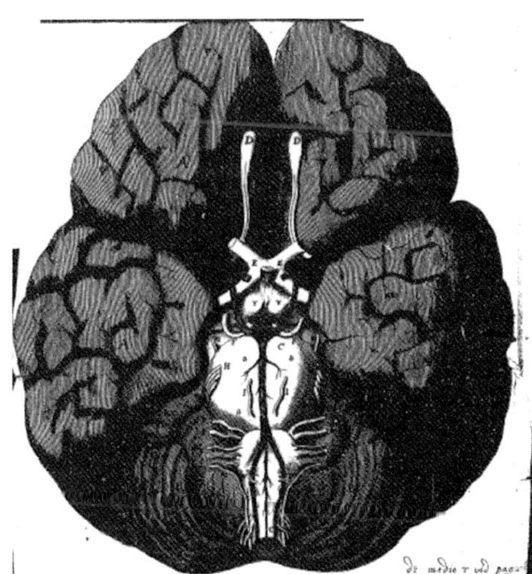

Fig. 4: Thomas Willis, Representation of the human Brain, 1664.

While the pyrotechnical visualizations initially emphasize that which is instantaneous and cast back by the reflex to a center, the comparison with a fountain also underlines the central position of the brain. Neither image is capable of appropriately capturing that the sensation and the movement occur in a sequence, one after the other – a concept important in 19th-century physiology. The components of the reflex cannot be comprehended as discrete events following one another by viewing the images from the early modern period you just saw. Instead, their discreteness seems to be lost to the instantaneous and the explosive. I hypothesize that only with the experimental practices of the 18th century did a sequence become established, albeit accentuated differently, which finally rounded out physiological knowledge about reflexes and also made the establishment of a reflex model of the brain in physiology possible.

## II

Against this background, let us first take a look at the stimulus-response experiments of the 18th century, including those that are not usually viewed in connection with reflexes. This is the second point of my deliberations. These experiments include decapitation experiments and stimulus-response experiments on intestinal tissue. The Scottish physician Robert Whytt described such experiments in his 1751 "Essay on the Vital and other Involuntary Motions of Animals." He was broadly interested in effects and stimuli. Hydrotechnical and pyrotechnical metaphors are replaced by detailed descriptions of experiments that encompass complex manipulations of bodies, for example stimulation of nerves by means of aromatic substances, heating and touching of body parts, or removal of nerves or individual organs.[17]

The fact that Whytt considered stimulation – as a manipulative intervention – to be of central importance, may well be linked to the career of the experiment in the 18th century, as Margarete Vöhringer has shown. Various experiments established stimulus-response sequences, which initially denoted the execution of actions – a very concrete concept. This requires practical knowledge, know-how. In other words, in the 18th century, stimulation was a practice that itself was varied and trained, academic efforts focused on mastering it. So stimulation was not only a means to an end. It became a subject of knowledge itself and did not only serve to test certain hypotheses.[18] An experiment log written by a student of Albrecht von Haller's provides some insights:

17 Whytt: *An Essay on the Vital and Other Involuntary Motions*, p. 83f.
18 Steinke: *Irritating experiments*; Vöhringer: "Hallers Köpfungen".

> Um 11 Uhr stach ich eine Nadel durch das Gehirn eines Frosches. Der Frosch krümmte sich, wenn auch nicht zu stark. Nachdem ich das Gehirn entfernt hatte wurde der ganze Körper des Frosches mehrmals von Konvulsionen erfasst. 15 Minuten danach stieß der Frosch ein lautes Geräusch aus, um 11.25 machte er drei große Sprünge. Um 12.40 warf ich das Tier, das auf dem Boden lag, auf den Rücken. Es drehte sich in seine Ursprungslage um und machte ein paar weitere Sprünge. Um 1.46, als ich den Frosch mit einem Finger reizte, versuchte er ein paar große Sprünge zu machen. Um 2.43 ließ er sich sehr stark von Reizen an den Füßen erregen. Um 3.13 reizte ich ihn mit kaltem Wasser. Der Frosch machte Sprünge, eher größere. Danach legte ich den Frosch ins Wasser – er wurde ganz steif.[19]

The experimenter documented individual stimulus-response experiments. As his notes show, the experiments were repeated frequently, but no concrete research goal was stated. Instead, the practices introduced and automated procedures. They were often exercises that were obviously mechanical and that developed a stimulation regime in its own right. In this way, practical knowledge was imparted that became important for the later reflex experiments. Not only did the experiments make it possible to make important observations. Above all, they permitted integrating the cascade of sensation and motion, which Willis had still thought to be instantaneous, in a temporal order and placing a different emphasis on the fact that it was conceived as a sequence. Without this form of a sequence, which was established only by means of experimental practice, we would not have gained knowledge about reflexes.

## III

This know-how now became theoretically relevant for the physiologist Marshall Hall, and this brings us to the next and last point in my deliberations. Initially, he included this know-how in his definition of the reflex. I would like to call to mind the passage I quoted at the beginning:

> This [new] property is characterized by being excited in its action, and reflex in its course: in every instance in which it is exerted, an impression made upon the extremities of certain

19 Zimmermann: *Mit Skalpell und Federkiel*, p. 28. ("Around 11 o' clock I took a needle and lanced it into the frog's brain. The frog bended a little, but not too much. After I removed the brain, the body was captured by seizures. 15 minutes later the frog made a loud noise. At 11.25 he jumped three times. At 12.40 I turned the animal that laid on the ground, on its back. Then I turned it around again and it jumped again a few times. At 1.46, when I stimulated the frog with a needle, he tried to jump again. At 2.43 he was agitated by stimuli directed to its feet. At 3.13 I irritated the frog with cold water. The frog jumped, rather high. After that I threw the frog into the water - its body became inflexible.").

> nerves is conveyed to the medulla oblongata or the medulla spinalis, and is reflected along other nerves.[20]

The word "excited" now pointed clearly to the experimental designs of the 18th century which I discussed just now. It no longer denoted a natural feeling, that is, a random sensation such as an itch. Instead, it meant an artificially created occurrence, a stimulation whose effect was intentionally produced and which was intentionally clocked. The instantaneity of sensation and movement that Willis had focused on was lost. Hall replaced it with a sequence of stimulation (he used the term "excited") and movement. It was only this sequence, conveyed by the practices of the 18th century, that could now also be delineated by theory.

Bell/Magendie's research described, inter alia, the anatomical structures of the medulla spinalis.[21] It is known that they consist of an efferent sensory nerve and an afferent motor nerve. Hall associated these structures with the reflex, which he now conceived of as a bending back along the structures and also as a sequence of stimulation and movement. Temporally speaking, the reflex now became linear; in spatial terms, it was eccentric; and as a bent-back occurrence, it now had two phases. Nevertheless, it no longer originated in the brain, as in Willis's model, but from the spinal cord. Here, the reflex distinguished itself precisely because it did not include the central structures such as the brain, but that it remained limited to the brain's periphery. In addition, no intermediate structure was necessary as the motor and the sensory nerves communicated directly to the spinal cord.

Now, let us take a look at the impact that this research had for the depiction and notion of the brain. For instance in the writings of psychiatrist Wilhelm Griesinger, in particular in his textbook "Mental Pathology and Therapeutics" and also in the study "Über psychische Reflexactionen" first published in 1845. I quote from the textbook:

> Dementsprechend sehen wir, wie alle aus dem Körper und durch die Sinne centripetal einfallenden Eindrücke im Gehirn sich sammeln, percipirt, assimilirt werden, die Geistesthätigkeit erregen und unterhalten, und wie von hier aus wieder Anlässe zu neuen, centrifugalen Acten, Beziehungen der Empfindung und der Geistesthätigkeiten auf die Action der Bewegungsorgane – Strebungen und motorische Reize für die Muskelapparate entstehen.[22]

20 Hall: "On the Reflex Function", p. 652.

21 Bell: *Idea of a New Anatomy*.

22 Griesinger: *Allgemeine Pathologie*, p. 23. ("In this sense we see how impressions that are transported through the body to the brain by centripetal senses and that are gathered, perceived and adjusted, stimulate the mind and how, from there, newly created events continuously contribute as centrifugal actions to the emergence of muscular movements via sensations and mind operations.")

Griesinger was obviously following Johannes Müller,[23] whose work he read as early as 1838, with his version of the 'reflex brain'. Some central figures of knowledge of the reflex are represented here. For one thing, the role of the brain as the center is obvious and it thereby resembles the role of the medulla oblongata. For another, the idea that the brain, as an active organ, is to be integrated in a temporal sequence of sensations and movements. And there is yet another obvious structural analogy. Wilhelm Griesinger's notion of centripetal impressions and centrifugal acts corresponds to Hall's model of afferent and efferent nerves. Apparently, the brain, understood in this way, is a locus of transfer, a place where conduits of stimuli are redirected. How such redirection occurs, and whether it is to be understood in a causal sense, remained an open question here. The fact that this model was taken on from research on reflexes is clearly shown by Griesinger's 1843 essay in which he spoke explicitly of the psychological function of reflexes and conceived of the brain as a reflex device. I quote:

> Dem Rückenmark kommt die Leitung der Empfindungen zum Gehirn, der Bewegungsimpulse vom Gehirn und nächste dem vorzüglich die Bildung der einfacheren Reflexe, die noch ziemlich directe Umsetzung von Empfindung in Bewegung zu. Es ist die graue Substanz, welche die Thätigkeiten vermittelt, die zwischen der centripetalen Zu- und der centrifugalen Ableitung in der Mitte liegen; die Reflexaction ist eine ihrer specifischen Energieen. [...] Das Gehirn ist aber auch ein großartiger Reflexapparat, wo von allen jenen wie immer beschaffenen sensorischen Erregungszuständen Bewegungsimpluse angeregt werden. Auch hier finden zum Teil noch einfache, unmittelbare Reflexe von Sinnesreizen.[24]

In this context, the reflex was considered to be a psychomotoric phenomenon. It is extended to the processing of sensory functions in the brain which were mediated via the periphery and were reflected back, in turn, to precisely this periphery. Anatomically speaking, the reflex model by no means remained limited to the periphery. It was applied to the brain and now characterized the relationship between the brain, the spinal cord and the individual peripheral nerves, a relationship which was considered hierarchical. In this context, both periphery and center were doubled: the relationship between the spinal cord and the sensory and motor nerves corresponded to the relationship between the brain and the spinal cord.

Also, anatomical descriptions of nerve fibers contributed to this hypothesis. The fact that the spinal cord does not end in the brain, but that its fibers continue inside the brain, and that fibers extend from there, in turn, to the periphery, could be detected even in the absence of special dyeing techniques, that is, by viewing the relevant specimens merely macroscopically.

The discourse about reflex brains was founded less on anatomically precise depictions, but rather – I hypothesize – on schematic drawings of reflexes as presented by Marshall Hall, for example. In figure 4 you see such a schematic

23 Müller: *Handbuch der Physiologie*, pp. 610, 613.
24 Griesinger: *Ueber psychische Reflexactionen*, pp. 73–113, 82.

drawing of a reflex. Experiments, i.e. measuring the time required to process stimuli, were carried out using such drawings as a basis.

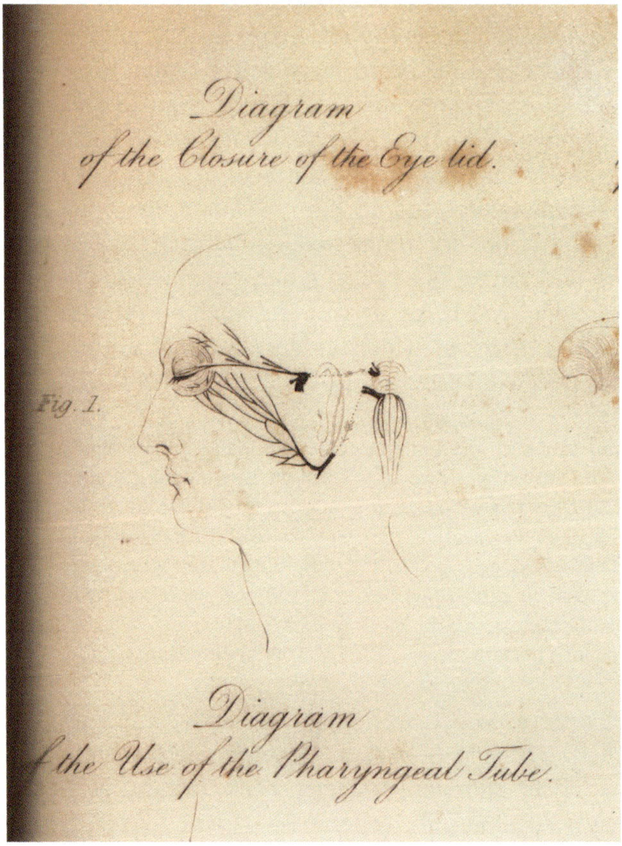


Fig. 5: Marshall Hall, Reflex arc of an eye lid, 1841.

A brief glance at the further developments during the 19th century, however, shows that reflex experiments produced increasingly complex ideas, also of accommodation and of feedback and inhibition mechanisms. For example, central phenomena of reflex inhibition or facilitation became known, and feedback mechanisms were assumed between the brain and the muscles innervated by peripheral nerves. One would assume that, in the end, it would have been difficult to hold onto the simple reflex processes.

In spite of these differentiations achieved by research on reflexes, the 'reflex model' of the brain remained the foundation of many areas of brain research. This was true especially of physiologists such as Sechenov. This was also true of psychiatrists who focused on anatomical work. In the essays on the pathology of the nervous system published in 1893, Carl Wernicke, for example, considered speech motion as following the pattern of reflexes.[25] Wernicke was aware of numerous peripheral reflexes and their modifications, for instance the blink reflex and the intensification of reflexes in the event of a stroke. Nonetheless, he still spoke of centrally controlled language reflexes, thus linking his work to Johannes Müller's and Griesinger's reflex model that was designed on the basis of simple stimulus-response patterns. Wernicke's concept of memory also used this simple model. He assumed that complex information was stored in individual cells that only needed to be activated like in stimulus-response-experiments. And here we can draw a parallel to ideas still current today. For instance, brain researchers such as Marco Iacoboni, who performed research in Gallese's laboratory and today focuses mainly on studying human mirror neurons, also refers back to such a model of memory.

Overall one can wrap this up: In the 19th century, the concept of reflexes remained an integral part of functional brain research, that is, part of research on speech and memory, where it maintained its central heuristic function. As Georges Canguilhem remarked, this concept refers back to Willis's definition, to "being cast back," and to the experimental practices of the 18th century. In addition, its historical components of meaning become accessible only if we include the images and practices in terms of their own epistemic accomplishments and not merely as a means to an end: Without the images of the early modern period that depicted explosions, Willis might not have included the idea of casting back in his definition of motus reflexus. Without the practices of the 18th century, the model of instantaneity would not have developed into one of a temporal sequence. Without the images and practices, a reflex model of the brain would not have developed, either. The images visualize the brain as a center, and motion is still related to that center. The practices made it possible to integrate the organ in a temporal sequence. Visualizations of the early modern period initially showed the brain as a central functional organ, the practices of reflexes established a temporal order. Both contributed to the understanding of the brain as the center of afferent and efferent nerve activity, and the place where such activity was redirected. Although the concept of the reflex was differentiated further in 19th-century experimental research, the simple reflex model of the brain still remained present in anatomically-based research for a relatively long time.

To conclude, permit me to summarize my results: Willis's concept of the reflex is based on spatial analogies that could be identified only by consulting visual representations from the field of pyrotechnics. Hence, a history of medical terms must include images, not just as illustrations, but as genuine media conveying knowledge: media that carry specific topographical or diagrammatic knowledge. In the experimental practices of the 18th century, in Whytt's work, a sequence of events is introduced as procedural knowledge. The practices generate knowledge

25 Wernicke: *Gesammelte Aufsätze*, and *Lehrbuch für Gehirnkrankheiten*, p. 203.

that is applied in experiments regarding reflexes and that is required in order to handle and then conceptualize reflexes. This aspect of knowledge about reflexes is not mediated via concepts and texts, either, but rather primarily via experimental practices. Only in this way does it become clear how Hall could formulate a concept of reflexes. He had practical knowledge at his disposal as well as a concept of temporal sequence and of casting back that were now applied to anatomical structures. This reflex concept was than introduced into brain research and remained present throughout the 19th century while practices and knowledge of the reflex were succeedingly differentiated.

## References

Bell, Charles: *Idea of a New Anatomy of the Brain* (1811).

Canguilhem, Georges: *Die Herausbildung des Reflexbegriffes im 17. und 18. Jahrhundert*, German translation by Henning Schmidgen, Munich (Fink) 2008.

Gowers, W. R.: *The Diagnosis of Disease of the Spinal Cord* (1880).

Griesinger, Wilhelm: *Allgemeine Pathologie und Therapie der psychischen Krankheiten*, (⁴1876).

Griesinger, Wilhelm: *Ueber psychische Reflexactionen, mit Blick auf das Wesen der psychischen Krankheiten, Archiv für physiologische Heilkunde*, Vol. 2 (1843).

Hall, Marshal: "On the Reflex Function in the Medulla Oblongata and Medulla Spinalis", in: *Philosophical Transactions of the Royal Society* 123 (1833), pp. 635–665.

Latour, Bruno: "Drawing Things Together. Die Macht der unveränderlich mobilen Elemente" in: Andréa Belliger und David J. Krieger (eds.): *Anthology. Ein einführendes Handbuch zur Akteur-Netzwerk-Theorie*, Bielefeld (transcript) 2006, pp. 259–307.

Machamer, Peter: "17th Century Demonstrations", in: Wolfgang Detel and Claus Zittel (eds.): *Wissensideale und Wissenskulturen in der frühen Neuzeit*, Berlin (Akademie Verlag) 2002, pp. 23–37.

Müller, Johannes: *Handbuch der Physiologie* (1844).

Secenov, Ivan: *Refleksy Golovnogo Mozga* (Moskow 1862/1952), English translation: *Reflexes of the Brain*, Cambridge, Mass. (M.I.T. Press) 1965.

Steinke, Hubert: *Irritating experiments. Haller's concept and the European controversy on irritability and sensibility 1750–90*, Amsterdam, New York (Rodopi) 2005.

Troemner, E.: "Ein neuer Reflexhammer, zugleich ein Beitrag zur Prüfung von Sehnenreflexen", in: *Berliner Klinische Wochenschrift* 21 (1910), pp. 997–998.

Troemner, E.: “Ueber Sehnen- resp. Muskelreflexe und die Merkmale ihrer Schwächung und Steigerung”, in: *Berliner Klinische Wochenschrift* 50 (1913), pp. 1712–1715.
Vöhringer, Margarete: “Hallers Köpfungen”, in: Tanja van Hoorn, Yvonne Wübben (eds.): *‘Allerhand nützliche Versuche’. Empirische Wissenskultur in Halle und Göttingen*, Hannover (Wehrhahn) 2009, pp. 105–121.
Wernicke, Carl: *Gesammelte Aufsätze und kritische Referate zur Pathologie des Nervensystems. Mit 19 Abbildungen* (1893).
Wernicke, Carl: *Lehrbuch für Gehirnkrankheiten: Schema des cerebralen Sprachmechanismus*. Vol. 1, (1881).
Whytt, Robert: *An Essay on the Vital and Other Involuntary Motions of Animals* (1751).
Willis, Thomas: *Five Treatises, The Second Medical and Physical Discourse, Of Musculary Motion* (1681).
Willis, Thomas: *De motu musculari* (1680).
Willis, Thomas: *The Anatomy of the Brain and Nerves*, ed. by William Feindel, 2 Vols. Montreal (McGill University Press) 1965.
Wübben, Yvonne and Margarete Vöhringer: *Phantome im Labor. Die Verbreitung der Reflexe in Hirnforschung, Kunst und Technik* (= *Berichte zur Wissenschaftsgeschichte* 32 [2009] 1).
Wübben, Yvonne: “Transhumane Physiologie. Bilder und Praktiken des Reflexes (Thomas Willis, Robert Whytt, Marshall Hall)”, in: Christoph Lüthy (ed.): *Early Science and Medicine*, Vol 25, Leiden (Brill) 2010, pp. 105–121.
Zimmermann, Johann Georg: *Mit Skalpell und Federkiel. Ein Lesebuch*, ed. by Andrea Langenbacher, Bern (Paul Haupt) 1995.

## List of Illustrations

Fig. 1 A reflex hammer ‘Modell Trömner’ (from: www.oeh-servicecenter.at/?s=medartikel).
Fig. 2 Anonymus, Pyrotechnica, etching, 17th century.
Fig. 3 Agostino Ramelli, Fountain (in: *The Various and Ingenious Machines*, 1620).
Fig. 4 Thomas Willis, Representation of the human Brain (in: *Cerebri anatome*, 1664).
Fig. 5 Marshall Hall, Reflex arc of an eye lid, (in: *On the diseases and derangements of the nervous system : in their primary forms and in their modifications by age, sex, constitution, hereditary predisposition, excesses, general disorder, and organic disease*, 1841).

# What Is It Like To Be *With* Bats? The Wisdom of Jean Painlevé

JAN SÖFFNER

Let me start with a Taoist Narration.

> Chuang Tzu and Hui Tzu were strolling along the dam of the Hao River when Chuang Tzu said, "See how the minnows [little fishes] come out and dart around where they please! That's the joy of the fishes!"
>
> Hui Tzu said, "You're not a fish – how do you know the joy of the fishes?"
>
> Chuang Tzu said, "You're not I, so how do you know I don't know the joy of the fishes?"
>
> Hui Tzu said, "I'm not you, so I certainly don't know what you know. On the other hand, you're certainly not a fish – so that still proves you don't know the joy of the fishes!"
>
> Chuang Tzu said, "Let's go back to your original question, please. You asked me how I know the joy of the fishes – so you already knew it when you asked the question. I know it by standing here beside the Hao.[1]

The question asked by Hui Tzu is the phenomenological question of what it is like to be a fish. This resembles the famous question brought up by Thomas Nagel, who asked "What is it like to be a bat?"[2] Nagel, like Hui Tzu, discussed the issue in terms of a consciousness-based phenomenology. The point is – first of all – about phenomenal experiencing. And therefore Nagel drew the conclusion that consciousness is not only human, but present in at least some animals too. Animals have experiences, about which you can ask "What is it like to…?" questions. In his eyes, though – again like in the eyes of Hui Tzu – it is this very fact that makes it so problematic to approach the phenomenon of other species' experiencing properly. When thinking about bats, it might indeed be possible to imagine what it would be like to have wings and fly around, and one can at least try to imagine what it might be like to have a sensorium allowing for a spatial orientation by acoustics. But this attempt never leaves behind the anthropomorphism of human imagination. Therefore it is only possible to imagine what it is like to be a bat for a human – one cannot experience what it is like to be a bat *for* a bat.

1 *The Complete Works of Chuang Tzu*, pp. 188–189.
2 Nagel: "What Is It Like To Be a Bat?"

The problem of the experience of another species is hence discussed in a similar way to the way in which the problem of other minds is discussed in Philosophy of Mind.

This is also the issue Chuang Tzu ironically picks up on when asking back: "You're not I, so how do you know I don't know the joy of the fishes?" But this does not help his argument. Hui Tzu points to the difference between himself not being Chuang Tzu and Chuang Tzu not being a fish. He introduces the consideration that a human being knows what another human being's sensorium is like. Therefore he is able to build a mental *model* of what Chuang Tzu *can* experience and what he *can't*. Hui Tzu *can* know that Chuang Tzu *cannot* know the joy of the fishes.

This, too, shares some traces of what Nagel proposes as an alternative phenomenology. He tries to push the boundaries of this kind of knowledge by bringing accumulated scientific knowledge about bats into play. Hui Tzu does not think about this option. Chuang Tzu also refrains from it, and so he loses the dispute. Nevertheless the narration would not be a Taoist narration, if it had this – or any – definite conclusion. And indeed Chuang Tzu restarts it by asking the question about the joy of the fishes on an even more basic level: a level without *models* of reality. He accordingly does not ask about the joy of the fishes by asking "what is it like to be a fish?": His point is neither about simulation nor about accumulated knowledge. It is about shared embodied interaction. He asks what it is like to be with Chuang Tzu and what it is like to be *with* fishes. By being with Chuang Tzu, Hui Tzu already *somehow* knew what he is now asking, and Chuang Tzu also *somehow* knew the joy of the fishes.

This argument, instead, resembles Vinciane Despret's approach on what she calls "isopraxis",[3] i.e. the shared embodied interactions between humans and animals. Despret argues that e.g. riding a horse is an isopraxis of a mostly unintentional embodied communication that makes the horse's movements enter what one could call the body image and the body schema,[4] and the same goes vice versa for the rider's movements becoming a part of the horse's embodied coordination. The effect is a kind of emergence of a shared existence, a "becoming-

3 Despret: "The Body We Care For".

4 The concept of a conscious body image and its distinction from a subliminal system of sensorimotor coordination, the body schema, was first proposed by Henry Head (*Studies in Neurology*). In phenomenological terms the concept of a body schema (*schéma corporel*) was rendered in a more precise way by Maurice Merleau-Ponty (*Phénoménologie de la perception*), and the most precise description of this opposition has been developed by Shaun Gallagher (*How the Body Shapes the Mind*). Gallagher and Alva Noë (*Out of Our Heads*), moreover state that the body schema is not monadic, it does not concern the body as a discrete and self-related entity, but always concerns the space this very body shares with the world in which it is situated. If a driver extends her body schema, e.g. to the car she is driving (sensing the ground under the wheels as part of an extended self), this fact becomes clear – and even clearer it becomes when the body of an avatar in a video game is corporally experienced. Something very similar, indeed, seems to occur in horse-riding as well.

with", as Despret calls it; and she conceives of this as a state in which the rider and the horse start to "embody each other's mind."[5]

But even taking this "becoming with" for granted, the question of knowledge *about* the other species is limited. The rider cannot know for sure what it is like to be a horse for a horse. Like Chuang Tzu – she can know what it is like to be with the animal. But not what it is like to be this very animal for the animal. Neither the rider nor Chuang Tzu can transpose the shared knowledge from their actual situatedness into the knowledge *about* the other species. The sharedness of their knowledge cannot provide for a model or a simulation of the fishes' experience. This is enough for Hui Tzu to not consider it as a real kind of knowledge. And indeed, one ought not to disregard the fact that Chuang Tzu has lost the first part of the dispute. Chuang Tzu cannot and will not understand what it is like to be a fish for a fish.

But nevertheless, one question remains to be resolved for the Hui Tzu / Nagel stance as well: When talking about the joy of the fishes and when talking about what it is like to be a horse, is the question what it is like to be an animal *for* this particular animal the only question to be asked, in any case? It would not be the right question to ask Chuang Tzu about joy, because the joy he 'knows' is shared. It is not his personal joy at all. And the same is true for the horse. Riding, too, is a shared experience. Its focus does not lie on the experiencer as a discrete entity. It lies in the shared interaction. It lies in the with. Chuang Tzu does point to a dimension of the question.

Hui Tzu does not reply, but Nagel has an answer. He argues that all experiencing of "what it is like to" needs a conscious focus of attention. Hence, as a human being one can perceive only *as* the conscious human being. Chuang Tzu, though, questions the exclusiveness of this stance. Despite the fact that he is located as a body near the Hao River, he can sympathetically share the joy of the fishes. He *shares* a perception that is not just centered on his body. It also has the fishes as a center of the experience. What else could give Chuang Tzu pleasure when watching the fish if not the experience of sharing in their swimming, as the rider shares in the movements of a horse? Hence the focus of the experience does not lie on the discrete entity only. It can also lie on the shared situation. Chuang Tzu's point, like Despret's, is that a "what is it like to" question does not only depend on self-experience. It also needs enactive embeddedness, which then allows for sharing a focus instead of just being a centered focus.

The question what it is like to be a fish *for* a fish, is thereby, yes, unsolvable for a human being. But it is not the only one to ask. The question what it is like to be *in a situation* is and remains a kind of other side of this question. And since this very situation can be shared, Chuang Tzu has access to it. Chuang Tzu seems to conceive of this shared side of phenomenal experiencing as another side of cognition. And thereby he realizes the knowledge of a Chinese *wise* master: And

5 Despret: "The Body We Care For", p. 115.

as the Sinologist François Jullien put it: In Ancient China *Un sage est sans idée.*[6] Wisdom does not consist in having the right thoughts about things: wisdom is not *about* anything, not even qualitative experiencing. It consists in adequately sharing situations.

I am not a philosopher. And so I do not wish to make any philosophical claim about Chuang Tzu. What I wish to say, though, is that the point the Chinese text addresses is of a certain interest for cultural phenomena. Making animal films, indeed, faces similar problems. For example, Jamie Uys' hilarious classic *Animals Are Beautiful People* has been widely criticized for the anthropomorphism that made it both hilarious and a classic. One famous scene is the one depicting animals eating the fermented fruits of the Marula tree and then behaving like drunken humans. Evidently the film makes people out of the animals in order to build a bridge between human experiencing and animal experiencing, thereby giving an easy account of what it is like to be an animal. Usually this kind of anthropomorphism is criticized because it lacks the adequate alterity, the relation of otherhood between humans and animals. The critique concerns the fact that the film is not concerned enough with what it is like to be an animal for an animal. Everything seems to be about what it is like for a human being to be an animal.

Nevertheless, anthropomorphism is perhaps the wrong term. Does human experiencing, indeed, really have a fixed shape; is there a stable *morphē* of the *anthropos*? And if there is not, but if humans become what they are by shaping or reshaping themselves, and, moreover by being shaped and reshaped in their interactions, then the question is also about becoming human while interacting with animals, which is the issue Despret calls "Anthropo-zoo-genesis". Seen from this angle, animal films are, in principle, not just about anthropomorphizing animals. They are also about theromorphising humans.

It is here that the interesting question for cultural studies also sets in. If one looks at different animal films from different times and cultures, one can easily grasp the fact that anthropomorphism highly diverges according to diverging cultural formations. Indeed, if animals are anthropomorphized in animal films, this fact takes part in the formation of what *humans* are like. Animals can therefore be presented as figurations partially *establishing* what it is like to be a human being. Anthropomorphizing animals takes part in forming human experiencing and developing a *habitus*. And this does not only concern the *habitus* of our way of acting with animals. Much more than this, presenting animals as people is also a work on the theromorphism, the animal-shape, of humans. Anthropomorphization of animals can thereby become a means of establishing what human beings *are* as animals – and Jamie Uys' movie implies that as *animals* they are *beautiful* people. As humans they are perhaps less beautiful.

6 François Jullien: *Un sage est sans idée.*

But when thinking this way, we are still very much following a Nagelian phenomenology, in so far as we have not considered the reciprocal shaping of humans and animals as a being-*with*, but rather as a being-*like*, i.e. a mimetic representation of forms (human forms in anthropomorphism, animal forms in theromorphism).

Before now proposing an alternative style of animal film, I have to deepen the thoughts on sharedness, on a phenomenological level. This is why I have to turn to the third major theoretical reference of my thoughts: Giorgio Agamben's approach on humanism as exposed in his famous work *The Open*.[7] Here things are about being-animal and being-human as two different forms of being-in-the-world. Agamben, indeed, does not conceive of the human being as something to be defined in opposition to or similarity with animals. Instead he focuses on the productive processuality of this very opposition. He conceives of the difference between humans and animals under the condition of what he calls a "humanist machine". By the work on this difference, humans are not just *understood* – they are rather *produced.* They are produced in the sense that humans are the very animals working on the difference between being animals and humans. And this very work *is* humanism in so far as it is the production of humans.

In conceiving of this difference, Agamben phenomenologically draws on (and simplifies) Heidegger's thoughts on world openness.[8] In Agamben's eyes, producing a human being equals producing a different way of relating to the world. While animals, in his eyes, do not have anything but an enactive stance, which makes them nothing but an embedded part of their world, humans can gain a stance on this very relation. Thereby they can disclose their own animalism. So, they can *form* this very animalism instead of living and experiencing it as a closed instinctive chain of reactions with their environment. The question about a *human* habitus in the *human* habitat, for Agamben, is therefore marked by the fact of leaving behind the very embedded stance which Chuang Tzu focused on. And by producing only *one* animal that has a stance on its own animalism, humanism is a kind of mono-animalism.

But, as Chuang Tzu shows us, this is not all there is. Agamben *is* indeed focusing on environmental embeddedness too. At the same time as gaining a human stance upon our animal being, we remain animals as well, and have embedded and embodied experiences, like dwelling alongside the Hao River. Agamben know this. His book, indeed, is about deconstructing the humanist machine, i.e. putting the humanist machine out of order and leaving the human animal "out of being", i.e. out of the humanist stance forced upon it.

This approach phenomenologically has some advantages, even when considering Despret's concept of anthropo-zoo-genesis. Despret, indeed, focuses on the environment, and the *significational* processes concerned. She grounds her

7 Giorgio Agamben: *L'aperto*.
8 Heidegger: *Die Grundbegriffe der Metaphysik*, pp. 244–388.

thoughts in the "Umwelt" in the Uexküllian sense of the word,[9] i.e. the world as it is lived and experienced by a particular animal, by focusing on the significances or meanings certain stimuli have *for* this particular animal.[10] And hence some aspects of the Nagelian questions still play a role. It is taken for granted that *something* can appear *to* an animal *as something* and therefore *mean something*, i.e. be *about* something. This means that somehow, for Uexküll and Despret even the animal is *with* an idea (i.e. with a meaning).[11] In following Heidegger, though, Agamben does not point to the *surrounding* world (Um-Welt), but to the world. And he does not point to significations, but to shared enactions, not meaning something to somebody, not reciprocally embodying "minds" (see above), but having their own, interactionally shared focus.[12] And this very fact of talking about *the* world (which is its own centre or better has none) – not the *surrounding* world (with a focus on the experiencing entity) – gives more power to Chuang Tzu's stance. To say it again: A wise master is without idea – and so is an animal. It is – so to speak – the humanist stance that imposes ideas upon the animal. And this is what Agamben makes his point.

What is strikingly absent in Agamben's approach, on the other hand, is the question of being *with* concrete animals. And with this, I finally turn to the real subject of my chapter: Jean Painlevé's movie *Le vampire*. The title already makes clear that Painlevé does not deal with animals as people. He deals with them as vampires. They are not presented on the verge of an individually grounded anthropomorphism, but rather on the verge of storytelling. The film begins by exposing a variety of astonishing animals to the music of Duke Ellingtion. The text spoken in a narrative tone introduces us to: "Animals in suits of armor [a cricket], strange and terrifying animals in form and movement [aquatic animals], hieratic living sculptures [a sea horse], frightening gestures full of grace [an octopus swiftly discloses a human skull]: The inspiration of legends and artists." Animal behavior is exposed on the threshold of cultural practice – and it is this very threshold the film now focuses on, by showing how diseases can be transmitted from animal bites and animal vampirism – Painlevé displays fleas and ticks. The question of anthropomorphism and theromorphism, here, is pointed to by *contagion* – instead of *identification*; it is about shared corporality, not about producing anthropomorphic or theroporphic likenesses; it is about sharing a common ground of interaction, not about empathy (feeling oneself *into* the shoes of the other) but sympathy (feeling *with* the animal in a shared situation).

This is also true for the film as such. Painlevé substantiates the inspiration of legends by phenomena shared with animals. His question is what it is like to be

9 Uexküll: *Umwelt und Innenwelt der Tiere*.

10 Cf. also Despret: *Bêtes et hommes*, pp. 42–47.

11 For a critique of meaning see: Gumbrecht: *Production of Presence*; concerning animals his theory of presence has been elaborated by Abram: *Becoming Animal*.

12 Fuchs and De Jaegher: "Enactive Intersubjectivity"; Gallagher and Zahavi: *The Phenomenological Mind*, pp. 171–196.

*with* vampire animals. Being with animals, though, is not just something natural. From the tick, Painlevé turns to "why the vampire came to be imagined as a human being" – and he shows selected scenes of Murnau's famous *Nosferatu*. Nosferatu's gestures find many striking parallels with the animal movements, when the vampire bat is presented sucking the blood of a guinea pig, literally exhausting this poor creature.

By drawing these parallels, Painlevé presents legends not only as inspired by a *nature* shared with animals. The direction of narrative contagion can be literally inverted, so that the animal's behavior shares the *legend* as well: The common ground of humans and animals is hence both natural and cultural, both imaginative and corporeal, both enactive and narrated. The habitat, as presented in this film, is all of this at once. Besides sharing the same music, the bat and the vampire also share mythical or legendary narrations. And sharing this phenomenal habitat means sharing a habitus as well. The bat's behavior in relation with its made-up natural habitat is parallelized with the vampire's gestures and, most of all, the actions in the imaginary habitat of Murnau's film.

The legend, hence, is not just something told or delivered. Narration is instead conceived of as myth – in a similar sense to Georges Bataille's concept of myths (indeed, Painlevé had a working relationship with Bataille). Myth is not just fiction in so far as those participating in it enact it as a living reality. Myths are not just told, but are intrinsic in social action. In this, Painlevé is very concrete. He opens up the concept for an embedded enactive relation concerning both nature and culture as the intricate convolute that is a human world. Here, myths are not a set of meanings, organized by narration, but are intrinsic in embodied enactions. Or to say it in more biological terms: They are not an 'Umwelt' with significations, but an intrinsic part of the world. They are without 'meaning' and thereby they are without idea. The myth of vampirism is accordingly presented as an essential aspect of participatory sense-making – it is not just something told and afterwards enacted; even the very narration shares in (natural) vampirism as a shared embodied experience; it is one of the "inspirations of legends and artists", and it lives on in shared enactions of humans with animals as much as it lives on in the meaningful narrations, or rather: Mythical narrations of vampirism become meaningful by participating in shared experiences of animal vampirism humans can have by being *with* animals. Myths and embodiment are exposed on the very same layer of experiencing. Myth, hence, is not introduced as a fictional *model* of the world according to which reality is organized and given its meaning. It is rather part of the shared interaction from which enactive meanings emerge. Just as the experience of natural vampirism gives an emotional background orientation to the myths narrated, so narrations of vampires give an emotional background orientation to the experience of natural vampirism. Meaning emerges in a shared world in which nature and culture are amalgamated.

This kind of experiencing, though, is not only a humanist experiencing, but one that can also leave both the human and the non-human animal "out of being".

Humans share the vampirism of bats, and in this shared experience the myth is as present as the instinctive interaction. Painlevé is concerned with how culture and nature share in each other – where there is no humanist machine producing stances upon one's own being animal.

Accordingly the voice of the 'narrator' does not draw the spectator into identification with *one* particular animal. The viewer identifies as much with the guinea pig as he identifies with the vampire: Or rather he identifies with none of them. Meaning derives from and is part of being drawn into a shared space of narrative action. And imagination accordingly is not conceived of as something projected upon other creatures, but rather something intrinsic in a perceptive encounter. Painlevé's focus is on action *in* a shared environment rather than on the action *of* a specific actor. More than anthropomorphism and theromorphism, the question is therefore about mythomorphism – the form of narration and action giving meaning to the embedded relation with animals.

This changes the question about animal films. The terror of bats does not lie in the fact of knowing what it is like to be a bat. Nor does it lie in the fact of experiencing one's humanity as reflected by animal behavior. For Painlevé it lies in the fact of being *with* bats and sharing something that is both, embodied interaction and narration.

Painlevé's phenomenology, though, is an interesting challenge for the phenomenology implied in Agamben's concept of the open too. As I mentioned, Agamben, following a Heideggerian concept of world-openness, finds the openness of human experience in the act of gaining a stance on one's own participatory environmental relation. And this fact, for Agamben, produces the humanist machine. Gaining a stance on one's animalism is no longer a fact of being an animal. The stance itself is human. At first glance, Painlevé seems to engage a similar phenomenology too. He makes vampirism appear *as* vampirism and makes the beholder gain a stance *on* vampirism. The film itself is not just sharing the mythomorphous environmental relation which I have just traced. It also is *about* this very relation. Especially the scientific correctness of explaining the experiment makes this more than clear. A pioneer of science films, Painlevé explains the constructedness of what he is showing. (Indeed he always used as many observational techniques as were available in his time – for example, anatomic dissections or microscopic images.) After displaying the suggestive parallelism of bats and vampires, the speaker's voice turns to explaining the experiment executed by the film-makers. In order to have enough light, they could not film at night. So they had to make a guinea pig fall asleep artificially by a substance. Thereby the illusion of seeing something just natural is undermined. But what in Berthold Brecht's poetics would have been an alienation effect does not disturb the esthetics of the film at all. This esthetics is not about deconstructing the humanist machine to leave the animal out of being. All these are techniques to gain a stance on animals (both human and non-human animals). In Agamben's terms they would thereby be part of the humanist machine.

But is this true? Painlevé, in doing this, is not only concerned with gaining a stance on the *human* animal alone. And accordingly he is neither asking what it is like to be a bat for a bat, nor what it is like to be a bat for a human. His film is about what it is like to be with bats in a habitat that is formed both by nature and by myths. Gaining a stance on this mythomorphous shared interaction therefore does not equal gaining a stance on human theromorphism (and producing anthropomorphism as this very stance). It is rather about gaining a stance on isopraxis and shared interaction. It implies gaining a stance on cultural vampirism sharing in natural vampirism, and vice versa.

Thereby the presumed 'humanist' question of what it is like to be a human animal is opened up for a different relation: One that is not just about being in the world, but rather about being in a world *shared with animals*. It is not by keeping animals out of being that Painlevé defies humanism. His point is about defying the humanist mono-animalism. The human animal, in his film, is no more as alone on earth as it would have to be in order to be concerned with its own being-animal alone. Humans are *with* bats.

## References

Abram, David: *Becoming Animal – An Earthly Cosmology*, New York (Pantheon Books) 2010.

Agamben, Giorgio: *L'aperto – L'uomo e l'animale*, Milan (Bollati Boringhieri) 2002.

Despret, Viviane: *Bêtes et hommes*, Paris (Gallimard) 2007.

Despret, Viviane: "The Body We Care For: Figures of Anthropo-Zoo-Genesis", in: *Body and Society* 10 (2004), pp. 111–134.

Fuchs, Thomas and Hanne De Jaegher: "Enactive Intersubjectivity: Participatory Sense-Making and Mutual Incorporation", in: *Phenom. Cogn. Sci.* 8 (2009), pp. 465–486.

Gallagher, Shaun and Dan Zahavi: *The Phenomenological Mind – An Introduction to Philosophy of Mind and Cognitive Science*, London and New York (Routledge), 2008.

Gallagher, Shaun: *How the Body Shapes the Mind*, Oxford (Oxford University Press) 2005.

Gumbrecht, Hans Ulrich: *Production of Presence – What Meaning Cannot Convey*, Palo Alto (Stanford University Press), 2004.

Head, Henry: *Studies in Neurology*, Vol. 2, London (Oxford University Press) 1920.

Heidegger, Martin: *Die Grundbegriffe der Metaphysik. Welt – Endlichkeit – Einsamkeit* (1929/30), Frankfurt am Main (Klostermann) 2004.

Jullien, François: *Un sage est sans idée*, Paris (Seuil) 1998.
Merleau-Ponty, Maurice: *Phénoménologie de la perception*, Paris (Gallimard) 1945.
Nagel, Thomas: “What Is It Like To Be a Bat?”, in: *The Philosophical Review* 83 (1974), pp. 435–450.
Noë, Alva: *Out of Our Heads: Why You Are Not Your Brain, and Other Lessons from the Biology of Consciousness*, New York (Hill and Wang) 2009.
Uexküll, Jacob von: *Umwelt und Innenwelt der Tiere*, Berlin (Springer) 1909.
Watson, Burtonn (ed.): *The Complete Works of Chuang Tzu*, New York (Columbia University Press) 1968.

# *Control and its Limits*

# "The Limits of Control" Understanding Cinema Beyond Signs and Meaning

FABIENNE LIPTAY

In the history of philosophical aesthetics the senses have only very gradually received recognition.[1] The effort to re-evaluate the senses, which were and are still often considered to be inferior to the mind, continues to the present day. Recent studies in the fields of philosophy, art history, literature, and film have put forward strong arguments in favour of a sensuous and bodily experience of aesthetic phenomena, drawing our attention to certain aspects of art which meaning cannot convey.[2] Growing interest in the sheer materiality and presence of art works, in their contribution to or subversion of meaning, has fundamentally called dominant modes of interpretation into question. Literature, painting, and cinema are no longer exclusively conceptualised in terms of signs and meaning.[3] Subsequent to the earlier materialist conceptions of cinema, such as those of Sergej Eisenstein, Walter Benjamin and Siegfried Kracauer, a number of contemporary film scholars have focused on bodily responses to film, e.g. Tom Gunning, Christian Mikunda, Steven Shaviro, Laura Marks, Linda Williams, and Vivian Sobchack. This theoretical move to "the other sides of cognition" may be considered as a paradigm shift not only confined within film studies.[4] It corresponds to an epistemological turn in cognitive science: the questioning of computational and representational models of cognition through theories of the embodied mind.[5]

Rather than aiming at another attempt to approach the mind-body problem with general assumptions, I consider a dynamic relation between the senses and the intellect, depending on their specific involvement in the perception of individual works of art. By focussing on Jim Jarmusch's film *The Limits of Control*

1 Gottfried Boehm speaks of philosophical aesthetics as an approval history of the senses ("Anerkennungsgeschichte der Sinnlichkeit"). Boehm: "Bildsinn und Sinnesorgane", p. 119. For the gradual rise of the senses in the history of philosophical aesthetics see also Naumann-Beyer: "Sinnlichkeit", pp. 546 ff.

2 Here, I refer to the title of Gumbrecht's study *Production of Presence. What Meaning Cannot Convey* (2004). For an anti-hermeneutic approach to cinema grounded on a critique of interpretation see Bordwell, *Making Meaning*; and Bordwell/Carroll: *Post-Theory*.

3 This is another reference to a book title, namely to Peter Wollen's *Signs and Meaning in the Cinema* (1969).

4 Elsaesser: "Erfahren, erleben, entgrenzen", p. 35.

5 For a discussion and critique of computational and representational models of cognition see, e.g., Varela: *Kognitionswissenschaft – Kognitionstechnik*; and Münch: *Kognitionswissenschaft.*

(USA 2009), I hope to provide evidence of three corresponding ideas: (I) that changes and epistemological turns in aesthetic theory should be considered as responses to changes in art practice, (II) that works of art actively engage in aesthetic discourse rather than being its passive object, (III) that films display and provide multiple forms of aesthetic experience in which carnal and cognitive responses interrelate in different ways.

## I

Art practice doesn't only proceed from art theory, but also effects and interferes with it. Therefore, significant changes in the theory of aesthetics cannot be regarded separately from the changes in the domain of art itself.[6] The turn towards aesthetic phenomena of presence and materiality, towards a sensual and carnal experience of art, indicates a crisis of an intellectual tradition in art theory that became increasingly unsuitable for the understanding of modern and contemporary art. Abstract painting, atonal music, modernist literature, post-dramatic theatre, performance art, avant-garde and experimental cinema dismiss classical representation and narration, the grounds on which metaphysical approaches to art were built. Methods of interpretation that seek to understand art as texts communicating meaning suddenly proved themselves to be inappropriate to grasp the essence of modern art. They seemed to miss the central point: the highly visible evidence that art had begun to substitute immaterial meaning with materiality, representation with presence, text with texture, and to make noise instead of sense.

Regarding the fact that the changes brought about by avant-garde films of the 1920s as well as experimental and modernist films of the 1960s and '70s are anything but new, current theories of embodied film experience seem rather belated. We may ascribe this to the "old" problem of writing about contemporary phenomena, of lacking the historical distance that enables a sustained and deliberate judgement. However, we may also look for evidence in our present time, tracing the possible reasons that may have had an impact on film theory's growing attention to the senses. Obviously enough, technical advances in the fields of sound design and special effects, for instance, have added to the experience of

6 See the introduction to Küpper/Menke: *Dimensionen ästhetischer Erfahrung*, p. 14. "Es wird überdies sichtbar, daβ sich dieser Wandel im Feld der Ästhetik gleichzeitig mit einem Transformationsprozeß in ihrem Gegenstandsfeld, zunächst und vor allem dem der Künste, darüber hinaus in Kultur und Gesellschaft, vollzogen hat; nicht nur die Theorie, die Verfassung ihrer Objekte hat sich verändert, und deshalb auch die Theorie. Trifft dies zu, würde der Hinwendung zur ästhetischen Erfahrung eine zumeist implizite und unausgesprochene Annahme über eine tiefgreifende Veränderung im Feld der Künste selbst zugrunde liegen: die Annahme, daß die Künste eine so grundlegend andere Verfassung anzunehmen beginnen, daß sie nicht mehr mit Hilfe traditioneller Werkkategorien gefaßt werden können."

films as spectacles or events, retransforming narrative cinema into a post-classical "cinema of attractions" (Tom Gunning).[7] Yet, at the same time, we are witnessing a growing "material and technological crisis of the flesh," turning living bodies into "ghosts in the machine" (Vivian Sobchack).[8] It seems that cinema in the digital age covers the span between carnal *stimulation* and *simulation*, contributing to an embodied and disembodied experience at the same time. This dual structure is what Raymond Bellour calls the "double-helix" of the new image, in which signs and sensations, codes and bodies are inseparably intertwined.[9] In opposition to the common diagnosis that we are virtually drowning in a flood of images, Bellour argues that the image has begun to withdraw: "We have gone beyond the image, to a nameless mixture, a discourse-image, if you like, or a sound-image ("Son-Image," Godard calls it), whose first side is occupied by television and second side by the computer, in our all-purpose machine society."[10] Traditionally, the image, especially the cinematic image, was thought to belong to the sphere of emotions, passions and sensual attractions, ranking low in the hierarchy of cultural production predominated by language. The subordination of images to words is nothing but a variation of the dominance of reason over the senses in a Western philosophical tradition that can be traced back to Heraclitus. This tradition is crystallised most clearly in Descartes' conception of human existence, which relies exclusively on the ability to think. Despite repeated objections, "Descartes' error" still persists today and has challenged Antonio Damasio and others to argue that in fact the body is the genesis of thought.[11] In a strange way though, this traditional hierarchy of word and image has collapsed in the age of the digital image. Bellour is convinced that the sensual experience of art has survived the digital revolution: "There is no visual image that is not more and more tightly gripped, even in its essential, radical withdrawal, inside an audiovisual or scriptovisual (what horrid words) image that envelops it [...]. In the long run, we'll have to invent a name for this new art, or – why not? – simply go on calling it 'cinematography.' On condition that *graphein* embraces the power of the voice as well as the physical quality of words, and that *kinema* includes the touch of the hand and all kinds of time."[12]

The increasing convergence of media has not completely annulled media specificity.[13] The availability of films on DVD, iPod, mobile phones and the Internet has not forced cinemas to close down, and cinematographers, on the

7 Gunning: "The Cinema of Attractions", p. 70. Gunning's thesis that the "cinema of attractions" is still alive within the special effects of narrative cinema is taken up for discussion in Strauven: *The Cinema of Attractions Reloaded.*

8 Sobchack: "The Scene of the Screen", pp. 161, 162.

9 In this sense, the graffiti, which figures prominently in Jarmusch's film, resembles Bellour's "double-helix," forming a hybrid of image and words purely visual sensation and graphic sign.

10 Bellour: "The Double Helix", p. 199.

11 Damasio: *Descartes' Error.*

12 Bellour: "The Double Helix", pp. 198 f.

13 For the convergence of media see Jenkins: *Convergence Culture.*

whole, still avoid the use of digital cameras unless it is necessary for special (mainly economic) reasons. There is at least one evident explanation for the filmmakers' preference of film material: the softness of blurred images, the tactile quality of the grain, the texture of film is still missing in digital images – despite the considerable efforts that have been made to simulate these defects or flaws amounting to sensual experience. We may consider our attachment to 35mm as pure conventionalism, as another case of "nostalgia" similar to the one which Erwin Panofsky attested himself while bemoaning the end of the silent film era.[14] However, in the midst of a digital and electronic society, cinema has all the more become an enclave of sensuous film experience.

The flipside of media convergence is a fruitful competition of cinema and new digital media. Christopher Doyle, the cinematographer of *The Limits of Control*, explicitly expressed this idea in an interview, stating that the distribution of images on TV, on the Internet or on the phone pushes cinematography to excellence, to even more precise and articulate images.[15] What he calls a "celebration of the image" can be attributed to a heightened susceptibility to the sensual world – to colour and light, to skin and texture, to composition and movement. *The Limits of Control* seems something like an anthem on this genuine capacity of cinema: by placing a seductive, but merely looked at nude (Paz de la Huerta) on a blue velvet bed sheet, by letting her dive into the blue water of a swimming pool, Jarmusch seems to stage the triumph of cinema over new media. These blue surfaces explicitly echo the blue video screens surrounding the film's villain, transforming technical devices of "military" power into the sensuously experienced images of cinema. In this context, even the main protagonist's laconic rejection of mobile phones serves as like a self-reflexive comment on the rivalry of cinema and new media.

14 Panofsky: "Style and Medium in the Motions Pictures", p. 116.

15 Doyle in an interview with Rüdiger Sturm at the Berlinale film festival, included in the extras of the DVD *Last Life in the Universe*, Alive 2003. Answering the question, how he sees his job in the era of digital filmmaking, where everyone can be a cinematographer, he says: "The push of young people making films on their phones, on the Internet, of people having access to pirate DVDs, you know, all that stuff actually pushes us to excellence, I think. [...] So, I think it's a great period of film making, especially visual film making. I mean, the relationship between the image and the word, the image and the idea is becoming much more concise than it could have been without karaoke, without 7,000 channels of TV, without the Internet."

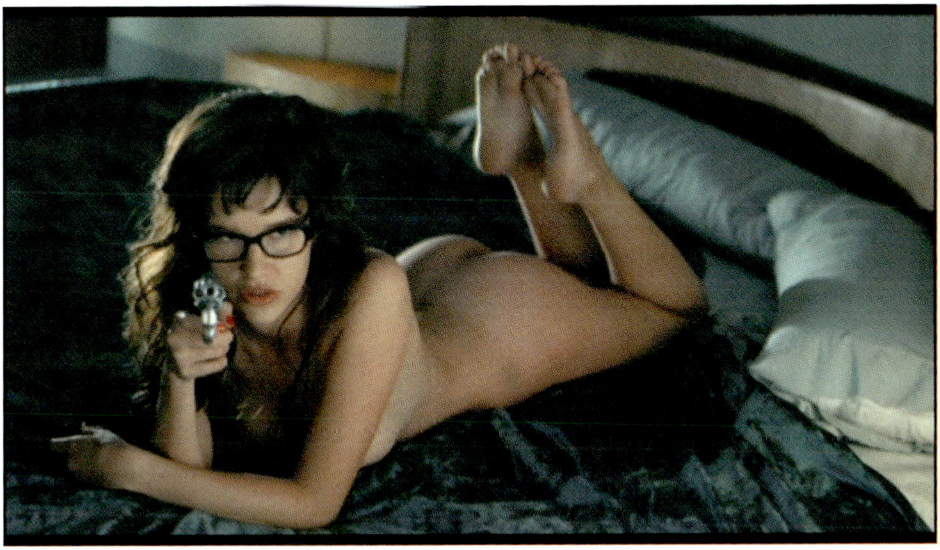

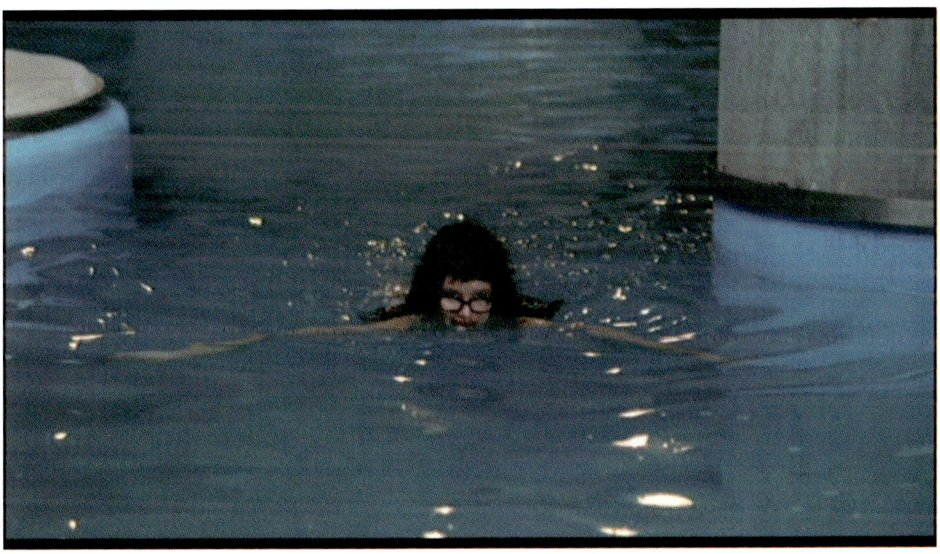

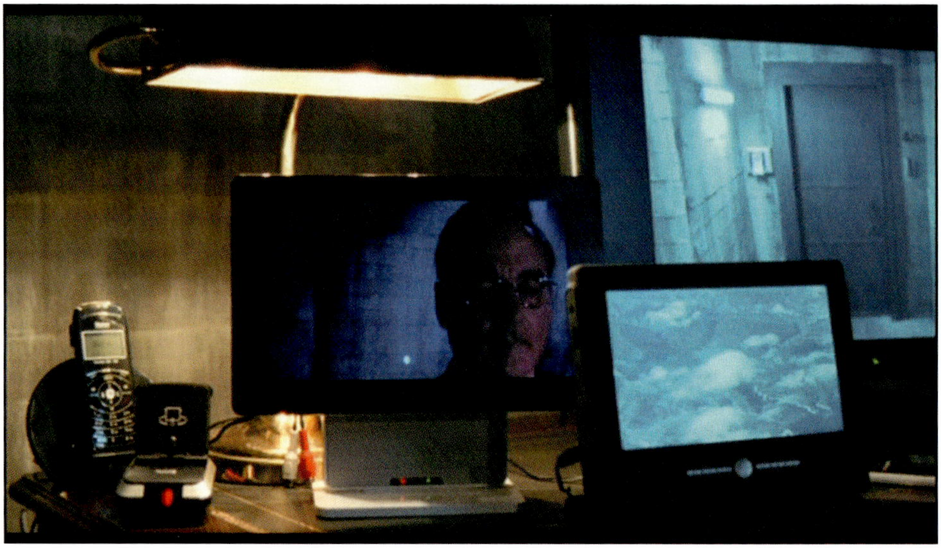

Fig. 1–3: Jim Jarmusch, The Limits of Control, 2009, The 'blue screens' of cinema and new media.

## II

Works of art are not merely the object of theory, but also actively engage in aesthetic discourse. Adapting Hegel's idea of history as a cognitive progress towards self-understanding, Arthur C. Danto argues that modern art has taken the role of philosophy by providing its own theory.[16] Recently, this idea has been expressed by W.J.T. Mitchell in his essay on metapictures, where he confronts the conception of "theory" as something that is primarily conducted in linear discourse, in language and logic, with pictures playing the passive role of illustrations, or (in the case of a "theory of pictures") serving as the passive objects of description and explanation. As an alternative, he recommends to advance the search for a "theory of pictures" by considering what he calls "pictures of theory."[17] Looking back on the history of film, we can see how dominant modes of film practice closely correspond to the development of film theories in the same period. This is the reason why Thomas Elsaesser and Malte Hagener, in their introduction to film theory, have suggested that films be regarded as extensions or continuations of theory and vice versa.[18] This is especially the case when it comes to an investigation of the sphere beyond signs and meaning. In art theory, the view that images exceed the capacity of language is frequently held, particularly in regard to

16 See the chapter "The End of Art" in Danto: *The Philosophical Disenfranchisement of Art.*

17 Mitchell: "Metapictures", p. 82.

18 Elsaesser/Hagener: *Filmtheorie zur Einführung*, p. 20.

questions concerning the specificity of visual as opposed to verbal expression.[19] Film theory has only occasionally participated in the debate on language failing the image. Kristin Thompson's concept of "cinematic excess"[20], which refers to Roland Barthes' notes on an obtuse or "third meaning"[21] in film, is one of few examples. If these arguments concerning the deficiency of language are valid, the image itself proves to be the most adequate medium to reflect on its visual potential: its capacity to produce an aesthetic surplus, which has frequently been described as material or sensual quality.

In this context, *The Limits of Control,* a film that triggers a sensual experience and its recognition at the same time, seems to be an exceptional example. The film clearly indicates a scepticism towards words, borrowing its title from an essay by William S. Burroughs, in which he aligns all efficient mechanisms of control with the power of words: "Suggestions are words. Persuasions are words. Orders are words. No control machine so far devised can operate without words, and any control machine which attempts to do so relying entirely on external force or entirely on physical control of the mind will soon encounter the limits of control."[22] Like the "drunken boat" in Arthur Rimbaud's poem of the same title (its first lines are cited at the beginning of the film)[23] the camera sets off shore to carry the spectator beyond "the limits of control" – into a trance-like sphere of images that flood visual perception and drown verbal interpretation.

If the film has a story at all, it is about a Lone Man (Isaach De Bankolé) on a secret mission in Spain, which leads him to "the American" (Bill Murray), an agent of evil, whom he kills in the end. The reasons for his mission remain obscure, although there are hints which suggest a conspiracy of the bohemian society against capitalism, or even more explicitly, art cinema's revenge on Hollywood. However, the thriller plot (inspired by John Boorman's *Point Blank*, USA 1967) serves only as a pretext to an essay on aesthetic experience centring on the protagonist's recurring visits to the Museo Reina Sofía, Madrid's museum of contemporary art. In his four visits he picks only one piece of art at a time, immersing himself successively in Juan Gris' cubist painting *El Violin* (1916), in Roberto Fernández Balbuena's modernist nude *Desnudo* (1932), in Antonio López García's realist cityscape *Madrid Desde Capitán Haya* (1987–94) and Antoni Tàpies' assemblage *Gran Sábana* (1968). Once he leaves the museum, his

19 Max Imdahl should be named here, who assumed that the genuinely visual aspect of visual arts – what he considered the 'iconic' content of images – could not be adequately or fully translated into words. Significantly, it was the confrontation with modern non-figurative art that inspired his post-iconologic approach, calling for an understanding of painting beyond the identification of objects, actions, and stories and the decoding of their different levels of meaning. More recently, the scepticism towards the reliance on language in art historical discourse has been expressed, e.g., by James Elkins in his study *On Pictures and the Words that Fail Them* (1998).

20 Thompson: "The Concept of Cinematic Excess".

21 Barthes: "The Third Meaning".

22 Burroughs: "The Limits of Control", p. 117.

23 "Comme je descendais des Fleuves impassibles, Je ne me sentis plus guidé par les haleurs…"

his enriched aesthetic experience expands into the everyday world. Gradually, he comes to perceive everything in the way he looks at paintings.[24]

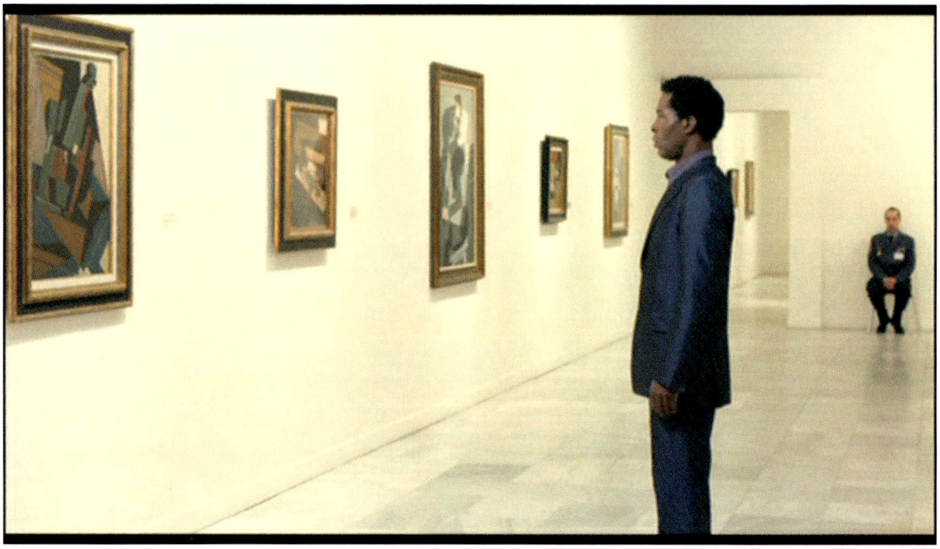

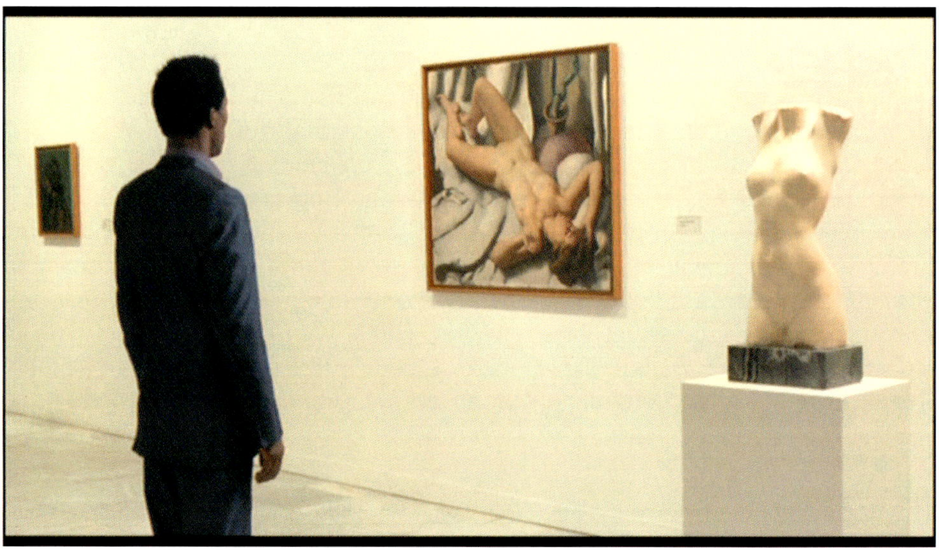

24 See Jarmusch's commentary in an interview: "So the idea was that he looks at *everything* in the way he looks at paintings. The way he watches the nude girl swimming in a pool. There's a scene where there are pears on a plate, and I wanted that to look like a painting. The way he compares the Tower of Gold to a postcard. Even the moving landscapes, when he is travelling by train." Dawson: "A Cultural Glossary to *The Limits of Control*".

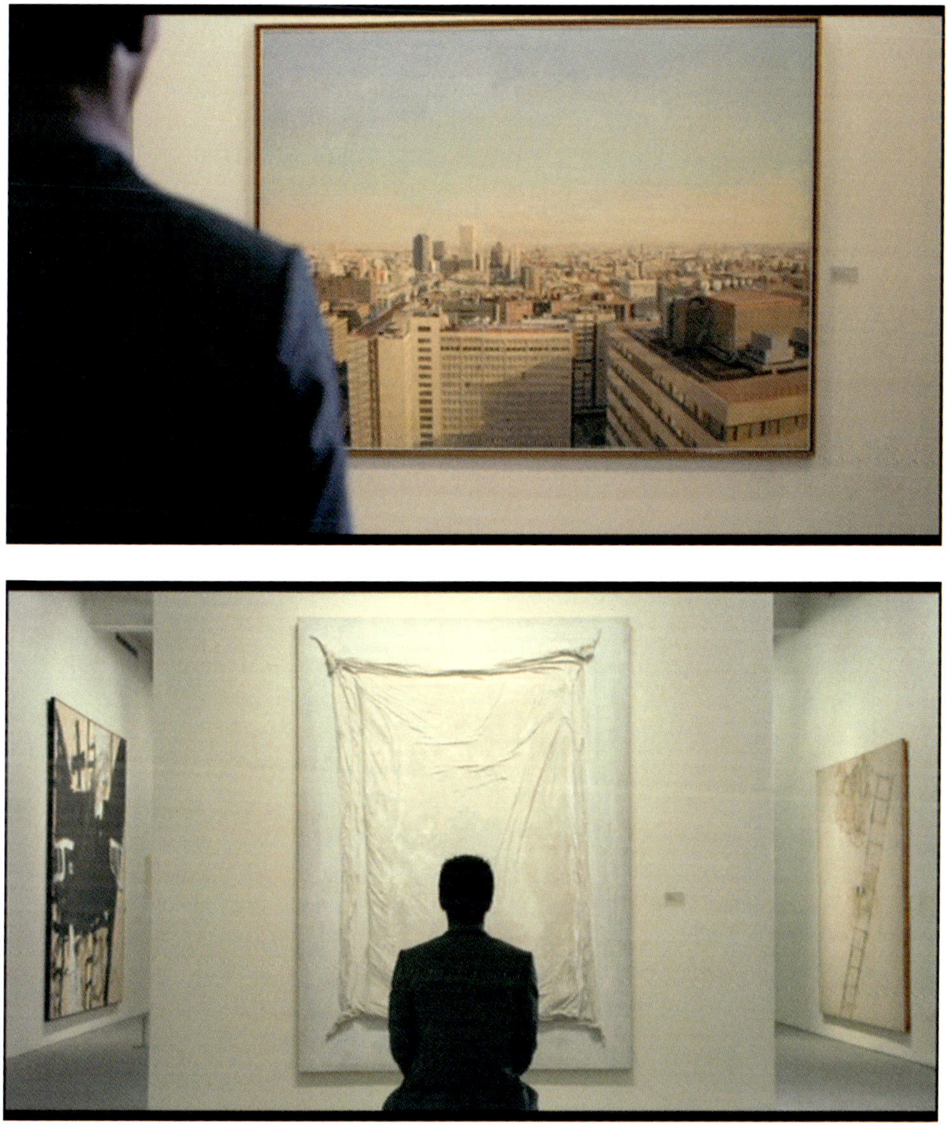

Fig. 4–7: Jim Jarmusch, The Limits of Control, 2009, The four visits to the Museo Reina Sofía in Madrid.

Regarding the film's general potential to engage in aesthetic discourse, one aspect of *The Limits of Control* seems of particular interest: repeatedly, the Lone Man meets a stranger from whom he receives a secret note in a matchbox. After having read the note, an enigmatic code consisting of letters and numbers, he chews and swallows the slip of paper by taking a sip from his double espresso (which he habitually orders in two separate cups). This recurring scenario does not merely show the concealment of a secret document following a convention of the thriller genre; it also demonstrates the transformation of an arithmetic code into a material thing: the reading of an abstract sign is replaced by the carnal appropriation of an object. This gesture initiates a transition between two different cultural modes, which Hans Ulrich Gumbrecht, in his book on the *Production of Presence*, has identified as "meaning culture" and "presence culture."[25] They correspond to different types of world-appropriation ranging from "interpretation and communication as exclusively spiritual ways of understanding" to "eating the world as the most direct way of becoming one with the things of the world in their tangible presence."[26] In this context, the Lone Man's gesture of eating the note expresses a break from "meaning culture" and its attachment to semiotic or hermeneutic methods of interpretation. It calls into question the dominant idea that meaning is something immaterial or mental to be discovered underneath the material surface in the depth of the text.

Yet, the sensuous appropriation of the world performed in *The Limits of Control* doesn't simply dismiss meaning, it rather embraces the possibility that *having* and *making* sense are the same thing. In cinema, looking out of the train's window and watching the landscape passing by has often indicated a self-referential moment, in which the camera contemplates on the nature of the moving image. Here, the train view takes on an additional connotation, as an emblem for an aesthetic experience that reintroduces our senses to the making of meaning. Significantly, the German word for meaning, "Sinn," etymologically includes the notion of "traveling."[27] It originally meant a directional movement or focused experience, in which sensation and signification were not yet divided. The traveling sequences in *The Limits of Control* remind us of this former unity of sensorimotor and conceptual inference, which is acknowledged by recent studies on the embodied mind. Amongst others, George Lakoff and Mark Johnson claim that reason is not disembodied: "The locus of reason (conceptual inference) would be the same as the locus of perception and motor control, which are bodily functions. If this seems like a radical claim, it is radical only from the perspective of faculty psychology, a philosophy that posits a radical separation from the point of view of the brain, which is the joint locus of reason, perception, and movement."[28]

Significantly, the last note, which the Lone Man receives on his journey by train, is completely blank: a little "white screen" that may remind us of all its famous predecessors in the history of modern art, ranging from Kasimir Malevich's *White on White* (1918, New York, Museum of Modern Art) to Robert Rauschenberg's *Erased De Kooning Drawing* (1953, collection of the artist). The Lone Man places the paper on his open palm, watching instead of reading it.

25 Gumbrecht: *The Production of Presence*, p. 79.

26 Gumbrecht: *The Production of Presence*, p. 87.

27 Sybille Krämer points to the etymology of the word "Sinn" as it is recorded in Jakob and Wilhelm Grimm's German Dictionary in order to question the dualism between "Sinn und Sinnlichkeit". Krämer: "Sinnlichkeit, Denken, Medien", p. 29.

28 Lakoff/Johnson: *Philosophy in the Flesh*, p. 20.

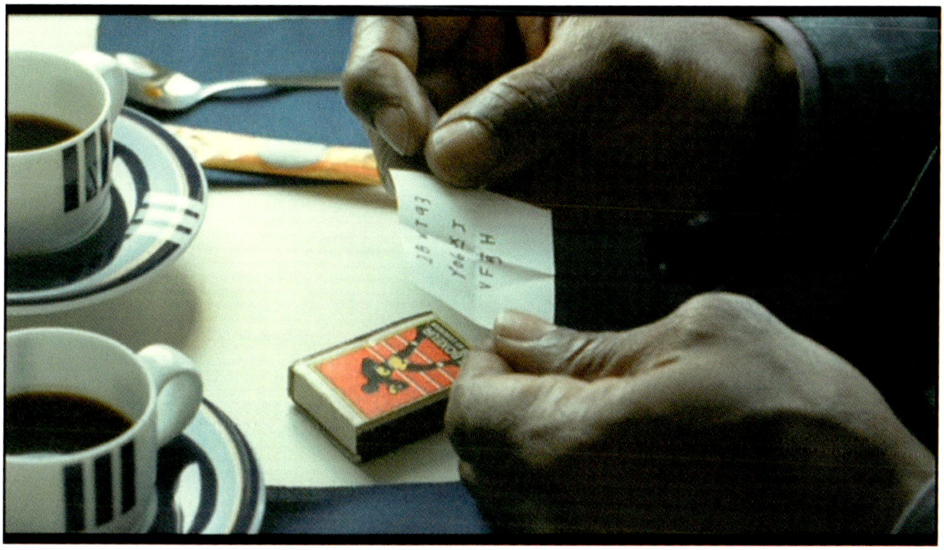

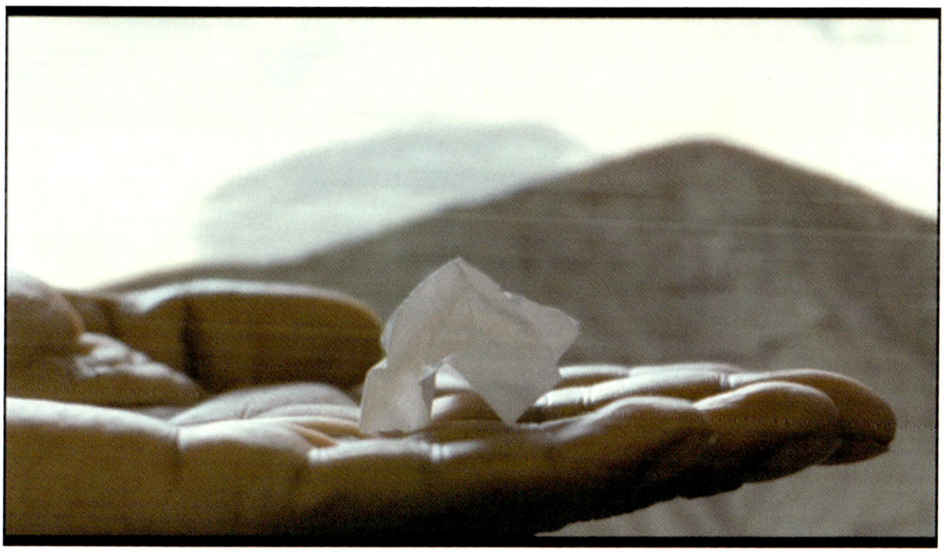

Fig. 8–9: Jim Jarmush, The limits of Control, 2009, Transformation of signs into images.

Against the backdrop of a mountain seen through the train's window, the sculptured piece of paper seems to mirror the view, resembling a small mountain itself. Here, the character has successfully completed his actual mission: he no longer decodes meaning, but senses the materiality of images. In his final visit to the Museo Reina Sofía, he is thus prepared to confront Antoni Tàpies' *Gran Sábana*, a big white sheet arranged plastically on a white canvas, with each corner tied in knots. The sheet, which pretends to hide or veil an actual image underneath, has confidently taken the place of this image, substituting figural representation with the sheer presence of art as object. Finally, at the end of the journey, something new seems to enter not just the museum, but also the art of cinema: the beginning of the end of images – at least in a conventional understanding.

## III

Films display and provide multiple forms of aesthetic experience, in which carnal and cognitive responses interrelate in many ways. Following the common distinction between mainstream and art cinema as opposing modes of production, we may also ascribe them different modes of perception. At first sight, an embodied film experience seems to be privileged either by technically advanced mainstream and blockbuster films, or by genre films that display eccentric body dramas: tears in weepies, blood in splatter films, orgasms in pornography, sweat in action films, adrenaline in thrillers etc. A discreet and subtle (some might say boring, fatiguing or tedious) art film such as *The Limits of Control,* in which nothing much happens, does not fit in either of these categories of mainstream films with event character or body genre films with shock potential. The film's withdrawal from bodily action can be seen as a challenge to many of the existing theories of an embodied experience, which focus on transgressive or action-packed cinema. Needless to say, theories of embodied film experience have taken diverging directions, depending not only on the methodological framework but also on the selected corpus of films on which they are based.

Torben Grodal, in his cognitive approach to film, has characterised mainstream and art cinema in relation to their cognitive appeal to the audience. For him, the key difference between art films and mainstream films rests on their specific treatment of concrete bodily and abstract mental aspects, respectively. "Films with higher meaning are often characterized by a certain 'disembodiedness,' in striking contrast to the typical mainstream film, which is based on embodied interaction with an online reality."[29] By drawing on Antonio Damasio's identification of different levels of consciousness (in *The Feeling of what Happens*, 1999), Grodal associates the mainstream film with the so-called "core self," which is responsible for "the basic interaction between the embodied mind and the world." He links the art film, however, to the higher level of the "autobiographical self," which is equipped "with an extended consciousness that interprets the online present in the context of past memories and future goals and aspirations."[30] According to this view, we could make the rather simple distinction between two modes of filmmaking that involve our bodies and our minds to different degrees.

29 Grodal: *Embodied Visions*, p. 208.
30 Grodal: *Embodied Visions*, pp. 213, 214.

Recalling my own film experiences, I don't quite agree with Grodal's interpretation of art films as representations or displays of disembodied qualities, be they mental, transcendental, spiritual or whatever. It seems to me that art cinema has provided various examples for heightened sensuous and embodied experiences on the side of the characters as well as the audience. Even Jarmusch's protagonist, who adheres rigidly to the rules "no guns, no mobiles, no sex," cannot entirely be regarded as a character lacking a sense of his body and his desires. The way he looks at paintings and the corresponding way the camera looks at the world suggest a strong sensitivity to the phenomenal aspects of perception, illustrating Maurice Merleau-Ponty's idea that "to see is *to have at a distance.*"[31] By gradually moving closer to the things he is looking at, the camera suggests an immersion, through which the protagonist virtually drowns his gaze in the image, just as the nude girl, equipped with a big pair of glasses, lets her body sink into the pool water.[32]

Considering *The Limits of Control*, Grodal is absolutely right to note that the main characters of art films "are more often observers than participants" and that "art film narration is often phenomenological" compared to the more action-focused and goal-oriented classical narration.[33] But does this phenomenological, perceptive quality of art films necessarily entail the impression or experience of disembodiedness? Are the "streams of perception," as Grodal suggests, really "disembodied, insofar as they are isolated from any pragmatic concerns that might link them to action"?[34] Considering Merleau-Ponty's emphasis on the body (*le corps propre*) as the constituent of perceptual openness to the world and its influence on recent positions of embodiment in cognitive science and film studies, I would say no. On the contrary, and this is my thesis, it is precisely *because of the elimination or displacement of the plot* that art cinema allows for an *intensified embodied experience of film*. It is significant that a great number of film theories, focusing on the physical sensations and material qualities of film, share a scepticism regarding the central status of narration. This scepticism towards narration is echoed in Jarmusch's film, which was shot without a common script, rejecting story in the interest of style. Just a sketch of about 25 pages served as the basis for the shooting,[35] enhancing the performative power and sheer presence of the image: Tilda Swinton's elf-like make-up and Paz de la

31 Merleau-Ponty: "Eye and Mind", p. 166.

32 As a nude with black-framed glasses, she is unmistakably characterised as an object *and* subject of visual pleasure, which does not entirely fit in the scopic regime of classical cinema and its critique in feminist film theory.

33 Grodal: *Embodied Visions*, p. 221.

34 Grodal: *Embodied Visions*, p. 221.

35 See Jarmusch's commentary to the notebook of production designer Eugenio Caballero. "My script for this film was initially only a 25-page story, but throughout that story it said, maybe 15 times, 'He looks at so-and-so as though looking at a painting at a museum.' I was going for a kind of trippiness, a way of looking at everything in a different way. I kept accumulating things as we went along, without a completely drawn map from the beginning. We had more of a sketch of a map, which was the idea – to have freedom to expand it." Jarmusch: "*Limits of Control*. Diary in Pictures", p. 2.

Huerta's transparent rain coat, an old woman sitting at a train station and two building workers carrying a bath tub, graffiti in the streets and the still life of a pear on a plate – these are the film's main attractions. Within the framework of aesthetic experience, even the ordinary landscape passing by the train's window magically transforms into an edited (!) sequence of cinematic art. With every cut on the window's screen, the false colour landscapes change in an almost psychedelic way, reminding one from far of the stargate trip near the end of Stanley Kubrick's *2001: A Space Odyssey* (UK 1968).

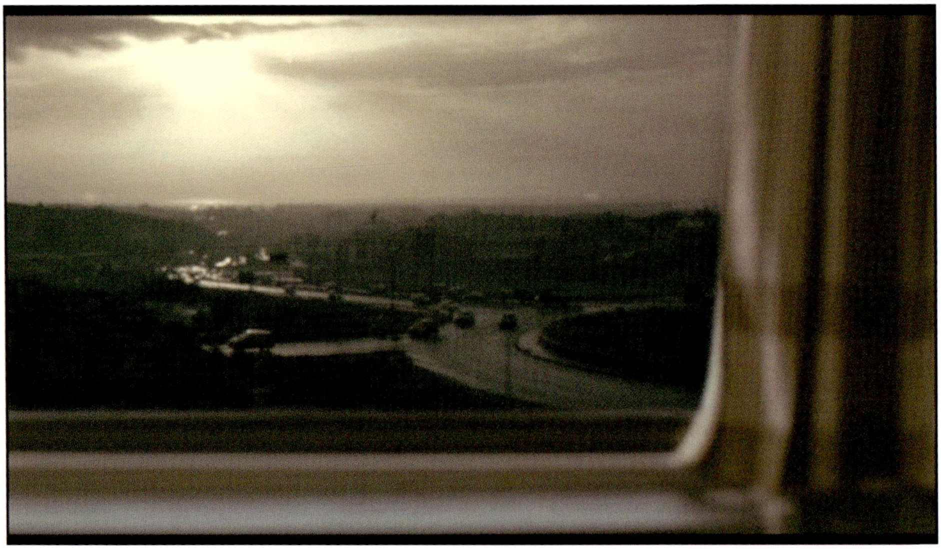

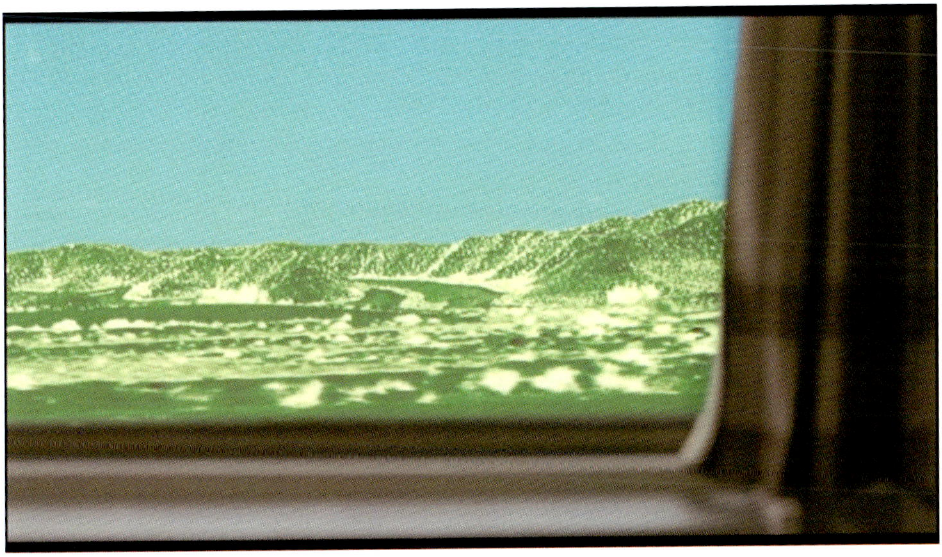

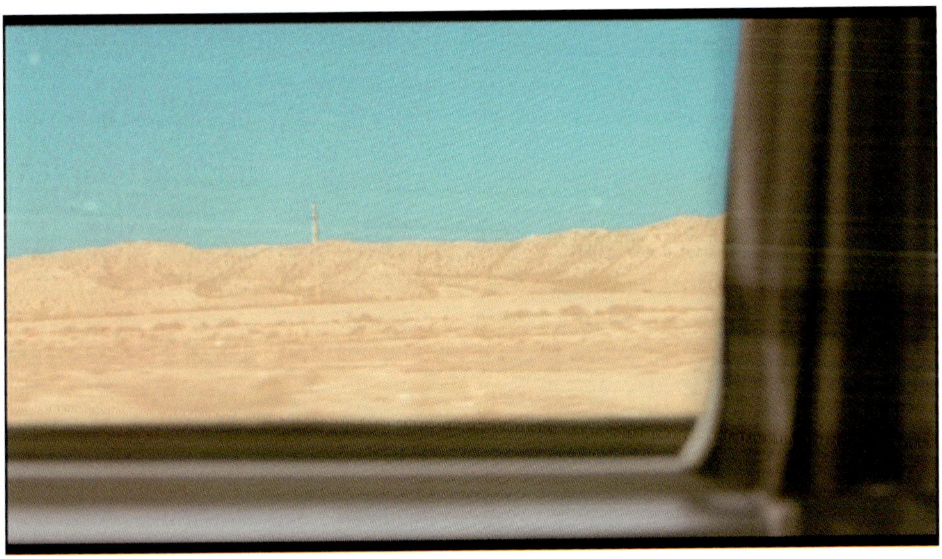

Fig. 10–13: Jim Jarmusch, The limits of Control, 2009, The train window as film screen.

I suppose that the intensification of an embodied experience is caused by an increased awareness of our senses and their active engagement in the film. According to John Dewey, aesthetic experience, unlike ordinary experience, is characterised by awareness.[36] For Dewey, the domain of aesthetics is not radically autonomous, but constitutes a heightened form of experiencing the world. Therefore, like Jarmusch's protagonist, Dewey doesn't distinguish between the aesthetic experience of art and the aesthetic experience of everyday situations. For Jar-

36 Dewey: *Art as Experience*.

musch's character, a girl swimming naked in a pool has the same aesthetic appeal as Fernando Balbuena's painting of a nude. When he sees her for the first time lying naked on his bed, he opens the jacket of his elegant suit with one hand, not to get undressed, but to look at her; it is a nonchalant gesture he casually performs in front of the museum's paintings.

The thesis I would like to put forward here is that our awareness (which Dewey considers as the condition of aesthetic experience) correlates with the degree of our involvement in the plot. Following sequences of dense action, which are typically characterised by fast editing and a maximum of suspense, reduce the awareness of our aesthetic experience. We simply don't get the time and space to reflect on our embodied film experience, even though we might be caught in the grips of a melodrama, a horror or even a pornographic film (just to name the most popular examples of Linda Williams' category of "body genres"[37]). Our body will display a physical reaction, but this reaction will not necessarily become a focus of our interest or occupy our mind.

On the contrary, art cinema's tendency towards "dysnarration"[38] creates the space, which allows us to become aware of our embodied experiences, insofar as we do not only consciously recognise, but also reflect on them. Annette Michelson has very convincingly argued in this direction in her reading of Stanley Kubrick's *2001: A Space Odyssey*, a film which seems to have more in common with an opera than with classical narrative cinema. Michelson sees the film as being in line with avant-garde and modernist attempts to provide "therapy for an intellectual tradition"[39] through the substitution of action by scenes of perceptions. Her concise essay, published as early as 1969, can be considered as a contribution to cognitive film theory *avant la lettre*. For her, Kubrick's film serves as a "Primary Structure, forcing the spectator back, in a reflexive gesture, upon the analytic rehearsal of his experience."[40] The constant mediation between sensation and reflexion, between carnal and mental modes of perception, thus requires a form of "athleticism"[41] on the part of the spectator: "The difference between the two qualities and intensities of response is the difference between things seen and things felt, between situations visually observed and those sensed haptically, between a narrative emblem and a radically formal embodiment of spatial logic."[42] And as if she had read Lakoff's and Johnson's contributions to a "philosophy in the flesh"[43] before these were even published, Michelson concludes her article with a definition of film as carnal knowledge: "Seeing films, in general,

37 Williams: "Film Bodies", pp. 2–13.

38 Other than avant-garde or experimental films, art cinema doesn't completely resign from storytelling. It is characterised by "dysnarration," a term that Francis Vanoye uses to describe "an operation of a *récit* (narrative) voluntarily challenging itself." Vanoye: *Récit écrit, récit filmique*, p. 199.

39 Michelson: "Bodies in Space", p. 57.

40 Michelson: "Bodies in Space", p. 56.

41 Michelson: "Bodies in Space", p. 59.

42 Michelson: "Bodies in Space", p. 60.

43 Lakoff/Johnson: *Philosophy in the Flesh.*

one gains an intimation of the link between the development of sensori-motor knowledge to that of intelligence itself."[44] For Vivian Sobchack, this perceptive athleticism is an integral part of what she calls the "cinesthetic experience." the ambivalent impression "of having both a 'real' (or literal) sensual experience and an 'as-if-real' (or figural) sensual experience," which relates to the interplay "of 'having sense' and 'making sense' – meaning thus constituted as both a *carnal matter* and a *conscious meaning* that emerge simultaneously (if in various ratios) from *the single system of flesh and consciousness that is the lived body*."[45]

Following Annette Michelson's and Vivian Sobchack's arguments, I would like to read *The Limits of Control* as a contribution to a theory of aesthetic experience in which the spectator gains awareness of his or her physical being, provoking an intersection of reflexion and sensuality in the process of viewing "so that pleasure is informed with the shock of recognition."[46] The Lone Man's exposure to art as a means of training his senses mirrors our own exercise in viewing the film. Just like his, our aesthetic experience is disembodied and embodied at the same time: we merely watch without touching or interacting with the objects of our contemplation. At the same time, we undergo a sensitisation of our senses, which increasingly respond to the image. In this case, cinema provides a privileged form of aesthetic experience, which allows for an analytic rehearsal of our physical response. The result is a paradox: *our mind becomes occupied with our senses.*

This theory of aesthetic experience extracted from Jarmusch's film does not only disagree with Grodal's interpretation of art films as disembodied; it also diverges significantly from a tradition of film theory that has aligned an embodied experience with a surrender of intellect and has equated cinema's address of the senses solely with notions of shock, excess, attraction, and spectacle. The idea of cinema's numbing bombardment of the senses informs the writings of Walter Benjamin,[47] Siegfried Kracauer[48] and others, who have placed film and its radical impact on perception in the centre of modern life. Just like the roller coaster, the factory, and urban traffic, film was assumed to virtually attack the spectator's senses, nerves and whole physical condition. This anaesthetic potential attested to cinema refigures prominently in Steven Shaviro's study of *The Cinematic Body* (1993), where he investigates the "ways in which film renders vision tactile, short-circuits reflection and directly stimulates the nervous sys-

44 Michelson: "Bodies in Space", p. 62.

45 Sobchack: "What My Fingers Knew", p. 73.

46 Michelson: "Bodies in Space", p. 59.

47 In his artwork essay Benjamin speaks of the "chock" experience of film, a concept he develops further in his essay on Charles Baudelaire. Benjamin: "Das Kunstwerk im Zeitalter seiner technischen Reproduzierbarkeit". See also Benjamin: "Über einige Motive bei Baudelaire".

48 According to Kracauer, the material elements of film virtually attack the spectator as a subject, finally leading to the decomposition of the self: "Das 'Ich' des dem Film zugewandten Menschen ist *in ständiger Auflösung begriffen*, wird unablässig von den materiellen Phänomenen gesprengt." Kracauer in his Marseille notebooks, quoted in Bratze-Hansen: "Dinosaurier sehen und nicht gefressen werden", p. 265. See also Hansen: "With Skin and Hair", pp. 437–469.

tem."[49] Referring to Benjamin's tactile apperception of film, Shaviro understands film viewing as an experience of shock and an over-stimulation leaving no time for semiosis. A similar view, which simply inverts the hierarchy between body and mind, is expressed by Wolfgang Welsch, who holds media responsible for a postmodern condition of a trance-like insensitiveness, in which aesthetics and anaesthetics are dialectically joined.[50] *The Limits of Control* clearly contrasts these half euphoric, half technophobic visions of embodied cinema as aggressive, harming and loud. The aesthetic experience displayed in the film allows for a sensuous and reflexive encounter with images at the same time, portraying a highly alert and disciplined character that is self-trained in his capacity of distancing himself in order to get deeply involved in what he sees. If this experience echoes modernity and its tendency towards an "intoxication" of the senses, it succeeds in anaesthetising not through numbing, but through intensifying sensory experience. Like Benjamin's *flaneur*, Jarmusch's protagonist travels and strolls the streets in search for "l'éternelle du transitoire." Rather than being caught up in the big spectacles of mass entertainment, he slows his pace in order to make sense of the little perceptions isolated from the flow of life. Here, and not only in this film, cinema displays and provides an aesthetic experience beyond the simple dualism of body and mind – a questionable basis on which conventional conceptions of mainstream and art cinema are often built.

49 Shaviro: *The Cinematic Body*, p. 53.
50 Welsch: *Ästhetisches Denken*, pp. 14 f.

## References


Barthes, Roland: "The Third Meaning. Research Notes on Several Eisenstein Stills" (1970), in: *The Responsibility of Forms. Critical Essays on Music, Art, and Representation,* Berkeley (University of California Press) 1985, pp. 41–62.

Bellour, Raymond: "The Double Helix", in: Timothy Druckrey (ed.): *Electronic Culture. Technology and Visual Representation*, New York, NY (Aperture) 1996, pp. 173–199.

Beugnet, Martine: *Cinema and Sensation. French Film and the Art of Transgression*, Edinburgh (Edinburgh University Press) 2007.

Benjamin, Walter: *Das Kunstwerk im Zeitalter seiner technischen Reproduzierbarkeit. Drei Studien zur Kunstsoziologie*, Frankfurt am Main (Suhrkamp) 1977.

Benjamin, Walter: "Über einige Motive bei Baudelaire" (1939), in: *Charles Baudelaire. Ein Lyriker im Zeitalter des Hochkapitalismus*, Frankfurt am Main (Suhrkamp) 1990, pp. 101–150.

Benjamin, Walter: *Das Passagen-Werk*, 2 vols., ed. by Rolf Tiedemann and Hermann Schweppenhäuser, Frankfurt am Main (Suhrkamp) 1991.

Boehm, Gottfried: "Bildsinn und Sinnesorgane in Anschauung als ästhetische Kategorie", in: *Neue Hefte für Philosophie Göttingen*, 18–19 (1980), pp. 118–132.

Bordwell, David: *Making Meaning. Inference and Rhetoric in the Interpretation of Cinema*, Cambridge, MA (Harvard University Press) 1989.

Bordwell, David and Noël Carroll (eds.): *Post-Theory. Reconstructing Film Studies*, Madison, Wisc. (University of Wisconsin Press) 1996.

Brandt, Stefan L.: *The Culture of Corporeality. Aesthetic Experience and the Embodiment of America* (1945–1960), Heidelberg (Winter) 2007.

Bratze-Hansen, Miriam: "Dinosaurier sehen und nicht gefressen werden: Kino als Ort der Gewalt-Wahrnehmung der Benjamin, Kracauer und Spielberg", in: Gertrud Koch (ed.): *Auge und Affekt. Wahrnehmung und Interaktion*, Frankfurt am Main (Fischer) 1995, pp. 249–271.

Buck-Morss, Susan: "Aesthetics and Anaesthetics. Walter Benjamin's Artwork Essay Reconsidered", in: *October* 62 (1992), pp. 3–41.

Burroughs, William S.: "The Limits of Control" (1975), in: *The Adding Machine. Selected Essays*, New York (Arcade) 1993, pp. 117–121.

Clark, Andy: *Supersizing the Mind. Embodiment, Action, and Cognitive Extension*, New York (Oxford University Press) 2009.

Crowther, Paul: *Art and Embodiment. From Aesthetics to Self-Consciousness*, Oxford (Clarendon Press) 2001.

Dawson, Nick: "A Cultural Glossary to *The Limits of Control*", in: *Film in Focus* April 28, 2009, www.filminfocus.com/article/a_cultural_glossary_to__em_the_limits_of_control__em_/.

Damasio, Antonio: *Descartes' Error. Emotion, Reason and the Human Brain*, New York (Putnam) 1994.

Damasio, Antonio: *The Feeling of what Happens. Body and Emotion in the Making of Consciousness*, New York (Harcourt Brace) 1999.

Danto, Arthur C.: *The Philosophical Disenfranchisement of Art,* New York (Columbia University Press) 1986.

Dewey, John: *Art as Experience*, New York, NY (Perigee) 1980.

Dyson, Frances: *Sounding New Media. Immersion and Embodiment in the Arts and Culture*, Berkeley (University of California Press) 2009.

Eisenstein, Sergej M.: "Montage der Filmattraktionen" (1924), in: *Jenseits der Einstellung. Schriften zur Filmtheorie*, ed. by Felix Lenz and Helmut H. Diederichs, Frankfurt am Main (Suhrkamp) 2006, pp. 15–40.

Elsaesser, Thomas: "Erfahren, erleben, entgrenzen: Das Kino der (zu starken) Körper und Gefühle", in: *Hollywood heute. Geschichte, Gender und Nation im postklassischen Kino*, Berlin (Bertz + Fischer) 2009, pp. 35–52.

Gallagher, Shaun: *The Phenomenological Mind. An Introduction to Philosophy of Mind and Cognitive Science*, London (Routledge) 2008.

Grodal, Torben: *Embodied Visions. Evolution, Emotion, Culture, and Film*, Oxford (Oxford University Press) 2009.

Grodal, Torben: *Moving Pictures. A New Theory of Film Genres, Feelings and Cognition*, Oxford (Clarendon Press) 1999.

Gumbrecht, Hans Ulrich: *Production of Presence. What Meaning Cannot Convey,* Stanford (Stanford University Press) 2004.

Gumbrecht, Hans Ulrich and K. Ludwig Pfeiffer (eds.): *Materialität der Kommunikation*, Frankfurt am Main (Suhrkamp) 1988.

Gunning, Tom: "The Cinema of Attractions. Early Film, Its Spectator and the Avant-Garde", in: *Wide Angle,* 8 (1986) 3–4, pp. 63–70.

Hansen, Miriam: "'With Skin and Hair'. Kracauer's Theory of Film, Marseille 1940", in: *Critical Inquiry,* 19 (Spring 1993) 3, pp. 437–469.

Jarmusch, Jim: "*Limits of Control.* Diary in Pictures", in: *New York Magazine*, April 26, 2009, http://nymag.com/arts/articles/09/04/limitsofcontrol/.

Jenkins, Henry: *Convergence Culture. Where Old and New Media Collide*, New York (New York University Press) 2006.

Kracauer, Siegfried: *Theory of Film. The Redemption of Physical Reality*, New York (Oxford University Press) 1960.

Krämer, Sybille: "Sinnlichkeit, Denken, Medien: Von der 'Sinnlichkeit als Erkenntnis' zur 'Sinnlichkeit als Performanz'", in: Bernd Busch, Annett Müller and Jutta Seligmann (eds.): *Der Sinn der Sinne,* Göttingen (Steidl) 1998, pp. 24–39.

Küpper, Joachim and Christoph Menke (eds.): *Dimensionen ästhetischer Erfahrung*. Frankfurt am Main (Suhrkamp) 2003.

Lakoff, George and Mark Johnson: *Philosophy in the Flesh. The Embodied Mind and Its Challenge to Western Thought*, New York, NY (Basic Books) 1999.

Marks, Laura U.: *The Skin of the Film. Intercultural Cinema, Embodiment and the Senses*, Durham, NC (Duke University Press) 2000.

Merleau-Ponty, Maurice: "Eye and Mind", in: *The Primacy of Perception*, ed. by James Edie, Evanston, Ill. (Northwestern University Press) 1964, pp. 159–190.

Mérö, Lázló: *Die Grenzen der Vernunft. Kognition, Intuition und komplexes Denken*, Reinbek bei Hamburg (Rowohlt) 2002.

Michelson, Annette: "Bodies in Space. Film as 'Carnal Knowledge'", in: *Artforum,* 7 (February 1969) 6, pp. 54–63.

Mikunda, Christian: *Kino spüren*, München (Filmland Presse) 1986.

Panofsky, Erwin: "Style and Medium in the Motions Pictures", in: *Three Essays on Style*, ed. by Irving Lavin, Cambridge, Mass. (MIT Press) 1995, pp. 91–128.

Mitchell, W.J.T.: "Metapictures", in: *Picture Theory. Essays on Verbal and Visual Representation*, Chicago (The University of Chicago Press) 1993, pp. 35–82.

Münch, Dieter (ed.): *Kognitionswissenschaft: Grundlagen, Probleme, Perspektiven*, Frankfurt am Main (Suhrkamp) 1992.

Naumann-Beyer, Waltraud: "Sinnlichkeit", in: Karlheinz Barck (ed.): *Ästhetische Grundbegriffe. Historisches Wörterbuch in sieben Bänden*, Stuttgart/Weimar (J.B. Metzler) 2003, vol. 5, pp. 534–577.

Plantinga, Carl: "Cognitive Film Theory. An Insider's Appraisal", in: *Cinémas* 12 (2002) 2, pp. 15–37.

Robnik, Drehli: "Körper-Erfahrung und Film-Phänomenologie", in: Jürgen Felix (ed.): *Moderne Film Theorie*, 2nd edition, Mainz (Bender) 2003, pp. 246–280.

Shaviro, Steven: *The Cinematic Body*, Minneapolis, Minn. (University of Minnesota Press) 1993.

Sobchack, Vivian: "The Scene of the Screen. Envisioning Photographic, Cinematic, and Electronic 'Presence'", in: *Carnal Thoughts. Embodiment and Moving Image Culture*, Berkeley/Los Angeles/London (University of California Press) 2004, pp. 135–162.

Sobchack, Vivian: "What My Fingers Knew. The Cinesthetic Subject, or Vision in the Flesh", in: *Carnal Thoughts. Embodiment and Moving Image Culture*, Berkeley/Los Angeles/London (University of California Press) 2004, pp. 53–84.

Sobchack, Vivian: *The Address of the Eye. A Phenomenology of Film Experience.* Princeton, NJ (Princeton University Press) 1992.

Strauven, Wanda (ed.): *The Cinema of Attraction Reloaded*, Amsterdam (Amsterdam University Press) 2006.

Thompson, Kristin: "The Concept of Cinematic Excess" (1977), in: Philip Rosen (ed.): *Narrative, Apparatus, Ideology. A Film Theory Reader*, New York (Columbia University Press) 1986, pp. 130–142.

Vanoye, Francis: *Récit écrit, récit filmique,* Paris (Nathan) 1989.

Varela, Francisco J.: *Kognitionswissenschaft – Kognitionstechnik. Eine Skizze aktueller Perspektiven,* Frankfurt am Main (Suhrkamp) 1990.

Varela, Francisco J., Evan T. Thompson and Eleanor Rosch: *The Embodied Mind. Cognitive Science and Human Experience*, Cambridge, Mass. (MIT Press) 1991.

Voss, Christiane: "Filmerfahrung und Illusionsbildung. Der Zuschauer als Leihkörper des Kinos", in: Gertrud Koch and Christiane Voss (eds.): *...kraft der Illusion*, München (Fink) 2006, pp. 71–86.
Welsch, Wolfgang: *Ästhetisches Denken*, 6th, enlarged edition, Stuttgart (Reclam) 2003.
Williams, Linda: "Film Bodies. Gender, Genre, and Excess", in: *Film Quarterly,* 44 (Summer 1991) 4, pp. 2–13.
Wollen, Peter: *Signs and Meaning in the Cinema*, expanded and revised edition, London (British Film Institute) 1998.

## Screenshots

All Screenshots are taken from the DVD *The Limits of Control*

# Excerpt Neuropower[1]

WARREN NEIDICH

## 1. Introduction

Today more then ever, it is culture with language that has replaced nature as the primary force of epigenesis. Epigenesis is defined as the means by which the unfolding of the genetically prescribed formation of the brain is altered by its interaction with the environment.

> [...] The most extensive modification to take place in human brain evolution – the disproportionate expansion of the cerebral cortex, and specifically of the prefrontal cortex – reflects the evolutionary adaptation to this intensive working memory processing demand imposed by symbol learning. So the very nature of symbolic reference, and its unusual cognitive demands when compared to non-symbolic forms of reference, is a selection force working on those neurological resources most critical to supporting it. In the context of a society heavily dependent on symbol use-as is any conceivable human society, but no nonhuman societies-brains would have been under intense selection to adapt to these needs. [...] This, then, is a case of selection pressure affecting the evolution of a biological substrate (the brain) and yet which is imposed, not by the physical environment, but ultimately from a purely semiotic realm.[2]

When one considers post-natal brain development in this context, the term neural plasticity is used. Neural plasticity refers to the ability of the components of neurons, their axons, dendrites and synapses plus their extended forms as neural network systems, to be modified by experience. The neurobiologist Marcus Jacobson defined neural plasticity as a process through which the nervous system adjusts to changes in the internal and external milieu.[3] Adjustments in the internal milieu can occur after brain injuries. For instance, a child is able to recover function of language production and reception after trauma or stroke to the left language hemisphere of the brain. The right hemisphere, not normally an active part of that system, is capable of being modified so as to assume these language

1 This essay is a slightly modified excerpt from a longer forthcoming text entitled, "From Noo-Power to Neuropower: How Mind Becomes Matter", in: Deborah Hauptmann and Warren Neidich (eds.): *Cognitive Architecture: From Biopolitics to Noo-politics*, Rotterdam (010 Press) 2010.

2 Terrence Deacon: "Multilevel Selection".

3 Jacobson: *Developmental Neurobiology*, p. 26.

functions with little deficit if the onset of left hemisphere dysfunction occurs at an early enough age. Adjustments can also be in response to changes in the external milieu. The heterochronous changes of the neurobiological substrate that occur in time as an unfolding of the genetically determined neurobiological timetable create what are called critical periods of development. Certain regions and systems of the neurobiological substrate are extremely sensitive to the conditions of, for instance, the linguistic milieu, which predispose it to language acquisition during a particular time window. And therein lies the bigger question of which language will be acquired of the 6,700 available in the world that the child's brain has the potential to learn. Which one is actually learned is dependent upon the close coupling of the child's brain-mind to his or her linguistic field which produces immaterial selection pressures upon the neurobiological substrate of those areas of the cerebral cortex with specific predispositions for language learning. As we will see in what follows it is this condition of neural plasticity that will be key in understanding the rapprochement of Rancière's distribution of the sensible and its concomitant regulation of the pluripotentiality of the brain's neural plasticity. It is the 'Institutional Stabilization' of the distribution of sensibility in designed space which is crucial to policing of that field and fulfills the necessary conditions with which to restrict the potential heterogeneity implicit in the pluripotential character of the neurobiological substrate by restricting what can be attended and remembered. This then has implications for the sculpting of a people and forms the basis of what Maurizio Lazaratto calls Noo-politics.

> In order not to name such different things with the same word, one could define the new relations of power which take memory and its conatus (attention) as their object… noo-politics. Noo-politics (the ensemble of the techniques of control) is exercised on the brain. It involves above all attention, and is aimed at the control of memory and its virtual power.[4]

Today in the age of information and tertiary economies, in which objects and thing-ness have been replaced by services and communication, power is not only focusing on what is remembered but how those memories are constituted in future schemata in planning of future actions.

## 2. Extensivity and Intensivity

As we advance historically from primary economies of extraction to those described as secondary, involved with manufacturing, to those involved in services defined as tertiary we also move through different assemblages of sensational fields. Consider for a moment the differences in laboring practices and the archi-

4 Maurizio Lazzarato: "The Concepts of Life", p. 186.

tectures that subsume them of, on one hand, a factory worker assembling and mass producing an automobile on an assembly line as compared to that of the prosumer designing computer games simultaneously with others on-line at distant locations or a college professor having discussions with students on skype from his lap top while drinking coffee at Starbucks. Stationed in a restricted spatial volume and hegemonous singular schedule of the conveyor belt, the laborer is a cog in the wheel of production whilst the prosumer and professor are active sites or hubs in a massive fluid global diagram in which multiple flows rule the day. These different conditions of the work place have repercussions for the society as a whole. As such each represents different sensational and experiential fields. The former can be described as extensive because it is divisible into equal parts and it represents the simplest distribution of singularities leading to the production of similar images and objects ad infinitum. The latter is best described as intensive as it occurs as distributed networks that create non-linear affects and effects and contain assemblages of nested systems within systems that act as attractors producing multiple solutions.[5] "An assembly process may be said to be characterized by intensive properties when it articulates heterogenous elements as such."[6] Extensive systems create stable, typologies of essences while intensive ones are described instead as topologies, as states in the process of becoming. Intensive systems are under normal conditions subsumed into extensive ones. In order for them to manifest their full complexity as intensive systems, large differences in intensity must be maintained by external constraints.

> A non-linear system with multiple attractors, on the other hand, continues to display its virtuality even once the system has settled into one of its alternative stable states, because the other alternatives are there all the time, coexisting with the one that happens to be actualized.[7]

Extensive systems as they concern, for instance, architecture, are represented by a homogenized geographical spread like that found in Le Corbusier's identical units of habitation and the grid city model of New York. Conceptual practices of the sixties and seventies are extensive as they used rules and systems as instructions to produce similar products in varied aesthetic contexts. As we mentioned above extensive labor is the model of late 19th century production of real objects tethered to the actions of the physical body working along an assembly line while intensive culture is the culture of the network. Extensive Culture is driven by the

5 De Landa: *Intensive Science*, pp. 59–61. "Thermodynamic properties can be divided into two general classes, namely intensive and extensive properties. If a quantity of matter in a given state is divided into two equal parts, each part will have the same value of intensive properties as the original, and half the value of the extensive property. The first modification, which must be made to the standard definition of intensive property, is that the intensities defining a particular physical system may indeed be divided but the differences that result change the system in kind from an equilibrium to a non-equilibrium."

6 Ibid., p. 64.

7 Ibid., pp. 59–61.

production of exact objects and is a culture of equivalence. Intensive Culture, however, is characterized by nonequivalence and difference. Intensive things are one-offs and singular. Whereas extensive culture produces the commodity as a form of equivalence, intensive culture is diagrammatic and is defined by multiplicitous, non-linear, rhizomatic processes nested together in complex assemblages, immaterial labor, and the idea of the brand.[8] The degree to which one form dominates as a cultural modifier and descriptor depends, today, first and foremost upon the degree to which a culture has embraced or has access to the information society. When the conditions of the information economy predominate over those of the industrial and agricultural or artisanal ones, as is the case in the Northern European economies and the United States, the emergent forms of, what Marx referred to as general machinic intelligence, to be explained below, reflect the conditions of that networked, non-linear distributed and intensive cultural milieu. The brain/mind that is coupled to this system results in a store of distributed networked memories that reflect those very conditions of remembering.

> From the perspective of distributed cognition, this sort of individual learning is seen as the propagation of a particular sort of pattern through a community. Cultural practices assemble agencies into working assemblages and put the assemblages to work. Some of these assemblages may be entirely contained in an individual, and some may span several individuals and material artifacts.[9]

An intensive culture calls out to the potentialities inherent in the developing brain to utilize intensive cognitive strategies to playback those remembrances.

Lets look deeper into the reasons why.

## 3. Cutural Intelligence

> It seems surprising that the science of psychology has avoided the idea that many mental processes are social and historical in origin, or that important manifestations of human consciousness have been directly shaped by the basic practices of human activity and the actual forms of culture."[10]

8 Lash and Lury: *Global Culture Industry*, p. 5. "In global culture industry this changes. Products no longer circulate as identical objects, already fixed, static and discrete, determined by the intentions of their producers. Instead, cultural entities spin out of the control of their makers, in their circulation they move and change through transposition and translation, transformation and transmogrification. [...] In global culture industry, products move as much through accident as through design, as much by virtue of their unintended consequences as through planned design or intention."

9 Hutchins: *Distributed Cognition*, p. 5.

10 Luria: *Cognitive Development*.

Two conditions have implications for how we might understand the idea of general intelligence. In the *Fragments on Machines*, Marx understands the idea of general intelligence as 'a machine intelligence.' In the transition from artisanship to mechanized production of the assembly line, the unitary consciousness necessary for the crafting of the unique object is now linearly distributed throughout an assemblage of laborers who function in concert to produce the replicated object now reproduced ad infinitum. This is extensive labor as it produces a similar product over and over again. The laborer is simply a cog in the wheel of production and is subsumed by the machine as simply conscious linkages between the machine's mechanical organs.

> But once adopted into the production process of capital, the means of labor passes through different metamorphoses, whose culmination is the machine, or rather, an automatic system of machinery (system of machinery: the automatic one is merely its most complete, most adequate form, and alone transforms machinery into a system), set in motion by an automaton, a moving power that moves itself; this automaton consisting of numerous mechanical and intellectual organs, so that the workers themselves are cast merely as its conscious linkages.[11]

Their labor is fetishized into a series of partial acts that together produce the object and the machine, binds all their minds together synchronously. Together, as a single entity, they produce similar objects as long as the machine functions correctly. However things can go wrong as comically dramatized in Charlie Chaplin's, Modern Times, where, while working on an assembly line, he becomes accidentally consumed by the machine. In the transition to a post-Fordist condition, this assemblage of individuals along with new forms of architecture that reflect it, break up and are dispersed horizontally, distributed across multiple times and spaces bringing forth products that are singular and unique. The reflective machine intelligence is therefore of a different kind; it is intensive. Today, the general intelligence – the machines and apparatuses that bind people together and the social processes thus engendered – are invisible, non-hierarchical and distributed. The information thus generated reflects the conditions of this production. Hence, the collectivity of the human intellect is ultimately also evident in the machine. In Marx's words they

> are organs of the human brain, created by the human hand; the power of knowledge objectified. The development of fixed capital indicates to what degree general social knowledge has become a direct force of production, and to what degree, hence, the conditions of the process of social life itself have come under the control of the general intellect and been transformed in accordance with it. To what degree the powers of social production have been produced, not only in the form of knowledge, but also as immediate organs of social practice, of the real life process.[12]

11 Karl Marx: *Grundrisse*, p. 692, quoted in Gerald Raunig: *A Few Fragments on Machines.*
12 Ibid., p. 3.

As we will see in the age of information and mass intellectuality, it is, in fact, information itself that sculpts neural plasticity. General intelligence here is then defined as information produced by these mutating conditions of labor available to any population. As we saw earlier, extensive and intensive labor produces very different kinds of information, and it is this information, especially in its intensive form, that today creates the conditions of neuromodulation. These conditions of distributed information are powerful attractors that can act as powerful regulators of attention and memory, they pump up their informational content, and thus are sites of Noo-power. This Noo-power is what forms the basis for Neuropower in which the brain's neural plasticity and its pluripotentiality to become, are the sites of power's interrogation. It is in this context that the sculpting of the neural plasticity, through assemblages of trajectories of attention, subsumed in the regulatory patterns of built space, its affordances, with its implicit temporality and representational and presentational rationality, can occur. Whereas Noo-power concerns people perceiving in the present, a kind of primary animal consciousness, Neuropower concerns the production of a people in the future. It uses the products of Noo-power to produce elaborate future trajectories of planned action. Extensive projections are linear and veridical, only one unambiguous answer exists whilst intensive ones are adaptive and ambiguous in which many right answers exist simultaneously. "In a nutshell, veridical decisions deal with 'finding the truth,' and adaptive, actor-centered decisions deal with choosing 'what is good for me' in the future."[13] Of interest for us here in the light of Neuropower is that the frontal lobes are "critical in free-choice situation, when it is up to the subject to decide how to interpret an ambiguous situation."[14] Like the Neuroplastic potential, the frontal lobes are the new sites of sovereignty s engagement with the subject.

In the conditions of intensive culture the representation of an object as something real and equivalent is substituted by its branded value whereby its nature is determined by the stories that orbit around and through it and the relations those stories form with other stories ad infinitum. In the end producing the complex non-equivalent conditions of its brand equity. The crunchy edible matter in a box of cereal is not what creates its value, rather it arises from the way that the information on the box design excites a concomitant 'considered' neural architecture sculpted over time by a complex assemblage of a previously designed and present multilevel contexts that the individual has experienced before in which other cereal boxes played a role and into which this new box is inserted as well as the overall molar context of the designed space it is linked to. In this case the breakfast table, milk cartons, sugar bowls and so and so forth. On one hand, there is a history of cereal box covers which that are related to each other and form nested, aesthetic and stylistic relations, an eco-aesthetic niche. On the other

13 Goldberg: *The Executive Brain*, p. 77.
14 Ibid., p. 77.

hand, there is an already formed memory structure which has developed in the young consumers mind through its experiences with other cereal boxes that it is coupled to. The cereal box is reinstalled ad infinitum into a system of recatagorical memory that creates an active site for its infinite retrieval in the minds eye as both real and imaginary. Rather than linear equivalence that organized and delineated the ecology of objects in an artisan economy and began to dissolve in a Fordist one, what defines the post-Fordist landscape of cultural objects is a non-linear condition of value that is formulated by conditions of communicative labor as it functions along the distribution channels of media and hypermedia. The act of eating the cereal, simultaneously with the reading of the cover of the box is conjoined with the media strategy of advertising the cereal on multiple platforms, such as TV and the Internet, creating a buzz that intensifies the emotional and affective content of the experience. This buzz operates on an individual and group level and is distributed to other minds through, for instance, gossip. In the end an individual experience and memory is reconstituted as a group experience and collective memory. As we will see shortly, general intelligence according to the model I would like to develop is a condition of the ratio between the apparatus of Cognitive Capital and Cultural Capital. Different cultural contexts allow different expressions of each thus having implications for the production of a people or multiplicity.

## 4. The Cognitive Capital/Cultural Capital Ratio

Cognitive Capital here is defined as that 'information distribution and production system' centered around knowledge and utilized by sovereignty and the conditions of the administration of normalcy which produces a system of homogenized thinking. Cultural Capital, was first designated by Pierre Bourdieu, but is used here in the context of the ways and means through which artists using their own materials, practices, histories, apparatuses, critiques, performances, spaces and non-spaces produce objects, non-objects and activities that, when assembled in the cultural landscape, mutate the conditions of that landscape and produce resistant paradigms, or, as we will see, abnormal epistemologic trajectories. It is at the intersection of these mutating conditions expressed as a resultant cultural referendum, that the brain and mind are hailed by different attentional concoctions activating different attentional neurologic tool-boxes. The 'Global Workspace Theory' elaborated by Stanislas Dehaene and Claire Seargent is a case in point. The global neuronal workspace theory tries to account for these essential properties by emphasizing the role of long-distance reciprocal connections among brain areas. According to this theory, conscious processing crucially involves a set of neurons, the 'workspace' neurons, which can work in synergy through long-distance reciprocal connections.

> Those neurons, which can access information, maintain it online, and make it available to virtually any other process, although particularly numerous in frontal-parietal areas, are distributed throughout the brain, thus constituting a 'global workspace.' This state of global availability is, according to the theory, just what is to be conscious of a piece of information. [...] The particular set of workspace neurons involved in this mutual amplification process at a given time, would code for the current conspicuous content, and would delineate the possibilities of conscious manipulation, intentional actions and reports.[15]

According to this theory, only a single representation can be processed sufficiently by the workspace at any time leading to its being conscious whilst the other competing stimulations remain implicit or unconscious.[16] Thus the relationship between cognitive capitalism and cultural capitalism, as it influences, first, the conditions for cultural attention – what is culturally important – and, subsequently, through activating specific conscious representations, as in the global neuronal workspace, has implications for what the brain and mind will remember and therefore how the brain itself will be formed. This, I would like to suggest, has implications for the production of the history of thought itself. The neuronal recycling hypothesis provides us with the next step in this logical process and is an important key as to how long term changes might occur in the presence of sustained cultural niches. Cultural acquisitions like, for instance, reading (don't forget writing and reading are a fairly new abilities occurring in Mesopotamia approximately 3,500 B.C.), must find their neuronal niche, defined here as a set of already exiting neuronal circuits which have functions that can be easily adapted to the newly required function and are sufficiently plastic, thereby able to change if need be.[17] At the crossroads of competition and cooperation expressed by this ratio, the brain and mind are formed.

15 Sergent and Dehaene: "Neural Processes Underlying Conscious Perception", pp. 379, 380.

16 Ibid., p. 381.

17 Dehaene and Cohen: "Cultural Recycling of Cortical Maps". The neuronal recycling hypothesis consists of the following postulates:
1. Human Brain organization is subject to strong anatomical and connectional constraints inherited from evolution. Organized neural maps are present early on in infancy and bias subsequent learning.
2. Cultural acquisitions (e.g., reading) must find their "neuronal niche," a set of circuits that are sufficiently close to the required function and sufficiently plastic as to reorient a significant fraction of their neural resources to this novel use.
3. As cortical territories dedicated to evolutionary older functions are invaded by novel cultural objects their prior organization is never entirely erased. Thus prior neural constraints exert powerful influence on cultural acquisition and adult organization.

## 4. Neural Plasticity and the Sculpting of the Neural Zoe into the Neural Bios.

How is the development of brain and mind linked to the history of objects, abstract knowledge, and to the production of the subject in the context of neoliberal capitalism with its emphasis on immaterial labor and knowledge industries? How might we formulate a theory of resistance in this context? In what follows, I would like to use ideas emanating from two theories to constitute, on one hand, the ways and means through which institutions might restrict the potential for difference and on the other, the way that culture might emancipate it. Importantly both the theory of neuronal group selection as formulated by Gerald Edelman and the theory of neural constructivism, formulated by Steven R. Quartz and Terrence J. Sejnowski, sculpt and choreograph the neural potential but in different ways.[18] I shall argue that these ideas, often considered contradictory, can be understood as complementary, especially in the context of this argument concerning as it does, the cultural sculpting of a becoming brain.

Edelman's theory and that of Quartz and Sejnowksi both ask a basic question: What are the determinants of postnatal neural development? Is it, as neural Darwinism would suggest, an unfolding of a prescribed neurobiological process, in which the formation of a stochastic, disordered postnatal neural architecture characteristic of the neonatal nervous system is best described by the early exuberant growth of neural elements followed by a period of pruning and regression. That as a result of a Darwinian survival-of-the-fittest regime powerful and omnipresent and powerfully stimulating environmental contingencies sculpt repeatedly stimulated neural elements into a finely tuned sensorial-perceptual-cognitive machine coupled to those patterns of stimulation? This theory has the benefit of parsimony and mimics in certain ways the concrete genetic and immunological systems already in place. According to Quartz and Sejnowski, the weakness of this theory lies in its dependence on the notion of prespecification, as this theory necessitates that, for instance, the network must build in the problem domain a priori. That it must know before hand what it must come into contact with and have neurons that are all pre adapted. That is to say that the world that human beings live in is constantly changing and, even though neural Darwinism might work in the controlled environment of the laboratory, where all the conditions can be controlled, the real world is in flux. Both agree in the early stage of massive exuberant growth of neural elements but neural constructivism proposes that instead of simply a regression of neural elements, development is rather "a progressive increase in the structures underlying representational complexity" and these changes depend on an "interaction with a structured environ-

18 Edelman: *The Remembered Present*; Quartz and Sejnowski: "The Neural Basis of Cognitive Development".

ment to guide development."[19] The creativity and pluripotentiality of culture as it unfolds is mimicked in the dynamic and static structural states that develop in the brain in relation to it.

Neural Darwinism and neural constructivism in the end rely on the conditions of epigenesis, and, in this case, a cultural epigenesis, to produce or sculpt the neurobiological substrate into the neurobiological architecture to change the skin of brain into the flesh of mind. Epigenesis refers to the influences on development that arise from other factors then genetic instructions and therefore in terms of my argument here, both theories are in agreement. The brain undergoes changes commensurate with the postnatal environment it is exposed to. In the early days of prehistoric man it was nature that formed those contingencies. Today as more and more people move to the city, it is designed space and information.

> Plastic human brains may nonetheless learn to factor the operation and information-bearing role of such external props and artifacts deep into their own problem-solving routines, creating hybrid cognitive circuits that are themselves the physical mechanisms underlying specific problem-solving performances. We thus come to what is arguably the most radical contemporary take on the potential cognitive role of nonbiological props and structures: the idea that, under certain conditions, such props and structures might count as proper parts of extended cognitive processes.[20]

As you will see, I view neural selectionism as the dominating force early on and neural constructivism more important later, keeping in mind that Darwinian forces may still play a role. All agree that a phenomenon of excessive growth of neurons in the early years of life is characteristically followed by a reactionary depletion. Neural constructivism attempts to account for what happens thereafter.[21]

The theory of neuronal group selection, the hallmark of neural Darwinism, is made up of three components. Simply stated there is the primary repertoire that is a product of developmental selection, the secondary repertoire that is produced by experiential selection and reentry that stabilizes the results of the first two processes through dynamic synchronous potentials. I will cover developmental and experiential selection now, leaving reentry for later.

This primary repertoire describes the condition of the initial variability of the anatomy of the brain at birth that is produced by a process called developmental selection. First, it relates to the variation that results from the combination of the DNA contributed by the father's sperm and the mother's egg as two very diverse genetic heritages. Secondly, it relates to the history of the species itself in its evolutionary journey and the conditions of the genes that reflect that history and produce variable primary neural architectures; forms of disparity that are the result of evolutionary experiments leading to both the explicit and implicit hu-

19 Ibid., p. 538.
20 Clark: *Supersizing the Mind*, p. 68.
21 Quartz and Sejnowski: "The Neural Basis", pp. 543–545.

man nervous system. The history of those experiments are archived like the archive of a library, which at times is made visible and at other times remains out of sight according to need. Such is the case of the human genome that under certain environmental stresses can become expressed from its previously latent form. Finally, it is the result of events that take place during the pregnancy. For example, the effects of smoking, drinking or cocaine use on the condition of the developing fetus's brain are well known. What results from these three processes is that each brain at birth, although sharing many commonalities, also expresses a tremendous amount of neuronal variability that afford the brain the opportunity to be affected by population dynamics in which evolution is the result of the changing compositions of populations of unique individuals from generation to generation. It is to this variation in its primordial and plastic state that makes the primary repertoire relatively unspecified and which the underlying and modifiable conditions of a changing cultural milieu can hail. I would like to call attention to the primary repertoire as the site of what is referred to as neural biodiversity and what I would like to refer to as the neurobiologic common or neurozoon. The neurozoon embodies the full extent of the possibilities that a human brain can become and awaits the moment of its unfolding not as a natavist series of heterochronous events emblazoned in the codon of the genome but rather an unfolding or becoming in the context of a duet between itself as the inherent structural and apparatic conditions of brain in the context of nature or as I am arguing today, designed culture. This neurozoon emerges as a subset of the zoe, which is then sampled to become the neurobios. The neurobios is the secondary repertoire with all the political implications contained therein.

The secondary repertoire is a result of epigenesis and neural plasticity during a process called experiential selection. The term repertoire often relates to musical performance and designates the full scope of a performer's abilities. In fact, Gerald Edelman, one of the founders of neural Darwinism, is himself a musician. The obvious connection to new labor as a virtuoso performance and its association with a number of possible activities that link labor and politics and which have repercussions for the material of memory interests us here.[22] Neuropower posits, in contradiction to the work of Paolo Virno in *The Grammar of the Multitude*, that the virtuoso performance does in fact leave a materialist residue.[23] Rather then the industrially formed products characteristic of secondary economies, performances of the tertiary economy leave lingering memory traces, which have the potential to mutate the conditions of the neurobiological architecture. My performance *In the Mind's I* is oriented towards this result as collaborative performances in which works of art are created in the collaborating artists' mind's eye producing memory sculptures and architectures which the artist takes with him or her at its conclusion.

22 Virno: *A Grammar of the Multitude*, p. 70.
23 Ibid., p. 70.

A neural constructivist account could also concur. However, instead of resulting from a regression and deletion of neural elements, the secondary repertoire in this account is the result of a productive complexification and intensification. Epigenesis refers to the process by which the environment affects the patterns of stimulation and communication in the neurons and neural networks of the primary repertoire. Hebbian theory, which states that neurons that fire together wire together preferentially.[24] In the secondary repertoire such electrical activity is the result of linked objects and object relations in the world, both real and abstract, and, in the case of our world, the conditions of information and its distribution as dynamic codes in the real-imaginary-virtual interface. Network relations in the world stimulate and stabilize related and repetitively stimulated networks in the brain.

> The probability that neurons synchronize their responses both within a particular area and across areas should reflect some of the Gestalt criteria used for perceptual grouping. [...] Individual cells must be able to change rapidly the partners with which they synchronize their responses if stimulus configurations change and require new associations. [...] If more than one object is present in a scene, several distinct assemblies should form. Cells belonging to the same assembly should exhibit synchronous response episodes whereas no consistent temporal relations should exist between the discharges of neurons belonging to different assemblies.[25]

In an intensive culture made up of nested regularities operating at different time scales, diagrammatically rendered systems with multiple hubs acting as non-linear attractors that operate near phase transitions that sculpt dynamic coding systems of the brain. As noted above, Hebbian dynamics and neural Darwinism state that those neurons most intensely stimulated develop firing potentials that are selectively reinforcing whereas those not as stimulated undergo a process termed apoptosis and die out or manage to form connections with networks that are favored. Consequently, in the battle for limited neural space the stimulated neurons and their networked condition replace those that have receded. It is not a difficult intuitive leap to understand how branding and other tools of the global economy, which depend on the moment to moment relational changes of attention for instance, could create new gestalt relationships necessary to stimulate and stabilize global cell assemblies throughout the brain.

A third tenet of the theory of neuronal group selection is called reentry. Reentry is defined as the recurrent parallel exchange of neural signals between

24 http://en.wikipedia.org/wiki/Hebbian_theory. "Hebbian theory concerns how neurons might connect themselves to become engrams [...] If the inputs to a system cause the same pattern of activity to occur repeatedly, the set of active elements constituting that pattern will become increasingly strongly interassociated. That is, each element will tend to turn on every other element and (with negative weights) to turn off the elements that do not form part of the pattern. To put it another way, the pattern as a whole will become 'auto-associated'. We may call a learned (auto-associated) pattern an engram."

25 Singer: "Coherence as an Organizing Principle", p. 158.

neuronal groups or maps taking place at many different levels of brain organization: locally within populations of neurons, within a single brain area, and across brain areas. The importance of reentry as a mechanism of neural integration has been realized. Let us look at one example as an illustration. Area V4 of the occipital cortex, the visual cortex is divided into modules that are labeled as V1, V2, V3 and so on, samples the world according to color, that is, its' cells are wavelength selective, while those of V5 are motion selective.[26] We don't, however, see the world as disjointed patterns of color and motion but rather as a seamless whole. Why is this? It is through reentry's ability to temporally integrate these disparate regions linking them together in register in order to produce an integrated picture/image. Referred to as binding, these different registers are bound together. Reentry also plays a role in binding regions distributed throughout the entire brain which is referred to as global mappings.

> This suggests a close relationship between consciousness and binding. It seems that only those results of the numerous computational processes that have been bound successfully will enter consciousness simultaneously. This notion also establishes a close link between consciousness, short-term memory and attention.[27]

An understanding of binding may be a key to phenomenological immersion – the feeling that when reading a book, watching a movie, or actively engaged in a virtual reality program, that you are actually taking part in the action of the movie, book, or virtual reality program. Binding is not a process only occurring in the brain but in the world of objects, their relationships, and, today especially in conditions the abstract real relations that now capture our attention in the informational economy. The abstract real used here refers to the multiple stories and memories that orbit inanimate objects. Binding in the brain is not a constantly elaborated phenomenon, but one that is immanent. Neoliberal cognitive capitalism, through the elaboration of a set of epistemological trajectories, linked and bound stimuli that coerce the mind along prescribed routes of contemplation in time during conscious perception, creates fields of bound signifiers in the form of brand alliances that call out to the brain-mind of its collective subjects producing, as we shall see shortly, synchronous discharges in the neurobiological architectures that are its correlates. This is medium through which it organizes a people from the multiplicity.

Architectures tuned to specific dispositions are sculpted upon this neural plasticity. A social group or culture can share these dispositions. This process may result in the formation of a people who share similar perceptual and cognitive ideas about the world. Thus, intra-cerebral binding that occurs underneath the skull, within the boundaries of local maps, and those occurring throughout the brain as global maps can be 'extended' beyond the brain/skull to engage as

26 Zeki: *A Vision of the Brain*, p. 126.
27 Metzinger: *The Ego Tunnel*, p. 67.

inter-cerebral binding in the social context. Thomas Metzinger, alluding to the work of Antonio Damasion, notes:

> We mentally represent ourselves as representational systems, in phenomenological real-time. This ability turned us into thinkers of thoughts and readers of minds, and it allowed biological evolution to explode into cultural evolution. The Ego is an extremely useful instrument-one that has helped us understand one another through empathy and mind reading. Finally, by allowing us to externalize our minds through cooperation and culture, the Ego, has enabled us to form complex societies.[28]

The epistemological apparatuses embedded in culture facilitate these conditions of mind reading and other-mind knowledge. This in fact is one of the most important conditions of the homogenization of mindedness, that it makes mind reading easier but also deception. As we will see later on, art and architecture can facilitate this process as well as subvert it.

## 6. Branding and Networks

Recently an image of a Pepsi Cola can occurred recurrently all over New York City on billboards of different sizes placed strategically for maximum visibility. The advertisement, not surprisingly, was effectively designed for maximum and rapid perception by both a slow walking pedestrian and a fast paced auto driving public. (Traffic jams slow automobile traffic to a crawl.) The color and design of the advertisement interestingly used strategies first found in the pop paintings of Andy Warhol, Roy Lichtenstein, and Robert Indiana. The advertisement was designed with a specific context in mind in which other products advertised within the same visual milieu reverberated together producing a network of stimulation. In other words, the advertisement itself and its relation to other similarly designed advertisements in combination produced a cumulative intense effect upon the viewer. Such individual forms and their combined effect in the network where they are embedded produce correlated learning resulting in temporal coincidence at pre and post-synaptic membranes in local and global cortical mappings that strengthen synapses in the brain. Further this advertisement occurred on multiple platforms distributed repeatedly on television screens, and computer laptops throughout the planet simultaneously. As members of the planet earth, we are stimulated by global franchised sensations without national boundaries. National mindedness becomes transnational consciousness. These new contingencies provide the new affordances of the planetary urban environment, to use a Gibsonian term. Those neurons that code for these newly engineered affordances

28 Ibid., p. 67.

are coupled with these repetitive, intense stimuli and are therefore more apt to be favored over other neurons and neuronal networks in future encounters with those stimuli. In fact these conditions of neoliberal capitalism makes future encounters probable!

These stimuli can also be grouped together into larger ensembles of stimulation that are persistently aligned in the environment and thus are always coded together as a form of cultural mappings. Pop Art created and still creates reverberations in not only in painting but in design, fashion, film, and architecture. Andy Warhol's factory was a creative facility that produced paintings and films but also elaborated styles and forms of behavior that corroborated with those occurring in the culture as a whole. Thus discovering the Velvet Underground and holding court with other art star dignitaries at Maxes Kansas City created non-linear informational trajectories that found other lives in newspaper and magazine articles elaborating the events occurring therein. In other words cultural mappings are intensive, delineated by a multiplicity of immanent social, historical, psychological, economic, and psychic relations that are collaged together forming a superstructure though which they can produce new conditions for understanding. Today, architecture and designed space, understood as both the physical conditions of built space and the immaterial virtual spaces of the internet, house and support these elaborate amalgamations tethering them to learned activity trajectories, whether they are in the form of walking, driving or surfing the web. Through practice of these routines and internalization they form the habits of organized thinking itself.

There is an ecological logic to the forms of immanent distributions that are produced.[29] Branded environments are one such example where through corporate agreements Nike Shoes, Post Grape Nuts, Hertz Rent Car, Airberlin, and Sony Music appear together in the commercial landscape of billboards and airline magazines. The Institutional Understanding and sovereignty for which it does its bidding is empowered by this network of cultural signifiers. What Paul Virilio had formerly referred to in the representational and extensive era as Phatic Signifiers today become Fields of Phatic Signifiers embedded in the intensive logics of emerging meaning produced by the new apparatus of global culture.

Each brand is made up of its brand equity and, what I would like to call its marginalities, both positive and negative, that together compete with other assemblages for the attention of the market place.[30] Brand equity is explicit; it is a

29 Tononi: "Reentry and Cortical Integration", p. 129. "Two of the main tenets of this theory are that neurons act together in local collectives called neuronal groups and that they communicate with each other and correlate their activity by a process called reentry."

30 I was first introduced to the idea of externalities and their relationship to Cognitive Capitalism in a lecture by Yann Moulier Boutang given at the conference I helped organize with Deborah Hauptmann called "The Mind in Architecture" at TU Delft School of Architecture in 2008. A related text will be published in *Cognitive Architecture: From Biopolitics to Noopower*, 010 Press, 2010.

real entity that can be quantified based on market studies, while marginalities are implicit and in the process of becoming. They are ineffable and incalculable only to become comprehensible and commodifiable.

Marginalities can under certain conditions become explicit. Vans shoes were originally just tennis shoes to be worn all day. Their appropriation by skate boarders and their resultant popularity could never have been imagined. It was a result of a burgeoning skate culture in Southern California that added to its explicit brand equity when later they were understood and advertised as skating shoes. They are overlaid or superimposed or embedded in already existing networks of cultural signifiers and as such inflect upon diagrams of attentional flow. They form selective pressures, which are coupled to analogous selective pressures in the brain/mind. The conditions of cultural intensivity integrate dynamic flows of hierarchical distributions together with folded rhizomatic distributions of sensibility that these branded environments are instrumental in producing. Already existing oscillatory potentials, important for the production of the dynamic environment of the brain, transmitting information throughout it, are piggy backed by dynamic gestalts and rhythms at play in the cultural environment and onto which branded equities are imbricated. It is these dynamic potentialities as they are phase locked in ensembles synchronously that create intense branded networks. These stimulate networks in the brain/mind that first pay attention to them and then memorize them as a result of registering them preferentially, in the end effecting the overall architecture of the brain/mind. In the competition for neural space during critical periods of development, neural networks selected for by these branded environments will out-compete those that are not selected for, which either wither away or are incorporated in other assemblages where they can continue to play a role and be stimulated.

Branded networks work directly and indirectly on the child's mind, which is especially malleable. Directly through sophisticated marketing techniques in which advertisements specifically engineered with the child's mind in mind are transmitted cross-culturally during Saturday morning cartoons. These specially designed advertisements are analogous to 'babyese,' in which parents prolong and exaggerate certain key phonetic distinctions coupled to the child's immature brain. The same is true of childhood advertisement. Bright colors, fantastic talking cartoon animals, speaking in 'babyese,' which the child already knows from Saturday morning cartoon programs, create an indistinguishable set of signifiers in a child who is as yet unable to distinguish himself/herself from others. This is where the Society of Control really begins in the inside/outside of the child's mind.

But there is another way that the conditions of capitalism are transmitted to the child and that is indirectly through the parents. As I mentioned in the introduction Neuropower is focused on the planning and attention capacities of the frontal lobe. Adults assist children in the routines of their daily life that are beyond the capabilities of their immature brain. At first through such activities as pointing adults are indispensible in the early process of object learning and then symbolic language formation. Later when these activities involve planned action, for instance, parents extend their children's abilities by acting as and being agents of their frontal lobe.[31] They are there to help them plan beyond the here and now. This coupling of adult and child is a necessary condition of the early neural sculpting of Neuropower. The parent is at the service of the institutional understanding, acting as its agent of neuromodulation. But perhaps in the future with more sophisticated computer interfaces and software agents the parent won t even be necessary as the following quote from Andy Clarks *Mindware* might suggest:

> Imagine that you begin using the web at age 4. Dedicated software agents track and adapt to your emerging interests and random explorations. They then help direct your attention to new ideas, web pages and products. Over the next 70 years you and your software agents are locked in a complex dance of coevolutionary change and learning, each influencing and being influenced by, the other. In such a case, in a very real sense, the software entities look less like part of your problem-solving environment then part of you. The intelligent system that now confronts the wider world is biological-you-plus-the-software-agents. These external bundles of code are contributing rather like the various subpersonal cognitive functions active in your brain.[32]

## References

Clark, Andy: *Mindware*, Oxford (Oxfort University Press) 2001.
Clark, Andy: *Supersizing the Mind*, Oxford (Oxford University Press) 2008.
De Landa, Manuel: *Intensive Science and Virtual Philosophy*, New York (Continuum) 2002, pp. 59–61.
Deacon, Terrence: "Multilevel Selection and Language Evolution", in: Bruce H. Weber and David J. Depew (eds.): *Evolution and Learning: The Baldwin Effect Reconsidered*, Cambridge, MA (MIT Press) 2003.
Dehaene, Stanislas and Laurent Cohen: "Cultural Recycling of Cortical Maps", in: *Neuron Review* 56 (2007), pp. 384–385.
Edelman, Gerald: *The Remembered Present*, New York (Basic Books) 1989.
Goldberg, Elkonon: *The Executive Brain: Frontal Lobes and the Civilized Mind*, Oxford (Oxford University Press) 2001.

31 Wexler: *Brain and Culture*, pp. 108–9. "Given the prolonged postnatal physical maturation of these structures in human beings, lasting until or beyond puberty, it is not surprising that adults must provide these functions if they are to be present in the behavior of infants and children. Essentially, then, the frontal lobes of parents are functionally linked with the lower brain centers and the sensory, motor and association cortices of their infants and children. While the child's frontal lobes are developing, the parents' brains provide frontal lobe functions for the child."

32 Clark: *Mindware*, p. 115.

Hauptmann, Deborah and Warren Neidich (eds.): *From Noo-Power to Neuro-power: How Mind Becomes Matter, Cognitive Architecture: From Biopolitics to Noo-politics*, Rotterdam (010 Press) 2010 (forthcoming).

Hutchins, Edwin: *Distributed Cognition*, in: *IEBS Distributed Cognition* (http://files.meetup.com/410989/DistributedCognition.pdf).

Jacobson, Marcus: *Developmental Neurobiology*, New York (Plenum Press) 1991.

Lash, Scott and Celia Lury: *Global Culture Industry*, Cambridge (Polity Press) 2007.

Lazzarato, Maurizio: "The Concepts of Life and the Living in the Societies of Control", in: Martin Fuglsang and Bent Meier Sørensen (eds.): *Deleuze and the Social*, Edinburgh (Edinburgh University Press) 2006.

Luria, A.R.: *Cognitive Development: Its Cultural and Social Foundations*, Cambridge, MA (Harvard University Press) 1976.

Marx, Karl: *Grundrisse: Foundations of the Critique of Political Economy*, trans. by Martin Nicolaus (http://www.marxists.org/archive/marx/works/1857/grundrisse/ch13.htm).

Metzinger, Thomas: *The Ego Tunnel*, New York (Basic Books) 2009.

Quartz, Steven R. and Terrence J. Sejnowski: "The Neural Basis of Cognitive Development: A Constructivist Manifesto", in: *Brain Sciences* 20 (1997), pp. 537–556.

Raunig, Gerald: *A Few Fragments on Machines*, (http://transform.eipcp.net/transversal/1106/raunig/en).

Sergent, Claire and Stanislas Dehaene: "Neural Processes Underlying Conscious Perception. Experimental Findings and a Global Neuronal Workspace Framework", in: *Journal of Physiology – Paris* 98 (2004) 4–6, pp. 374–384.

Singer, Wolf: "Coherence as an Organizing Principle of Cortical Functions", in: Olaf Sporns and Giulio Tononi (eds.): *Selectionism and the Brain*, San Diego (Academic Press) 1994.

Tononi, Giulio: "Reentry and Cortical Integration", in: Olaf Sporns and Giulio Tononi (eds.): *Selectionsim in the Brain*, San Diego (Academic Press) 1994.

Virno, Paolo: *A Grammar of the Multitude*, trans. by Isabella Bertoletti, James Cascaito and Andrea Casson, New York (Semiotext[e]) 2004).

Wexler, Bruce: *Brain and Culture*, Cambridge, MA (MIT Press) 2006.

Zeki, Semir (ed.): *A Vision of the Brain*, New York (Blackwell) 1993.

natur, wissenschaft und die künste
nature, science et les arts
nature, science and the arts

Edited by

Julia Burbulla, Bernd Nicolai, Ana-Stanca Tabarasi-Hoffmann,
Philip Ursprung & Wolf Wucherpfennig